The Healing Dimensions
Resolving Trauma In BodyMind and Spirit

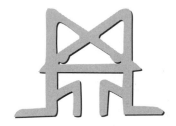

INTRODUCING HOLOGRAPHIC MEMORY RESOLUTION
FOR THE HEALING OF
PHYSICAL, EMOTIONAL, MENTAL, AND SPIRITUAL BLOCKAGES TO
HEALTH AND WELL-BEING

By
Brent M. Baum, S.T.B., S.S.L., I.C.A.D.C, C.C.H.

WEST PRESS
Tucson ◆ Arizona

The Healing Dimensions
Resolving Trauma In BodyMind and Spirit

Published by:
Healing Dimensions, A.C.C.
5675 N. Camino Esplendora #6137
Tucson, Arizona 85718
Phone: (520) 615-9247
Web Site Address: www.healingdimensions.com

Edited by Laura Orlich
Cover illustration and design by Dale Chaon
Cover photographs by Brent M. Baum
Portrait photograph by Philip Ramackers
Inside illustrations by Lynne M. East
Layout by Glen Weimer
Manufacture and reprint by West Press
Original Cover production by Artistocrat Printing
First Printing, 1997; Second Printing, December 2004
Printed in the United States of America

Library of Congress Cataloguing-in-Publication
Baum, Brent M.
The healing dimensions: resolving trauma in bodymind and spirit/ by Brent M. Baum – 1st ed.
p. cm.
Includes bibliographical references.
ISBN 0-9661990-0-6
Library of Congress Card Catalog Number (CIP): 97-91308
1. Self Help   2. Psychology   3. Spirituality
4. Mind and Body   5. Psychoneuroimmunology

I. Title   II. Author

*This book is dedicated to Doug Brantley
whose early departure inspired me to seek
a more effective and timely resolution
for the traumas that foster illness
in bodymind and spirit.*

Contents

Acknowledgments		vii
The "Yantra"		ix
Foreword		xi
Preface		xiii
Definition of Trauma		xv
Chapter One:	The Focus	1
Chapter Two:	The Journey of Empowerment	16
Chapter Three:	Holographic Space	32
Chapter Four:	Trauma Metaphors – The Keys to Healing	48
Chapter Five:	The Dynamics of Trauma Induction	69
Chapter Six:	"Triggers"– The First Glimpse of Trauma	83
Chapter Seven:	The Language of Healing	96
Chapter Eight:	The Electromagnetic Key	115
Chapter Nine:	The Physics of the Soul	138
Chapter Ten:	The Hierarchy of Healing	158
Chapter Eleven:	The Spiritual Implications of Trauma	180
Chapter Twelve:	Recovering Spiritual Awareness After Trauma: Twelve Principles	198
Chapter Thirteen:	The Healing of Dreams	269
Chapter Fourteen:	The Healing of Disease	280
Chapter Fifteen:	Creating the Future and Resolving the Past	299
Chapter Sixteen:	Conclusions	307
Notes		323
Bibliography		329

Acknowledgments

First, to each trauma survivor whose shared struggles have given me the gift of insight and validation, I remember and offer my tribute to you. Without your willingness to face your pain, the lessons and techniques contained herein would not be. I thank my angels, especially Michael and his associates: Gail Konz, Chris Oehrle, Mary Jo McCabe, Fran and Ray Lemkul, Ronnie and Betty Falgout, Tim Frank, Gay Mallon Frank, Rev. Reed Brown, Rosemary Vaughn, Tony Farano and Sue Pirrung, David Abadi and Martha Foy, Susan Holmen, Irene Anderson, Linda Prucha, Chris Russell, Bill Wigmore, Martha Hildreth, Ron Welch, Talbot Outpatient Center, Cottonwood de Tucson, Kathleen Fitzgerald, Rachel, Judy, Liz, all the "Light Bearers," Dr. Mariko Tanaka, Dr. Roger Cummings, Dr. Teri Daunter, Dr. Carol Arnoff, Dr. Fran Moore, Dr. Beth Shapiro, Dr. Lorraine Baillie, Dr. Jim Graham, Dr. George Nash. Acknowledging some other special friends and influences from near to remote past: Marty Zlatic, David Ulkins, Robert H. Jordan, Scott McLavy, Dare Nagy, Don Lavender, Daniel Moxley, Bobby Spell, Shawn Marsh, Peter Udall, Kirk Kupensky, James Efferson, Reverend Jaime Madrid, Reverend Janusz Ihnatowicz, Dr. Paul Jacobs, Dr. Harold Forshey, Dr. Joseph Seger and Patti Seger, all my friends over the thirteen years of digging at Tel Halif, Kibbutz Lahav, John and Nancy Stein, Gabriel and Alicia Stein, the Missionaries of Charity at Mansatala in Calcutta, Reverend John Naughton, Reverend Leo Guillot, Reverend Jean-Pierre Ruiz, I express gratitude. I recognize the Diocese of Baton Rouge for its twenty years of support. To my friends in Holy Family, St. Thomas More, and St. George Catholic Church Parishes, I express gratitude. I thank the "medical team in spirit" who has worked at least as hard as I. I thank you who are my "spiritual family."

I offer heartfelt gratitude to Laura Orlich for your friendship, support, and indefatigable editing skills; Dale Chaon, for your artistry and graphic design; Glen Weimer, for your assistance in layout, and Robert Odom, for your support and personal reflections.

Most profoundly I am grateful to my earliest teachers – my parents, my first gods, Mom and Dad. I thank the Divine. All is perfect; all is as it should be. I cherish my secondary parents – my sisters, Margie and Peggy, who so greatly enhanced the love and nurturing, and my one of a kind brother, Jerry. Keep on singing. I thank my younger sister Carole for all that we shared growing up and for making me part of her current journey; it is a privilege to share your "little angels."

To all the guiding influences, of many eons, who have contributed to this expression of hope and vehicle of healing, I say thank you.

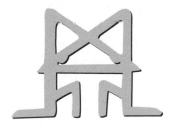

The "Yantra" – A Visual Meditation

"Unlimited Power in Service to Others"

A "Yantra" is a visual form of meditation. By looking upon the image one is drawn into its mysteries and messages. The design on this page contains a variety of images, including: two genuflecting "Ankh's" (⚲) – the ancient Egyptian symbols of "life," facing each other. These symbols were often depicted as persons to communicate special messages in the hieroglyphics and mythology of Egypt. In the Christian tradition, the figures resemble the combination of the Greek letters "Chi" (**X**) and "Rho" (**P**) which, when superimposed upon each other, combine to form the symbol for Christ; the "triangle" becomes the symbol of the "Trinity" – the "Father, Son, and Holy Spirit" of Christian belief. Whether Egyptian or Greek in derivation, the heads of these universal figures meet to form the mathematical symbol for infinity (∞), denoting eternity or absence of limitation. Their arms form a pyramid or triangle – ancient symbols of power and balance. These two figures of unlimited power are superimposed over two smaller human figures whose heads are bowed and are visible within the pyramid. The arms of the Divine figures are superimposed upon and render service through the arms and humble stance of the two small human figures who are overshadowed by the immensity of their "guides." The positioning of the heads and knees combine to form a four-pointed star, indicative of the four directions and four "spirits" of the Native American Medicine Wheel – inclusive of the four protectors invoked in the hierarchy of angels, the Archangels: Michael, Gabriel, Raphael, and Uriel. There is an arrow in evidence when looking upward from the bottom of the figure, a reference to Isaiah 49:2b, "He made me a polished arrow and in his quiver he hid me." The Greek letter "Tau" is also evidenced, signifying a new beginning. Together, these images communicate the abundant energy, life-force, and Divine support available for service to others. When you behold this yantra within the pages of The Healing Dimensions, may you be inspired to remember your true nature and the powerful resources available for healing self and others.

Foreword

All pain, trauma, addiction and disease are raw material from which our conscious awakening is formed. The experience of walking through the pain (utilizing the tools available, whether they be therapy, treatment, bodywork, journaling, etc.) is a journey of healing which moves us from darkness into light. This journey is multi-dimensional, transcending the limiting experience of pain and embracing the divine self within each of us. The journey through the "valley of the shadow" can bring us from the depths of desperate limitation to the heights of expressing the fullness of our humanity. This is our birthright.

The book you now hold in your hands is an extraordinary work. Through its pages you will embark upon your own journey of understanding. Brent Baum offers the gift of transforming your pain, trauma and addiction into emotional, psychological and spiritual gifts which have the potential to enrich you, your family, your community and the planet we all share. We are all one people. We are all inextricably bound together in our pain as well as in our wholeness. Therefore, as you heal, your brothers and sisters, in some way, participate. As I heal, a part of you heals. The great spiral of creation includes all of us, together, in the agony of our pain and the beauty of our healing.

My work with clients has convinced me that recovery from addiction and trauma is a communal experience. No one practices addiction or recovers alone. There are always others involved in our dysfunction as well as our healthy celebrations of life. It is imperative that we summon the courage to plunge headlong into the various dimensions of healing presented to us on our journey back to the Source.

The long history of human interaction proves the importance of honoring the communal nature of our lives. Every spiritual tradition emphasizes our interdependence. In fact, thousands of years ago, Lord Krishna said in the <u>Bhagavad Gita</u>, "When a person responds to the joys or sorrows of others as if they were his own, he has attained the highest state of spiritual union." Indeed, Lord Krishna taught that whether we perceive it or not, the joys and sorrows of other are ours as well. I believe this is a mandate to heal. This same teaching was echoed later in the message of Jesus. It is also found in the beautiful traditional spirituality of the Hopi and other tribes. We ignore this truth at our own great peril. It should also be pointed out that this journey is a continuing experience. I do not believe we are ever "healed," but, rather, that we are "healing." Healing and recovery are multidimensional processes, not isolated linear events. We have the opportunity to move ever deeper, from one level to the next, from the dimension of limited pain, higher and higher into the dimensions where balance and harmony are the hallmarks.

Brent Baum is a healer; he is a guide; he is a teacher. In <u>The Healing Dimensions</u>, Brent shares his experience, strength and hope. He shares his own knowing in ways which are accessible both to those beginning a journey of healing, and to professionals with years of experience.

I have moved deeper into my own healing through Brent's technique. I experienced a profound revelation of healing one snowy evening several years ago when Brent was a guest in my home in the mountains of northern New Mexico. I continue to marvel at that experience. Having worked with many healers in my career, this was one of the few times I actually experienced the healing dimension myself. I am confident that you will find the information and techniques in this book to be valuable tools in your own healing and in your work with others. May we continue to bless and enrich each other as we explore the healing dimensions.

God bless us all.

Robert Odom, M.Div.

Preface

*How do our bodies record what our minds
and emotions cannot handle?*

*Are our bodies continuously prompting us
to heal emotional wounds?*

*How can we safely access painful information
without retraumatizing ourselves?*

What Brent Baum has developed, in Holographic Memory Resolution, is a simple yet profound method of accessing memories and events from our lives that remain frozen in time, locked within an eternally present moment just waiting to be healed. This innovative approach to trauma resolution provides gentle, expedient methods for resolving those events in their totality, not simply addressing them mentally and emotionally, but discharging them from the nervous system where they are held in the body. The hallmark of this process is that it addresses trauma on the "cellular" level.

As we move into this work, it is important to understand how the term **trauma** is being used today by trauma therapists like Brent Baum. Trauma is not so much **what** happens. Of course rape, dismemberment, and incest, are all traumatic. Yet seemingly ordinary or common events can prove damaging as well: hearing one's parents argue, suddenly losing a loved one, being fired from a job. Trauma is determined by how a person *views* what is happening. At the moment of trauma, the individual is unable to handle what is happening, so the system internally records the entire event to be dealt with later from a safer, more resourceful state. At the moment of trauma, the person simply does not have the necessary tools or assets available to avoid the experience or resolve it. It is a conflicted moment in which the individual experiences a powerlessness to alter the external course of events. Emotionally, the message that reverberates in the victim's system is an overwhelming one: "Oh, my God! I can't deal with this! It's just too much to handle! I feel like I'm going to die!" By this definition, we have all been traumatized at some time in our past, overwhelmed by everyday life.

The implications of this work run deep: One is that we **can** reclaim those parts of ourselves that are still expending energy rehashing, reliving, or unsuccessfully trying to "forget" those old events (whether we remember those events or not), and come into the present as whole individuals truly "living in the moment." Another is that the lessons contained herein constructively challenge our very concept of self, reality, and our physical world.

This writing, through the use of the author's personal experiences, case studies, and references to the leading edge theories on body mind connectedness, examines the mechanisms that our system employs for holographically recording events internally and for retrieving and healing those events. Whether you are a therapist looking for body- centered techniques to address the bodymind component of verbal therapy or an individual looking for effective self-help techniques, I believe you will find this book to be thought provoking, enjoyable, and extremely enlightening.

Glen Weimer, RPP, Director
Arizona Polarity Institute

Trauma

A *"trauma" is a spontaneous state of self-hypnosis*, an altered state of consciousness which encodes state-bound problems and symptoms (Cheek, 1981). *Hypnosis occurs spontaneously* at times of stress and serves to contain the experience to prevent the subject from becoming overwhelmed. Psychological shocks and traumatic events are *psycho-neuro-physiological dissociations* and often result in "traumatic amnesia" or "delayed recall." This amnesia may be resolved by *"inner resynthesis"* (Erickson, 1948/1980). The *encoding* of trauma in the nerve cells of the body is facilitated by the *limbic-hypothalamic-pituitary system* and exercises a profound influence on the functioning of the *autonomic nervous system*, the *endocrine system*, and the *immune* system (Selye, 1976). At the moment of traumatization, all sensory perceptions are "paused" and stored holographically at one millisecond prior to the worst part of the event ("T-1" – David Grove, 1989). The event is encoded as a holographic fragment and is *stored in the nerve center(s)* of the body where the pain first became overwhelming (Baum, 1995). Focusing on such memory fragments provides access to the stored memory, as every fragment of a holographic scene contains the whole. The holographic nature of our perception (Pribram, 1977) forms the foundation for self-hypnosis and the containment of the overwhelming experiences of our lives. Whereas we could not "control" the *external* circumstances which led to traumatization, the *bodymind assisted us by seizing control of our internal* picture, a reality we could control through our creative act of perception – a creativity affirmed by quantum physics. A trauma is a moment when we utilize our creative resources of mind to "pause" our space-time perceptions to prevent overwhelm to the psyche. *The resolution of our traumas, therefore, requires that we address these powerful, encoded moments and states of consciousness.*

Brent Baum, 1997

Chapter One

The Focus

This book explores our power to transform reality itself. It is born from my own pain and that of other trauma survivors who, like myself, sense that life is intended to be more than victimhood or exile from one's own happiness, wholeness, emotional and spiritual "connectedness." Do not be misled by the word "trauma," for contained within this work is an important message for all. Each and every one of us has known some experience of trauma – that is, trauma as it shall be exposed within this work. At the same time, we shall discover that we each possess, within our remarkable design, an inherent capacity to deal with the overwhelming experiences of our lives by freezing them or pausing them until such time as we are able to release or resolve them.) Forgetting does not release this energy, and remaining in the victim posture or medicating pain necessitates its attention-getting emergence as illness, addiction, depression, nightmare, or flashback. This built-in capacity to deal with the critical moments of our lives has not been clearly understood or appreciated until now.

As individuals and as a society, we began to recognize the presence of trauma in our psyches by becoming conscious of our addictions, of the many faces of abuse, and of the "flashbacks" of our war veterans.

1

Slowly we gained a greater understanding of our mind's ability to protect us from the overwhelming pain of traumatic experiences. As a society that long ago learned to cope with pain primarily by medicating it, resistance to exploring the nature and origins of this pain is great. For the most part, the healing efforts of the medical profession have revolved around medicating symptoms in the physical body while missing the mechanisms underlying and sustaining the majority of our illnesses – the trauma induction process. Only now, with the emergence of quantum physics, "psychoneuroimmunology," (the new mind-body science) and spirituality, are we coming to understand the function of consciousness in rapport with the body and in defense against trauma. The case experiences that have been shared with me by thousands of trauma survivors over the last seven years have shocked and overwhelmed me. Working with the partners and children of these survivors has also moved me to report the truths that I have found. It is terrifying and confusing both to the trauma survivor and to family members to see the sudden and compelling emotional withdrawal, dysfunction, and even illnesses which result from carrying powerful traumas within our bodies, minds, and spirits. Some cases may surprise you. Many of them you will identify from your own experience, either personally, or in observation of others. All of them will stimulate your thinking.

In my own relationships I have felt the trauma-induced barriers to intimacy keeping me isolated and distant from those who reached out to me in love, and I have felt the anguish of those whose unresolved traumas prevented them from receiving my love and support. For so long, I, like most of us, lived in the belief that the past was essentially unchangeable – something that simply must be accepted as fact and "put behind" me. The shadows of my traumas, however, remained quite real and often close at hand. Triggered periodically, they continued to exert a profound impact on my self-esteem, my relationships, my health, and my occupation – and they frequently did so despite my best efforts to ignore them. It was this profound sense of frustration at the personal and interpersonal restrictions that were imposed from unresolved memories that stimulated my search for a more effective way of dealing with these blockages. After working with over five thousand trauma survivors, with more than twenty-five thousand memories, I am aware, not only that I am not alone in my frustration, but that an earnest search is under way for new solutions.

Individually and collectively we find ourselves discontent with having to settle for less than our full potential. Our attention is directed to that which is impeding our personal and professional lives. Focus is drawn to the fact that we are in an awakening stage – realizing that our lives have been programmed and influenced by experiences that, in the past, we felt powerless to change. This is the impact of trauma as I define it within this work. We are becoming conscious of everything from our addictions, to overt (obvious) and covert (hidden) forms of abuse. We are gaining a better understanding of the devastating impact of neglect and abandonment. Simultaneously, we are challenged to move beyond this stage – to not stop at the identification of our traumas and remain frozen in our victimhood, but to take the next step as well. We are invited to recognize our personal and collective power as creators. As creators, I assure you, we possess the ability to transform our traumas, overriding the power of the past. William Faulkner once said: "The past isn't dead; it isn't even past."[1] This truth will emerge more clearly as we explore the nature and resolution of trauma.

My work with trauma survivors has led to confrontations with a number of old beliefs that many of us have carried for generations. These involve our perceptions of ourselves – the nature of our bodies and the power of our minds. Imagine my great surprise when I realized that helping my clients resolve trauma memories also resolved their diseases as well! Their migraines, for example, turned out to be fragments of old trauma memories that were being triggered. By "trigger" I refer to the ability of a memory fragment to suddenly draw us back into an earlier, more emotionally potent (positive or negative) experience that is suddenly resurrected with all of its original intensity. Their pre-menstrual discomfort or "P.M.S." (Pre-Menstrual Syndrome) was simply the re-live of their first, traumatic experience of their own bodies at puberty. Their cancer was the manifestation of abuse or trauma memories surfacing to get their attention. Their arthritis was related to anger and pain from childhood abuse that they held repressed in their hands, unable to safely release. Their "anxiety attacks" were simply the re-experiencing of the original anxiety induced at a moment of trauma. Their "epilepsy" was the relive of an earlier seizure which encoded as trauma. Their chronic pain was the residue of the unresolved trauma memory that created it, not the result of any permanent nerve damage. In each of these cases, when the memory was resolved, the disease pattern yielded as well. These cases demonstrate the evidence emerging from scientific research that: 1) our nervous systems are so sensitive that they often, easily store traumatic experiences to protect us, 2) these traumas impact the functioning of the immune system, and 3) with such a connection, traumas have the ability to precipitate illness. This fact will become evident within this work. My contribution to this endeavor resides in my ability to identify and feel the primary site(s) in the nervous system where a trauma is stored – sites which become the habitation of migraines, arthritis, cancer, chronic pain, etc. I affirm here that there is an evident link between our traumas and the anxieties, diseases, depression, and dysfunction that we subsequently manifest. The most shocking implication is the demonstrable fact that we have been operating with impaired immune systems. In my practice I have encountered no one free of some encoding of trauma in the nervous system. It would appear that we have been struggling for health while holding tightly (on a subconscious level) to the traumas which repress the functioning of our immune system. It's quite simple: we have not known how remarkable and sophisticated our minds are at protecting us from the traumas of life, and, therefore, have been unaware of their impact on our health. Based on this premise, the resolution of our traumas should, therefore, produce enhanced immune system functioning. This is, in fact, what science is finding and which we are here to examine in detail. There is hope beyond our imagining. There are cures because most diseases are not independent physiological entities beyond the reach of our ability to self-heal; they are, more often than not, the products of our incredibly sophisticated consciousness manifest in body and mind – and given the power of this mind, which we are now exploring in this, the "decade of the brain," we have hope beyond anything that medical science has previously offered.

The title of this work, The Healing Dimensions, alludes to the place and manner in which we will reclaim our capacity to heal ourselves. Both science and spirituality are converging to bring this multi-dimensional experience to light. The findings of quantum physics and spirituality affirm our ability as creators. What has not been adequately appreciated until recently is our remarkable capacity to store intact the experiences that overwhelm us. This is part of our creative power, and it has been profoundly undervalued. The notion that we create both consciously and subconsciously, and that the mind possesses the capacity to freeze and store all perceptions at a moment of trauma, is only now receiving our full attention. Study of the dynamics of trauma induction allows us to operate more powerfully and responsibly as creators within these healing dimensions, as you will see. The power of our minds to move fluidly within and to alter our states of consciousness has unbelievably profound implications. Learning to move within these states of consciousness opens the door to the healing of illnesses, addictions, depression, compulsivity, nightmares, and many other painful life patterns.

The overall scope of this work is two-fold. On the one hand, it is my desire to provide you with very specific practical tools that will facilitate your self-healing and growth toward wholeness. The second goal is to provide the cognitive understanding and context for these tools to be used most effectively. Unless we understand these dynamics, we cannot take full advantage of them to facilitate the healing of self and others.

Personal Perspective

Above all else, I am a student of life. I have come to enjoy this learning process, having spent over half of my life in educational institutions. By nature I am an interdisciplinarian. In my evolution I have been a Catholic priest, a Near Eastern archaeologist, a seminary professor, a psychotherapist, and a facilitator of healing. While this may provide a glimpse into the influences that have shaped me and this work, there is a search, a continuity that underlies my entire journey.

As a child I wanted to be an archaeologist. This impulse was awakened during a vacation to New Mexico with Uncle Mel who was an amateur archaeologist. While visiting the Puye Cliff Dwellings in New Mexico, I was moved by the beauty, silence, familiarity, and overwhelming power of this civilization. Though only a child, this trip awakened a romance with the past and a craving to understand more about myself and my cultural placement in relationship to civilization's historic unfolding. Later, when I was chided by my best friend's father for aspiring to be an archaeologist in Louisiana (a state mostly covered with water), I found myself contemplating a more regionally respected occupation – that of a Catholic priest. Now I know that my serving as a priest was influenced by my family – a "family role assignment," and a way of subconsciously resolving personal and familial traumas. On a higher level, I know that it was my appropriate spiritual path. I began studying for ministry at the age of thirteen, long before I had any clear idea as to what I was undertaking. I seemed to thrive on the added spiritual component to my high school education and felt comfortable continuing on into the college seminary. While personally searching for some clear, secure experience of knowledge and truth, I found myself moving from a focus on mathematics to a major in theology in pursuit of more personally fulfilling knowledge. Much of this shift in interest was due to the influence of a brilliant theologian, Father Janusz Ihnatowicz, who nourished my spirituality and challenged my hungry mind. I completed my undergraduate degree in theology at the University of St. Thomas in Houston, Texas, and, subsequently, was appointed to continue my studies at the Pontifical Universities in Rome, Italy. My experience in Rome was profoundly nurturing both intellectually and spiritually. My first full day in Rome was the first day "in office" for Pope John Paul I. The events which transpired in the months that followed served to deepen my appreciation for my own spiritual heritage, while watching history in the making. To this day I am moved by my recollection of standing beneath the balcony of St. Peter's Basilica, watching the election of the first Catholic figurehead from a communist country and the first non-Italian Pope in several hundred years. A more global vision of my spirituality was one of the gifts of Rome, along with a certain appreciation for the political implications of spiritual change.

My time of study in Rome afforded me countless educational opportunities, and among them was the reawakening of my early childhood longing for a "hands on" experience of the past. With its proximity to the Middle East, Rome afforded me the opportunity to pursue my childhood impulse to do archaeology. One of my former college professors, Dr. Paul Jacobs, was involved in an archaeological research project in Israel. The summer of 1979, I joined the Lahav Research Project, an American-sponsored archaeological undertaking in Israel, and excavated an ancient site called "Tell Halif." My archeological work continued for thirteen years (1979-1992) – throughout my parish ministry and on into my transition to counseling. I did not know at the time that it was this very work that would provide a profound introduction to my future involvement in the trauma field. My archaeological work over these years would lay the foundation for developing the sensitivity in my hands necessary for my future trauma work while teaching me rigorous scientific discipline and providing me with profound motivation for gaining a deeper appreciation for the power of the past.

This was never more evident than in 1992 when, during excavation, I discovered the body of a man. Roughly the same age and height as myself, he had been trapped when a cave collapsed upon him and his family, entombing them around 3800 BC. I was the first to come upon the body with its hand raised upward to fend off the collapsing cave, his mouth opened in a cry of surprise and fear. Around the body were the treasures of his household – flint tools, potter's wheel, fired and unfired ceramics, red ochre, smashed jars of grain, a hearth, and countless other precious finds. I profoundly identified with this experience, having had an inexplicable fascination with the Chalcolithic Period (4500-3750 BC). I had studied this remarkably artistic and spiritual culture that had painted frescoes with spiritual representations literally thousands of years before any other civilization. The abrupt disappearance of the culture remains a mystery. Never in the history of Near Eastern archaeology had any "in situ" evidence (that is, in its original state of preservation) of this quality been found associated with the Chalcolithic Period. I still cherish the richness of the experience and the power I felt being able to recover the lives of those who lived over five thousand years ago. Ironically, the Chalcolithic culture was pre-biblical by over a thousand years and, therefore, pre-dated my theological field of study: Abraham, the patriarch of the Judeo-Christian tradition, didn't appear until around 2250 BC! Upon completion of the excavation of these finds, I felt that a chapter in my life was complete, and that I could now move on in my life. I had regained or acquired a "lost" part of myself in the process. I did not know at the time that Freud himself had used archaeology as a metaphor for psychoanalysis and emphasized the importance of "digging" into our past to understand who we are and why we live the way we do in the present.

I was ordained to the Catholic priesthood in 1982 and continued my studies with the Jesuits in Rome and Jerusalem, completing my post-graduate degrees at the Gregorian University and the Pontifical Biblical Institute. Even before ordination, however, following a profound spiritual experience during a retreat at La Storta, Italy, in March of 1979, I knew that my ultimate work would not be that of a "diocesan" priest. I became aware that my work would not simply be a ministry to the diocese or geographical region from which I had come and that, somehow, the implications of my work would be international. Having no sense of what direction this would ultimately take, I continued on the path that felt harmonious to me. I must humbly confess my ignorance that, at the time of this experience, I did not know that La Storta was the town where Ignatius Loyola had experienced his vision, his invitation to help "reform" the Catholic Church – an experience which led to his founding of the Jesuit Order. Recently, I have grown in understanding the implications of my experience there; it continues to unfold.

Among the most pivotal points in my life turning me toward my current work, were a series of traumas that occurred in 1983 which profoundly affected me and moved me in the direction of trauma research. These painful experiences included the emotional loss of my best friend, Marty, the death of my priest-friend, Joe, and the death of my mother from cancer. These were the three most powerful influences in my life at that time. To deal with my pain, I simply intensified my focus on my studies, not knowing how to deal with such profound sadness and grief, yet knowing that these feelings could better be addressed around family and friends. I completed my degrees at the earliest possible date and returned home to begin my ministry in Louisiana. My work in parishes of more than two thousand families allowed me to channel my sense of loss into constructive outlets, but it did not resolve the pain. One of my joys during this difficult time was the ongoing archaeological work which the diocese, with its increasing shortage of priests, hesitantly allowed me to continue. Within a few years of active ministry in Baton Rouge, I found myself "burning out" and feeling as though I were dying emotionally. Clearly, I was workaholic, attending less and less to my emotional pain. Because my peers were also struggling under increased occupational demands and were utilizing similar compulsive coping mechanisms, they were of little support. It was apparent to me that without changes in my life this sense of impending emotional death would intensify. I took a "leave of absence" in 1988 intending to identify the fundamental sources of my earlier anxiety. I began to delve into the underlying traumas which occurred within my family and religious system that had contributed to my unrest. My fascination grew as I discovered that childhood and adulthood trauma had profoundly shaped my choices in life. I was amazed at how unaware I was of the traumatic impact of certain childhood experiences. Immediately, some unique opportunities arose which, through following my intuition, validated what I had known all along – that I would, eventually, be specializing in a specific area of ministry. I began to perceive that, in light of my personal history and recent experiences, this service involved the integration of three of my life themes: trauma, science, and spirituality. These three themes had been evidenced throughout my life, whether in archaeology, ministry, or my everyday experience. I subsequently committed myself to the exploration of these personally historic themes.

I managed to delay facing the traumas that occurred earlier in my life by focusing on service to others in much the same way that my parents had modeled. I was surprised at the powerful feelings that remained from the traumas that had occurred years before. Facing the unresolved emotions that I had stored was a primary step toward the integration of my "life themes." From the liberation that I experienced through trauma resolution, I became motivated to help others get in touch with these peak emotional experiences that hold their victims captive until released. The trauma survivors that I met greatly facilitated my journey into exploring the interrelationship of trauma, science, and spirituality. Particularly through the guidance of some very intuitive women who were also therapists and healers, I began to see my path more clearly.

Some of the most spiritual people I encountered were recovering alcoholics and trauma survivors who had come face to face with their own deaths emotionally through their traumas. I could see clearly that there was a gift to be gained by embracing one's traumas instead of repressing, medicating, or avoiding them in other ways. Though not alcoholic myself, I had benefited greatly from the spiritual recovery model from programs such as The Twelve Steps of Alcoholics Anonymous and its off-spring self-help groups (e.g., Adult Children of Alcoholics, Al-Anon, Codependents Anonymous, etc.). I chose to become a Certified Addictions Counselor because of the spiritual nature of the approach to treating addictions, and soon found myself drawn into the histories of my clients who revealed powerful, antecedent forces that had precipitated their need to medicate. These forces originated in moments of trauma. As a result, I specialized in learning and developing techniques to resolve the trauma-induced triggers that fostered such compulsivity and relapse. I began to realize that the majority of my clients with addictions were also traumas survivors, often with extensive trauma histories. In even the least of my traumatized, addicted clients, the addiction itself had often managed to imprint as a trauma. Having medicated their feelings for long periods of time, emotional blockages had been erected; years of anger and hurt had been repressed through drink or other medicating agents. I also discovered that many of my clients had tried, like myself, to find ways of forgetting or releasing the pain of their traumas. And, like myself, they often found themselves recycling the same feelings over and over without release. Both for my own health and that of my clients, I began to investigate techniques that promised to more effectively resolve the feelings induced from trauma. I became acquainted with verbal techniques and approaches to trauma resolution like those of David Grove, a psychologist from New Zealand, and with electromagnetic field techniques like "Healing Touch," which, I found, when used in conjunction, greatly accelerated the trauma resolution process.[2] While creating the safety needed for my clients to resolve their trauma memories, I discovered a number of techniques which allowed me to support and enhance the functioning of their nervous systems during the process. When fully applied, these new principles enhanced their sensory access to memory, improving their ability to visualize and perceive the details of the experience without inducing a "relive" of the event. With these new tools in place, my own style and technique of memory resolution began to evolve very quickly. Soon I saw some amazing results:

- The negative feelings of a specific trauma could be fully resolved without having to relive the event and without subsequent recurrence.
- The need to medicate or "act out" a compulsive behavior often diminished considerably when the precipitating event or trauma was resolved.
- The "triggers" that had fostered relapse, flashbacks, and depression due to the presence of trauma in the body were no longer present.
- The physical symptoms and many illnesses of my clients completely disappeared when the original trauma scene was resolved, suggesting that eighty percent or more of the illnesses in evidence in the average person were trauma-induced and could be resolved using effective trauma resolution therapies.
- The spiritual impoverishment felt by many of my clients was directly related to their trauma and was pre-moral in its inception. This meant that there were profound spiritual implications to the induction of trauma.
- Many of the helping professionals who experienced the process reported that the effects were immediate and were cognitive, behavioral, and affective in their impact.
- Clients evidenced profound improvement in the functioning of the autonomic nervous system, the endocrine and the immune systems.
- Certain immunological problems, as the low T-Cell count in the HIV positive patients, showed considerable improvement once trauma resolution techniques were effectively incorporated. This was predictable from our current purview of the impact of trauma on the immune system.
- A positive correlation was found between the location in which a disease presented itself and the site storing the trauma memories. The location where the pain was encoded at the moment of trauma, quite often, became a site of illness. This was a predictable result of carrying distortions for years in the nerve centers of the body.

Though originally developed for my work with addicted populations, it became apparent that the underlying causes of many physical diseases as well as depression, perfectionism, compulsivity, and self-destructive behaviors had their origins in trauma. After working with a chemically dependent population in an inpatient setting, I was asked to extend my trauma work to dually diagnosed patients (for example, those with both alcoholism and major depression) and to those in the psychiatric unit. Here I found that many personality disorders originated in trauma, and, without a better understanding of the dynamics of trauma-induction, many of these patients were given psychiatric diagnoses while the Post-Traumatic Stress Disorder and the less evident traumas were missed during psychological assessment. With increasing success in the treatment of trauma and while working for an outpatient chemical dependency center, I also began to see the need to help survivors recognize the spiritual impact that trauma had in their lives and their relationships. They often berated themselves on a moral level for the dysfunction in their lives when, in fact, it was quite evident that the unhealthy behaviors and patterns were trauma related. To facilitate spiritual healing from trauma, I developed a spirituality tract that was used in conjunction with the treatment offered in the chemical dependency and psychiatric units. It was successful with patients and well received by administrators, due to its use of the more positively oriented trauma resolution model in place of the frequently shaming morality-based model.

As the technique continued to evolve and my effectiveness in treating trauma survivors increased, I was invited to bring my trauma work to a Catholic hospital. Incidentally, this was the hospital where I had been born. While my technique improved considerably during my work at this facility, it was unfortunate that well-researched and documented techniques like "Healing Touch" were suspect. The administration was bogged down religiously and politically in its efforts to introduce the proper protocols – those that had earlier been accepted in sister hospitals in other parts of the state. Before I could make further contribution to the discussion, I was invited to become Clinical Director of Cottonwood of Albuquerque, a treatment center to which I had referred clients due to its specialization in the treatment of acute trauma. Not long after my move to Albuquerque, New Mexico, Cottonwood Centers, Inc., decided to merge its Albuquerque facility with its larger Tucson, Arizona facility. Suddenly, I found myself in Tucson, developing the trauma resolution component as an adjunct to the treatment of chemical dependency, severe trauma cases, dual diagnosis patients, and a variety of other diagnoses. Word of the effectiveness of the technique I was developing spread through the experiences of both patient and therapist alike, and by the fall of 1994, I was asked to train therapists to use my approach for the resolution of trauma. Pressure began to mount for a more detailed description of my method, its history, implications, and underlying principles. As a resource for trauma survivors, therapists, and family members of survivors who were struggling to grasp what their loved ones were experiencing, I began to record my experiences in writing.

This book is intended as a tool for any of you who are desirous of gaining understanding and empowerment from experiences of trauma, whether this is your experience or that of a loved one. In its larger scope, I hope that this work reaches out to touch members of the population, especially children and adolescents, whose lives could be transformed at a younger age than has occurred for many trauma survivors. It is my belief that this process and its implications will provide new options for treatment of many diseases and disorders. Our findings suggest that many illnesses, some of which we are deeming "terminal" or "chronic," are being missed as the opportunities for healing that they are. Unresolved traumas manifest their presence in our systems by creating the imbalances which we come to label as "disease." These illnesses are the cues to healing our unresolved traumas which, when followed and resolved, leave us with no further need for such painful warnings or lessons.

About this Book

You will note that there is a strong spiritual component to this work. By "spiritual" I do not mean religious, for spirituality was evidenced in human evolution long before the advent of organized religion. The organized religions as we know them are, in comparison, fairly recent developments (this is the archaeologist speaking). Today we are coming to understand the profound role that trauma has played from humankind's inception. Rather than emerging as the victims of our past, we are on the verge of consciously claiming our identities as the "creators" of a new, emergent reality. The nature of trauma is such that it is profoundly tied into our spiritual nature – to the very question of our rapport with the "Creator," "God," the "Divine" or "Transcendent," though it is not my intention to define this for you. That is a personal journey which we each must undertake. Within this work, however, we will explore this question from the perspective of trauma. I feel comfortable stating that the most severe impact of trauma is spiritual, involving the actual containment and splitting of consciousness in such a way that our creative potential is necessarily diminished. Just as trauma is an altered state of consciousness – a fragment of consciousness that is separated by crisis from that greater unity that is self, so too is there a profound consequence for that greater unity we call spirit. Hence, if we fail to honor the power and invitation to heal the traumas of our lives, or are directed not to do so – perhaps to just "forgive and forget"— this is tantamount to spiritual abuse. From my own lessons and experience, born of the struggle to address trauma within my family, educational, religious and other social systems, I will discuss this notion of spiritual abuse. Much spiritual abuse has occurred from lack of knowledge and information about how traumas are induced and encoded. Our deepening understanding of consciousness and the mind's functioning assists us in this undertaking of healing. Within this work you will glimpse how influential are the states of mind that capture our traumas and our spirits. It appears that we have been, both individually and collectively, much like an adult with childhood trauma and the accompanying symptom of amnesia. Suddenly, we are awakening physically, emotionally, mentally, and spiritually to find the source of our loss of power – and it is all happening in concert! There is a growing appreciation for the intricacy of the human mind and its profound unity with the body. There is a spiritual awakening arising in conjunction with increased awareness of mind-body connection that directs us toward inherent unity.

I have structured this work to provide insight into the physical, emotional, mental, and spiritual implications of trauma. The format is designed to lead you through experiences and techniques from which I have learned the power of mind-body-spirit unity and its influence over the illusions of time and space. Hence, a brush with quantum physics is also contained herein. In the initial chapters we will explore the nature of the "Healing Dimensions" and the means of access and movement within this mysterious space. We will further examine the origins and principles underlying the trauma induction process, its encoding and resolution. I have also included some important reflections on how these principles manifest in the experience of diseases and dreams. I hope that the resources we share will facilitate your own healing process and provide you with valuable insights into the unlimited power for healing that you possess.

Chapter Two

The Journey To Empowerment

"Our deepest fear is not that we are inadequate. Our deepest fear is that we are powerful beyond measure. It is our light, not our darkness, that most frightens us. We ask ourselves, 'Who am I to be brilliant, gorgeous, talented, fabulous?'

Actually, who are you not to be? You are a child of God. Your playing small doesn't serve the world. There's nothing enlightened about shrinking so that other people won't feel insecure around you.

We were born to make manifest the Glory of God that is within us. It's not just in some of us. It's in everyone, and, as we let our light shine, we unconsciously give other people permission to do the same. As we are liberated from our own fear, our presence automatically liberates others."

— *From the Inaugural Address of Nelson Mandela,*
President of South Africa

16

As we embark upon this journey into the healing resources of body, mind, and spirit, I emphasize that the principal goal is that of empowerment. The power that I allude to is ever-present and is accessible to each of us. How is it, then, that we find ourselves powerless in certain moments of our lives? Through the traumatic episodes of our lives, each of us has been imprinted with illusions which foster a sense of powerlessness and dependency upon persons, systems, jobs, and ideologies. Yet, beneath it all is a profound, relentless craving for a wholeness and well-being that, somehow we know, must, ultimately, be found within the self. There is something that is constantly guiding us in the direction of this solution, whether we call it intuition, the subconscious, the Higher Self, the Transcendent, God, or the Source of All Things. For myself, I sought that security in the purity and truth of science. Later I found that science did not satisfy my craving nor my higher security needs; it did not answer my deeper questions.

I began studying to be a priest at age thirteen. I turned to what others had told me was spirituality, only to invest another thirteen years learning that religion was not the same as spirituality. Nonetheless, I am grateful for the lessons. In many ways, I have come to see that the journey has allowed me to identify a number of common threads woven through all of our lives. In some strange way, I write as "everyone." At the time of this writing, I have worked with a broad spectrum of trauma, evidenced in the lives of over five thousand survivors. I have understood each to some degree; I have learned volumes. These experiences have proven to be a most precious gift. I have been privileged to witness life-shaping events, to enter life's most critical moments of trauma and pain, and to participate in the healing of body, mind, and spirit. The fact that I am able to feel, literally, the emotional joys and pains of others as a physical sensation in my hands has added a dimension to my life that has demanded and promoted growth on many levels. A psychiatrist colleague asked me recently if I were an "empath" – that is, if I feel the pain of others as the same sensation in my own body. "Not exactly!" I responded, "I'm actually more of an 'inverse empath' – that is, as my clients access more and more of their pain, I become calmer; yet I do feel their pain as a distinct pressure or quality of discomfort in my hands; I see or locate their traumas with my hands." My mother apparently possessed the same ability, for when my siblings and I were in accidents, she felt a distinct physical change in her body, even over long distances. She described it as an "icy cold feeling," though she did not feel exactly the same sensation that we felt during the event. From my experience with this ability, particularly during the last five years, I have come to believe that we are each capable of developing this skill to some degree. I have had the privilege to teach many others, both nationally and internationally, to access this awareness within themselves. The simplicity of the healing process and techniques which I present to you reinforces for me the importance of not deifying nor externalizing our natural birthright. You are a healer. You are your own expert healer. That is precisely why this process is effective. You are doing it. I am a facilitator who can help to locate and activate the power you hold within. In this journey you are invited to explore your healing, creative power to assist in bringing yourself, others, nature, and our universe into oneness, into unity.

If I were to summarize for you the single most important lesson that I have gleaned from my "spiritual formation," it would be this: "**in**" – a two-letter word, a preposition even! Yet, it points to the single most important message of spirituality. In the Catholic spiritual tradition in which I was raised, it is called an "interiority concept." My experience shows that the effectiveness of any religious or "spiritual" system can be evaluated by the degree to which it has communicated effectively to its members the knowledge and the experience that the locus of divinity is **within** us. The power of this truth continues to be unrealized in our society and in our religious systems. This has not been, necessarily, intentional. For instance, it would appear that the message of Jesus that the individual is the Temple of the Divine – that the Holy Spirit now dwells within the psyche of the human person, has become sidetracked. This is due, in part, to the assumption that the blockages to the access and exercise of the "spiritual gifts" are linked to "sin" and "morality." It appears that we have not understood or have ignored the information about ways this Temple functions in times of stress and trauma. Trauma is pre-moral in its induction within the body, mind, and spirit, as we will see in the ensuing chapters. Once induced, it sets up barriers in the subconscious, which is the primary font for our spiritual thought.

Without an adequate understanding of the magnificence of this Temple of Consciousness and its ability to protect us from spiritual, emotional, mental, and physical threats, we are left with limited laws of morality. I have always known that my major spiritual obstacles were emotional and were largely in place before the age of moral decision-making at ages seven to eight. They were trauma-induced, leaving me with fewer moral options for use upon reaching moral decision-making age. To be promised spiritual enlightenment and healing but to be provided with inadequate tools for illumination and healing constitutes "spiritual abuse" by those systems claiming such power. Abuse need not be intentional. Without an adequate understanding of the ways my Temple of Consciousness functions, naturally I look outward for guidance and direction. Without this deeper grasp of the creator-healer potential within my psyche, my focus remains, like that of the needy child, outward. In this state of external attention, I remain vulnerable to outside influences which can easily lead to further dis-empowerment. Trauma reinforces this condition. Much of the empowerment, as intended by Jesus, for example, remains latent – buried beneath our subconscious blockages. In the meantime, we remain puzzled as to why our most sincere moral solution, our decision to "forgive," leaves us feeling little better when we recall the trauma experience. Proposing moral solutions for trauma experiences, many religious systems adamantly believe their brand of solution to be adequate for the task. Healing can and often does occur, in varying degrees, through woefully inadequate agencies. I can see now that, as a priest, I sometimes helped others in spite of myself and my limited thinking. While in ministry, I reminded others that it was Pope John XXIII who, with his sagacious wit, indicated that the Catholic church must offer authentic healing on some level because, he stated, "It continues to exist in spite of its priests." From my own experience I know that spiritually nurturing systems are here to promote our growth and expansion as primary, while unhealthy systems posit that we exist to make the system whole. It is the same in dysfunctional family systems. The spiritually nurturing system affirms that its purpose is to foster the child's growth – to allow the child to become empowered as the healer-creator that he is. (Please note: within the context of this work, masculine and feminine pronouns are used randomly to reflect that trauma knows no gender bias.) By this criterion our systems may be assessed. From such self-assessment, I chose to redirect my life and to step beyond the external constraints imposed by the well-intentioned systems. It was only then that the intuitive capacities I now exercise were free to emerge.

I believe that all of the traumatic experiences of our lives hold the promise of an equal, if not greater empowerment once we learn the means to approach them and use our inherent creative potential to transform and heal them. That is what we will be learning within this work.

I am a pragmatist at heart. There are many authors and researchers who are writing avidly of their understanding of the profound unity of body, mind, and spirit, but there are few who offer the answers as to how we can actually accomplish the hoped-for transformations. A nationally recognized physician and addictionologist once stated to me, despite my protestations that I had already taught several other therapists to do what I do, that, "I know that you have a gift – you're a healer; but the main problem I see is that what you do looks so simple and virtually painless that many people will find it hard to believe." He continued: "I've seen your work, and I know its results, but people have become accustomed to experiencing pain before they will believe that healing is occurring."

I responded by stating that I recognize that what I do involves a type of healing, particularly of memories. I added, however, that the "price of pain" has been more than paid by the trauma survivors who had to live with these immensely powerful scenes stored intact since the moment the trauma occurred. Many survivors and their family members have lived and relived their traumatic memories over and over, sometimes even at the therapist's prompting, hoping that these re-lives or "abreactions" would release them from the pain – only to find themselves triggered once again within a short time. No, the price of pain has already long been paid! I have worked with trauma survivors that have tried a multitude of trauma resolution therapies. And, speaking as one who is able to feel the stored emotional pain in the body of another, I can state that infrequently therapies achieve thorough resolution of trauma memories since they are stored in the cells and electromagnetic fields of the body. Few therapeutic approaches have reached the necessary levels to achieve the requisite release.

I was raised, as most of us, to be pain-avoidant. Fear taught me this. But, after living with pain for years, and after having client after client return to therapy sessions with me to re-live the same events repeatedly in a continuous re-experiencing of the pain, I became committed to the pursuit of a more effective way to resolve trauma memories and to find out what critical element or step we were missing in our approach. For many of my clients, their memories were triggered almost daily, leaving them with unexplainable fears, feelings of "dirtiness, unworthiness, inadequacy, failure, shame, guilt, shyness, incompleteness," etc. Some of them had panic attacks – with the same shortness of breath and pain that occurred at the onset of the original trauma; others came to see me while suffering migraines, stress headaches, chronic pain in their stomachs, backs, necks, and groin regions. Some had endured surgery repeatedly to alleviate the pain, only to find the pain return intact, even when the nerves were severed in the body. Frequently they reported the physicians' inability to explain why their pain continued. Many of the trauma survivors developed alternative and often compulsive or addictive coping mechanisms to compensate for the pain. Some compensated through work; others became chemically dependent. Many sought the alleviation of their suffering in relationships, sex, gambling, religion, food, exercise and a host of other behaviors. Human beings become very creative when attempting to stop pain. While trying to alleviate their discomfort, they became ensnared in and addicted to the "pseudo-solution." Nearly all experienced some depression and loss of self. No, I think that we are all too familiar with the pain of the many types of traumas and their impact upon our lives. We have come perilously close at times to accepting this type of pain-filled existence as the norm. This could not be more removed from the truth.

In the midst of our rapid advancement as a culture, we have become distracted and, in the process, surrendered much of our power to systems that have promised to heal us, guide us, support and secure us through transitional times. While there are systems that do support us, my experience teaches me that true security, ultimately, resides in trusting my intuition and in personal empowerment, not upon outside promises of safety. This also means that the healing process is always an internal or spiritual undertaking. There is no complete healing without bringing the spiritual and emotional aspects of self into the process. This has become even more apparent in my work with traditional healers – namely, physicians. Much of my work with physicians has involved educating them on an unpleasant issue: many of my clients induced trauma from their physician-healer while they were being treated. Sometimes the trauma was induced through insensitivity or due to the emotionally detached manner of the physician. In some cases it was the physicians own issues and traumas which were directed at the patient at a stressful moment. This raises a major ethical dilemma. Within the Hippocratic Oath is the mandate to never render harm to another. Since trauma, as we shall see in more detail later in this work, directly impacts and weakens the functioning of the immune system, the manner in which a patient is treated can profoundly affect the outcome. Just as trauma resolution enhances the functioning of the immune system and leads to an increase in the T-Cell count, so, too, trauma to the immune system diminishes its functioning. Only recently are medical schools considering the emotional and spiritual components of treatment by providing the training needed in order to prevent traumatization in the doctor-patient relationship. The other side of the picture that I see from my work with impaired (i.e., chemically dependent, emotionally ill) physicians, is the traumatization that can occur to them through abuse from their patients and from repeated exposure to crisis. Rarely have they been provided with the resources to process the profound emotional crises that arise from dealing day in and day out with life and death situations. As a priest arriving on the scene of tragedies and family crises, I found myself detaching emotionally and stuffing my feelings to prevent feeling overwhelmed. When I detached from my emotions, I lost something that could have enhanced my ministry to others, but I did not know how to remain in my emotions without moving into trauma. This skill has evolved through my work with many trauma survivors. Much of it has come from overcoming my fear of trauma itself.

Recent research into the functioning of the brain indicates that emotion is central to the process of rational thought; emotion is a key component of learning and decision-making.[1] When we eliminate emotional data from our interactions with others and from our decisions, certain vital channels will not be available to support the healing effort. Since emotions, as we shall see, are the primary bridge to our spirituality and relationships, these critical levels of interaction will also be impacted. I have worked with a number of cases where individuals were surgically intervened upon when the presenting issue could have been easily identified as emotional trauma had the physician been open to the emotional data evident in the patient's affect and presentation. Knowing what I now know about trauma, it is no longer an option for me to attempt to minister to or present myself to assist in the healing of others while shutting off my emotions. It is this very openness to emotion and my respect for the power of affect that allows me to do what I do and to feel what I feel in service to my clients. I have recovered a spiritual awareness in the process that was not even hinted at in my many years of training for ministry.

Let us examine the key question: What happens when intensely painful emotions are stored intact in the nervous system for prolonged periods of time as a result of trauma? These traumatic experiences will significantly color and shape our daily experiences until they are resolved. Merely talking about an emotionally painful experience will not always release the pain. I know this both from my personal resolution work, from having counseled others in ministry, and as a formerly frustrated therapist. The intellect cannot resolve what is emotionally imprinted. It is this imprinting process and its resolution that are the focus of this work. Just how powerful the imprinting process is will become clear in the remarkable cases we shall see within this work.

In learning the dynamics of trauma induction and in order to find more effective ways of resolving painful experiences, I first had to broaden my understanding of trauma. Originally when I was asked if I had experienced any traumas, I responded: "Well, no, I don't think so ... my family seemed pretty normal to me." Most of us assume that our upbringing was "normal." Well, at least it was normal for our family, wasn't it? Our parents or primary caregivers were, usually, the first to begin providing us with our language, our earliest notion of self, and the modeling needed to make our way through life. Their actions, speech, behaviors, and identities became our first definitions of love and normality. What was normal within our families, however comfortable, may not have been healthy. In addition to the natural vulnerability of a child whose learning is wholly dependent on what is imprinted from the caregivers, there is the issue of the nervous system's sensitivity. At last, in this decade, we are devoting our energy and attention to understanding the immensity of the brain, the mind, and the nature of consciousness. Through my capacity to physically perceive the pain-encoded transactions of trauma within the nervous system, I hold that we are dealing with an infinitely complex and sophisticated system that is living, interactive with all things, and profoundly sensitive on all levels. Trauma can, in such a system, be induced through oversight, accident, abandonment, neglect, through the witnessing of trauma to others, through one's degree of emotional sensitivity, and, of course, through more overt forms of abuse such as emotional, physical, sexual, mental, and spiritual abuse.

Oftentimes we deny any history of trauma out of fear that it will reveal something defective about us or our families. This is far from the actual truth. Trauma encoding and storage is demonstrative of our remarkable dynamics for self-healing — a manifestation of an immune system of consciousness. Events that overwhelm us are automatically stored by the interactive work of the autonomic nervous system, the endocrine system, and the immune system – all facilitated by the limbic-hypothalamic system. We will examine this in more detail in the ensuing chapters.

To a very young child, the refusal of a hug from a significant caregiver at a certain moment can prove traumatic. It does not take much to overwhelm a child. Similarly, we would expect some advantage to having such fragile boundaries. If trauma is so easily induced in us when we are young, should it not be able to be released easily as well? This is precisely what we are discovering. While I have not worked extensively with young children using this technique, I have worked with adolescents. They are remarkable. Irrespective of their presenting issues, because their boundaries are not well formed, they are able to access and resolve their traumatic memories in considerably less time than most adults. Who would think that there would be a therapy that chemically dependent adolescents would actually seek out and enjoy? In my current practice, the adolescents are my favorite group. Not long ago one of my adult clients brought her eleven year old son Robbie to address an abuse memory from some years prior. After "reframing" the memory from a negative scene to a positive one within just a few minutes, he left with his mother and brother in the car. While on the way home, his younger brother alluded to a fear that he was feeling. Robbie began using the trauma resolution technique to help his younger brother. His mother, who was familiar with the technique and had attended one of my training workshops, stated that she nearly drove the car off the road from the shock of realizing that he had learned the essential technique in a single session. The children, being less defended, heal more quickly and learn more easily.

Sensitivity works both ways, just as it does with boundaries and defenses. How many of us thought that blocking our negative childhood experiences would allow us to move forward free of the pain and trauma? Fortunately, our systems have built-in balances and safeguards that protect us from "stuffing" our feelings and traumatizing ourselves. These safeguards are rarely more evident than when we try to shut out or forget our "bad" memories, only to find that we have blocked out the good memories as well. The mechanism of repressing feelings is not a discriminatory filter allowing only the good to come through. I have worked with several individuals who, upon resolving two or three trauma memories, recovered numerous positive, nurturing childhood experiences that also had been repressed when the original trauma occurred. The walls that we build around ourselves do not discriminate. To blindly stuff or store our feelings creates the necessity for them to manifest in another manner, resonating to get our attention. There is a very real system of checks and balances. The emotional energy of our experiences is neither created nor destroyed; it just is. What form it takes in our nervous system is determined by our ways of coping with it. Traumas are simply holding patterns – patterns of energy pregnant with messages from other places and times when we were overwhelmed by strident life experience. These patterns emerge as part of our self-healing. It is through the resolution of such experiences that we unveil our true identities as the creators and sustainers of our realities. In my perception, there is a potent spiritual force at work here. Trauma is a powerful teacher. By consciously facing these stored moments of near-emotional-death we learn to utilize our power to transform these frozen, messages from blockages to bridges. These bridges enable us to explore our potential as creators of our reality rather than defining ourselves as its victims. This is a profoundly transformative spiritual process.

(The implications of this process are profound as well. It would appear that our tastes, dislikes, fears, phobias, relational patterns, comfort with our sexuality, capacity for intimacy – our very insecurities are directly related to the traumas that constrict us.) The fact that I have been able to take instances of dysfunctional or compulsive behaviors, ask individuals to focus on the precipitating feeling and, in each case, access a specific, relevant traumatic experience, reinforces the necessity of resolving our trauma memories if we are to freely promulgate our reality. None of us is without trauma as it is defined within this work and from what we have learned about the nervous system (See p. xv for the definition of trauma). The trauma induction/storage process is one of the main strengths of our spiritual psyche – the ability to manipulate our time and space perceptions until we are resourceful enough and safe enough for our traumas to surface and be healthily resolved.

I was privileged to facilitate the case of Jeremy, a young man who had no memory before the age of thirteen, who, I suspected, suffered from "traumatic amnesia." After resolving two horrific memories of sexual abuse, he suddenly recalled the majority of his childhood. Tearfully he thanked me and stated that he could now recall even his first birthday party. Another client, Sarah, sought treatment for addiction to pain medication due to acute physical discomfort that caused insomnia. She accessed and resolved feelings of leg cramps and abandonment while in her baby bed at age two, whereupon she released the pain trapped within her memory and was, thenceforth, able to sleep without the leg pain that had plagued her for forty-two years. But there are also the hundreds of traumatic moments when children overheard mom and dad fighting and arguing, unable to conceive how such a thing could be; or the many cases of a beloved or trusted family member touching them inappropriately or shaming them about their appearance or weight. There are the numerous memories of traumas by educators who employed disciplinary techniques that felt shaming, traumatizing, and abusive – some of whom were wearing attire that attested to a spiritual or medical origin or authority. In the context of this work, we will begin to examine the impact of spiritual abuse, particularly the impact of the seeming betrayals by our first gods – the first "higher powers" on whom we were totally dependent for life, love, and nurturing – our parents! There are also the traumas by our own religious representatives whom we blindly trusted to mediate God for us but whose love was tainted by their own unhealed traumas.

Having reached a level in our evolution where we can resolve memories without reliving them, we can revisualize or reframe feelings that have long controlled us and enlist them for the healing of our bodies, minds, and spirits. By "reframing," I allude to the ability that we each possess to change the emotional sense of a scene, eradicating the negative emotional content and substituting a positive perspective. In exploring these techniques within this work, I encourage you to keep yourself safe. As you read, some of the cases and examples may trigger memories of your own. While much can be done to foster safety, and while many memories can be reframed using the techniques detailed in this work, it should be noted that there are certain types of memories that our minds will not allow us to address alone. The intensity of some of these experiences demands the safety and aid of a facilitator. If such experiences begin to surface in your reading of this book, I counsel you to contact a therapist or facilitator to support you. It is true that many of us would prefer to heal ourselves in a private, quietly controlled manner. Since many of our traumas were induced interpersonally by others, however, a tremendous amount of healing emerges when we realize that there are other individuals who, rather than treating us as objects for their gratification and abusing us, see our inherent worth and integrity, while committing themselves to help us recover our personal power and nobility. While most of us would prefer the "quick fix" – to simply stay at home and fix it ourselves, it is far more efficacious to resolve certain traumas interpersonally when they were interpersonally induced. Trust can quickly and effectively be restored in this manner. Within the context of this work, we will explore the multidimensional impact of trauma on our relationships – to ourselves, to others, to nature – yes, and to our spirituality itself.

Trauma can be a painful and often frightening subject to examine. The degree of resistance to this journey often reveals the degree of necessity of making the journey back to health and freedom. I encourage you to open yourself to your feelings, your dreams, your self-talk, the patterns that emerge in your life today. This is the place where the fertile soil of empowerment and healing is found.

Safety is a prerequisite for trauma resolution and for overcoming any unnecessary resistance. Notwithstanding our most determined efforts to liberate ourselves from the influence of trauma, a trained facilitator can provide the safety and tools to overcome resistance and achieve resolution. The intensity, severity, and scale of trauma determine the need for outside facilitation. These factors figure significantly in determining the degree of overwhelm one experiences from trauma. As a society and as a culture, such overwhelm is far more prevalent due to a perceived, growing lack of safety. Given our virtually instantaneous access via "live media coverage" to local and global traumas within minutes of their occurrence, we are bombarded with traumatic experiences. Our families and educators did not prepare us to address this degree of exposure to trauma.

There is an appropriateness to the timing of this journey into the dynamics of trauma. Our media and mass communication are competitively focused on utilizing disasters and trauma to get our attention and their revenue. There seems to be a "no holds barred" mentality arising, with few cautions about the potentially traumatic nature of the manner in which a situation is presented publicly. In the case of the Oklahoma City bombing, for instance, I heard reports in the week that followed of several people whose traumatic memories had been triggered by the media presentation of this event. Is there a possible correlation between the media's sensationalizing presentation of traumatic events and the increase in our society's need to medicate pain? We are told that addictions are "on the rise." Media is adept at stimulating our "trauma triggers" to seize our attention. We are learning that stimulation of our memory triggers reproduces part of the original adrenaline (endocrine system) reaction and serves to focus our attention on events similar to our own traumas. Accessing such pain without knowing how to resolve it, we seek to medicate it. One such global trigger can be the catalyst for the surfacing of unresolved memories of thousands of "survivors" – each with her own emotional pain. With our current resources and competition in the field of mass communication, retraumatization is a common phenomenon. Scarcely a trauma exists that has not been converted into a film. Given the vivid access to events via live coverage, situations like the assassination of President Kennedy, the Challenger explosion, or the untimely death of Princess Diana will always present as global trauma. I become gravely concerned, however, when I realize that we have not really understood how these events have impacted our bodies, minds, and spirits until now. I vividly recall the words of one of my clients who, amidst her trauma work, discovered that it was the day of President Kennedy's assassination that she, as a seven year old child, stopped playing with dolls. She stated:

> *I just remember feeling like something died that day. I didn't really know what – I just knew that Mommy and Daddy were crying and were so upset … I was confused, but I could really feel the sadness. I didn't know what to do, so I just went outside and buried my doll. I don't remember playing with dolls after that.*

I have encountered many other individuals who, similarly, shared the vulnerability they experienced when, upon the assassination of President Kennedy, they saw their parents confused and grief-stricken. Now we are beginning to understand the impact of such global traumas. I witnessed this phenomenon most recently in preparation for my first workshop in London. Unexpectedly, the people of Great Britain and the whole world were faced with the shocking death of Princess Diana. Such events are global in their impact, serving to trigger countless reactions on an unimaginably large scale, resurrecting those feelings and issues that are closely tied to our personal histories. Such encompassing traumas profoundly impact our individual and mutual hopes and dreams, our collective consciousness, and, in doing so, our evolution.

In this "decade of the brain," we are glimpsing the depths of the magnificent and sophisticated system that imprints, stores, processes, and protects us from overwhelming experiences of our lives. For many of us, the actual healing of our traumas is, only now, commencing.

Exercise For The Creation of a "Safe Place":

This exercise is helpful for fostering a sense of security and assuring us that we are now capable of creating safety for ourselves. Safety is among our most basic needs. It is the prerequisite for all effective trauma resolution. Utilize this exercise as a resource during your journey through <u>The Healing Dimensions</u>.

1. Begin by taking a couple of deep breaths. As you exhale, picture yourself releasing all tension and stress from your body. As you inhale, draw into yourself light, well-being, and health.

2. Create for yourself the ideal Safe Scene. If you have already created such a place for yourself in present time, visualize this place now. If you have no Safe Scene, let us create one. Some favorite suggestions include: the beach or ocean, a field of wild flowers, the mountains, the woods, a cabin on a mountaintop or by a stream or river, a garden, a butterfly garden, walking in the clouds, a park, journeying in space, fishing, at the home of a beloved family member, in the presence of an angel or God. (These are some of the more frequently chosen safe scenes.) Take all the time that you need to find your safe place.

3. After you have chosen your safe place, use each of your senses to create and experience this peace (a favorite technique of Ignatius Loyola.) See it! Smell it! Feel the quiet, safe, calm atmosphere created by the scene. Feel what it is like to be completely safe from all harm, threat, danger or distraction. Some of us have never known such a place. See if there is anything or anyone else that you wish to accompany you in your safe place. Sometimes favorite pets, "animal guides," or spiritual guides are welcome. Remember that your Safe Scene is a living place that can always be improved or changed, as needed.

4. Photograph the Scene! When you have the scene as you want it for now, take a picture of it. If any of the details of the picture are blurry, something remains that you must "fix" in the picture to make it completely safe. When you can photograph it clearly, the essentials are in place.

5. Frame the Scene! After you have photographed the picture, place a frame around it of the color or colors of your choosing. (Note: If you had problems imaging a safe scene, you may find that you can simply use color to create the safety.) After determining the color(s) you want, move them through your whole body from head to foot. Frequently this is achieved by visualizing the colors flowing through the body like water, floating through (avoiding any blockages through which they simply cannot pass), or moving through the body like an X-ray scanner beam. These colors communicate to your nervous system, through frequency, the content of the picture. The movement of the colors through your body is an expedient, effective way of notifying the cells and fields of your body that this is now your chosen reality. As you move the color(s) of the frame through your body, you will experience an increased sense of relaxation and calm. Sometimes your hands and feet will tingle due to the energy displacement from these nerve plexes (centers). These colors can be utilized at any time that relaxation and calm are needed during the day. If, for some reason, your safe scene should begin to feel unsafe, a memory or issue may have been triggered. In the following chapters we will discuss techniques to resolve such memory triggers so that safety may be restored. Visualizing the colors as water flowing through the body helps to secure the image and, additionally, helps to relieve chronic pain or discomfort.

6. Record or Depict the Scene: If you are artistically inclined or feel creative, you may wish to draw or create some type of visual depiction or reminder of your safe scene. Any outstanding color, image, or feature from the scene can be used to cue you to its presence and return you to its security. Typically, upon completion of this work, clients trace the essentials of the safe scene in their journals and note the colors for future reference. Any anchor that helps to secure the new safe scene as a reality reinforces this new perception within the nervous system.

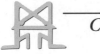

Chapter Three

Where is the love, beauty and truth we seek,
but in our mind?

> *Percy B. Shelley (1792-1822)*

Holographic Space

This work's primary goal is to support your recognition of the part of yourself that understands, dialogues with, and constantly abides within that space where all healing occurs. It is not an imaginary place, and it has often been ignored due to our eagerness to find security in the concrete and material realities presented to us by our five primary senses. Our eyesight, for instance, while incredibly sophisticated, generally renders images from the reflection of photons of light off of the denser particles and waves which constitute "matter" – photons which then imprint on the retina of the eye, upside down, and are subsequently organized and reinterpreted by the brain right-side-up. Once organized and "reduced," these images appear solid, although, in fact, all is comprised of living waves and particles of energy. Even as young children we learn to become comfortable with these 3-D images. While most of us are taught to become trusting of our five senses, few of us are taught to move beyond them or to use them "internally." Moving beyond the limitations of our five senses is also, I assure you, quite natural to us. Initially when I asked trauma survivors about the locations and descriptions of the feelings which remained after their traumas, I noticed that immediately they began to provide detailed three-dimensional descriptions of what seemed to be geometrically shaped objects or symbols. These were usually located at the nerve center nearest the physiological site of the trauma – where the intrusion or violation was felt most intensely. The extraordinary detail that they provided and their certainty about the presence of these internal images surprised me. What exactly were these 3-D images that they were "seeing" in their nerve centers, and how were they able to perceive them? Exploring these strange perceptions within myself and my clients, I noticed that the effort to describe a headache pain – a common complaint, often yielded intricate pictures or symbols. Headaches and other somatic pains, appearing in geometric forms, were usually trauma-related. The survivors that I interviewed reported little difficulty with accessing and visualizing these "objects" derived from their traumas, as though this was a normal phenomenon. Perhaps, I thought, these internal 3-D images were the standard vehicles for encoding trauma. This insight was to prove more valid than I would have ever imagined.

Who of us has not experienced, at one time or another, a "lump" in our throat, a "knot" or "butterflies" in our stomach, a "burning" anger ready to explode inside our chest, the "pressure" of sadness and unshed tears trying to emerge from behind our eyes, a "pounding headache" like a drum inside our head? We have been taught to discount these perceptions or to assume their origin in the physical body. It has been estimated that it takes approximately thirteen trillion nerve cells to present these pictures to us within a matter of seconds, but if we placed these parts of our bodies under an X-ray machine, nothing would appear; the exception is when our traumas have begun to manifest in the physical body as disease. Although we are developing the technology to assess these more subtle electromagnetic distortions in and around our bodies, nothing exists that is comparable to our mind's own capacity to enter and assess this elusive realm within seconds. What precisely is this mysterious reality or dimension that we can access so easily?

The "dimensions" where healing occurs constitute what I refer to as "holographic space." A hologram is a three-dimensional image that appears in space through the action of light waves interacting with one another (See Figure 1, p. 37).[1] In his remarkable work, The Holographic Universe, Michael Talbot pointed out that University of

London physicist David Bohm, a protege of Einstein and one of the world's leading quantum physicists, and neurophysiologist Karl Pribram of Stanford University, simultaneously and independently arrived at the conclusion that the universe itself and the brain both function holographically.[2] According to Bohm, all of the inexplicable phenomena found in nature and encountered by quantum physics begin to make sense when we realize that the universe is a kind of giant hologram.[3] Similarly, Pribram indicates that the holographic model provides an understanding of memory, perception, and various neurophysiological puzzles that standard theories of the brain were unable to explain.[4] To refer to reality as "holographic" may give us the impression that it is less than real. This is not an accurate assessment. The truth of the holographic nature of reality provides a more integrated and interconnected way of perceiving reality. If my body is not as "solid" as I once thought, then, perhaps, I can see these fragments of trauma stored within my system. The implications of this new model are much larger than this, however. The holographic model is now being used to explain everything from near-death experiences to dreams and flashbacks. It is the most significant concept for understanding how we might emotionally freeze and become stuck in the painful realities created at moments of trauma. Scientists are beginning to understand that we are really discovering our ability to shift our consciousness from one level of the hologram to another. As you will see from the contents of this text, this is particularly true in the study of trauma and its impact on the physical, emotional, mental, and spiritual levels of being.

This underlying unity – the holographic model, and the realization that we all possess the ability to move within "holographic space," has profound implications. Within the context of this work we will see how this shifting of consciousness has been used to cure cancer, to heal memory with all of its accompanying symptoms and painful emotions. Further applications include resolving chronic pain, healing dreams, resolving the flashbacks and triggers that impair daily life, and alleviating common complaints such as stress headaches. These shifts of consciousness can be used to restore the sense of wholeness and integration that is lost from physical, emotional, mental, sexual, and spiritual abuse. The holographic model reveals our ability to access and utilize virtually unlimited resources through the subtle focusing of our minds. Our capacity to alter our states of consciousness is the birthright of our holographic nature. In studying the functioning of holographic space, we will explore our capacity to move, shift, and change within the holographic universe. This is a profoundly empowering and exciting journey. It is the discovery of hitherto unknown or forgotten options that are being brought to bear in what many consider to be a profound period of awakening.

The initial case that indicated to me the healing properties of holographic space occurred during my work at an inpatient psychiatric facility. At that time I had developed a spirituality tract for use in the chemical dependency and psychiatric units. At the start of one group session, I simply polled the group members asking them how they were progressing in treatment. One of the patients, Lorraine, who was in treatment for alcoholism, indicated that she was being discharged in two days. When asked how she felt about being discharged, she responded:

"OK, I guess, but something is not finished."

"What do you think it's about?" I asked.

She responded, "It's about shame!"

"And when you feel this shame," I asked, "where do you feel it physically, in your body?"

She immediately responded: "It's over my mouth, throat, and chest like a hot metallic triangle – I can feel it getting hotter (grabbing her throat) … can you see it?"

Her face became slightly flushed as she accessed these feelings. Her response also shocked me. Not only was the image very specific and detailed, but its intensity seemed to be strongly evidenced in her body, producing an overwhelming sensation which, she was convinced, was visible to others in the room. It was very clear that she perceived her "triangle" to be very "real" and somehow related to her unresolved feelings of "shame." I have come to refer to these holographic fragments that encode and store trauma as "metaphors."

These metaphors are vehicles, derived from our personal experience, which serve to articulate and contain the overwhelming sensations. Formally, "metaphor" has been defined as "the transfer of the name of one object to another through a relationship of analogy."[5] The concept is particularly useful, with respect to trauma, when we see that the metaphor that one uses is often a substitution based on a relationship of extension – part for the whole, and contiguity – container to content. The "hot metallic triangle of shame" was a fragment of the original shame experience and was the holographic form in which her traumatic episode had been contained in its entirety and stored intact within her nervous system. Such metaphors, as fragments of the larger memory, actually contain the whole and are the vehicles of healing and transformation.

After Lorraine had identified this memory fragment in her body, she became intensely aware of this distortion and was anxious to resolve it. Being, however, in a large group setting, I was hesitant to encourage a process that could go well beyond the time allotted for the group and, moreover, would not involve the rest of the group. Instead, I asked her to obtain an order from her psychiatrist and to schedule an individual therapy session for the next day; she did so. Immediately upon entering my office, before I could explain what she could expect from the process, she resumed her commentary on the metaphor: "Well, the metallic triangle isn't as hot as yesterday, but it's still there."

We proceeded to define the metaphor as it continued to impose itself within her awareness. After completely defining it, I checked to see if its point of origin was in present or past time: "And when you feel a hot metallic triangle like that over your mouth, throat, and chest areas – how young might you be when you first feel a triangle like that?" I asked in a quiet, non-threatening voice.

"Seven years old," she replied.

"And where might you be when you first feel this hot triangle when you're seven years old?" I questioned.

"I'm in the garage," she answered.

"And what happens then, when you're seven and you're in the garage?" I inquired.

"I see daddy, and I go up to him to ask him a question," she indicated.

"And what happens next when you go up to him to ask him a question?" I delved, mirroring her own language and tone while gently supporting her recollection.

Figure 1: The Hologram

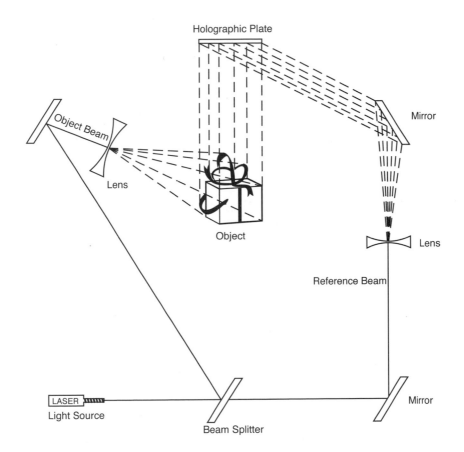

Figure 1: The hologram is produced when a single (laser) light is split into two separate beams: the reference beam and the object beam. The first beam is bounced off the object to be recorded: in this case, the "gift' pictured above; the second beam, the reference beam, is allowed to intersect with the reflected light of the first beam. The interference pattern created by the intersecting beams is then recorded on the holographic plate.

"He won't look at me, and he won't answer my question – it's like I'm not even there – he just ignores me," she added tearfully.

She proceeded to provide a historical narrative detailing the specifics of the trauma. When she was seven years old, her father lost his job. She and her father had been very close. Her father became depressed after having to take a lesser position with another company in order to remain in town. One day she approached her father to simply ask him a question. Her father did not respond to her question; in fact, he ignored her completely. At that instant, this seven year old girl found, as she stated: "I couldn't talk; I couldn't swallow; and I couldn't breathe." Tracking the feelings of hurt and shame that were induced in her mouth – expanding into her throat – and finally broadening out into her chest, I could see the exact dimensions of the shame feelings – a "hot, metallic triangle" of great intensity captured within her nervous system. Upon reaching this part of her history, Lorraine responded to my question by regressing into the unresolved, frozen feelings of the seven year old girl, sobbing and repeating, "I really thought that he just didn't love me any more … that he didn't want anything to do with me." She sobbed for several minutes. After she had released the feelings of sadness and the tears stored up for twenty-two years, I asked her if there was anything else about the event that she needed to describe. She proceeded to a description of how she became extremely self-conscious and afraid to perform in public anymore. She also shared that, at about this same time, she began to suffer migraine headaches. When asked what the migraine was like, Lorraine stated that it was "a vise on the outside of my head … it's heavy and gray."

Assuming the obvious, that this new metaphor had some relationship to the former metaphor, I simply followed her cue and asked, "Would a vise that's in your head be interested in a hot metallic triangle that's in your mouth, throat, and chest?"

At this point her eyes became large and a look of awe dawned on her face. "Yes," she said, "it is."

"And what happens then?" I continued.

"The vise takes hold of the triangle, and they both float away."

"And what happens when they float away?" I asked.

"Then I'm free," she stated.

"And how is the hot metallic triangle now, Lorraine?" I

continued, curious to see the outcome.

"It's gone!" she responded.

She elaborated that for the last twenty-two years she experienced this feeling whenever she approached males. Additionally, this made practicing a program such as Alcoholics Anonymous very difficult since a preponderance of males attended A.A., and she was easily shamed. With her trauma memory intact, she could not ask a male for help without triggering the triangle. This dilemma precipitated the emotional "relapse trigger" which contributed to her multiple inpatient hospitalizations.

In our efforts to resolve the original trauma, which had manifest in her mouth, throat, and chest, we proceeded to create a scene of emotional comfort and safety – holding and nurturing her seven year old self. Next, we framed the scene and placed it in her body where the original triangular metaphor had been felt. This placement is important, for when something is taken from a system, something else must replace it or a secondary addiction could be developed to fill the void created by the release of the old metaphor.

As a final note, just as Lorraine was walking out the door of my office, she turned to look at me and asked: "I wonder if this had anything to do with my becoming a speech pathologist to help children who had trouble speaking and expressing themselves?" Is it possible that we even choose our occupations as an attempt to heal ourselves? After witnessing the choices of trauma survivors in situations similar to Lorraine's, it is evident that our entire life often revolves around this singular task. Our "free choices" are greatly colored by our stored, subconsciously encoded traumas. We shall discuss this further in this work when we examine the nature of subconscious intentionality.

I had the opportunity to see Lorraine some months later. When I asked about her "triangle," she indicated that there had been absolutely no recurrence. When metaphors are actually resolved, there is no recurrence.

Interestingly, this process is second nature to us. A "prepared briefing" was not necessary for Lorraine. From the moment she entered my office for her individual session she appeared to know the process; she needed little prompting and did not need to be briefed on its mechanics. I simply followed the cues she presented to me and allowed her internal form of resolution to proceed. The entire resolution process took less than forty minutes. It is clear that individuals who have worked intensely on themselves, whether through individual therapy, Twelve Step programs, or some other healing modality, have enhanced capacity to access and utilize this type of holographic resolution. They are sensitive to their own holographic space and can look inward with little effort.

From this experience with Lorraine and thousands of other "walking wounded," I learned the following valuable lessons about trauma:

♦ *We each possess the natural ability to locate our encoded traumas.*

I have rarely encountered anyone unable to locate stored traumas. Each of us possesses the capacity to locate and define these memory fragments stored within our nervous system and, thereby, to access the whole memory as needed and appropriate. This occurs within a matter of seconds. In studying the physics of holograms, we discover that each fragment of the hologram contains the picture of the whole. This metaphor, therefore, contains the entire trauma scene. In light of this, it becomes evident that each and every one of us has the capacity to access the level of information needed and available in holographic space to bring about resolution and wholeness. We will see this truth emerge more clearly in the cases presented in this writing.

♦ *Stored traumas possess a "reality" which we bear intact until resolved.*

On a deeper level we are already aware of the reality of our invisible traumas or metaphors encoded within our nervous systems. Lorraine was immediately convinced that her trauma was visible to all in the room. These metaphors show us that we can, indeed, perceive beyond the limitations of our five senses, particularly within the confines of our own bodies. Within our own nervous systems, at least, we are somewhat accustomed to working within holographic space, but we have not, generally, thought of extending this perceptual ability outside the confines of our physical bodies.

This is often the result of the false impressions that we obtained from the old Newtonian physics that left us with the impression that "physical" meant "solid." Our bodies are not solid, as physics has now shown us. Once we realize that our bodies are not solid, why, then, can we not perceive these distortions in the bodies of others, just as we have in our own? As we shall see within this text, we can; in fact, we already do. The reality of the traumas of others have become all too real to me as the sensitivity in my hands has increased. This ability has allowed me to experience, in a limited manner, the authenticity of the painful memories of others and to witness the impact in the bodies of these survivors. The power of these encoded experiences will become apparent as we examine the trauma induction process within the context of Lorraine's case and others. The power of memory is revealed to us.

◆ *Trauma metaphors are created as part of our natural healing process and serve to "contain" and store our overwhelming experiences.*

Trauma metaphors like Lorraine's "hot metallic triangle" serve the purpose of containment. They are holographic fragments of the original scene and are created by the subconscious process of bringing the overwhelming impulses of the nervous system to stasis, or, in other words, to a static state. This containment process allows the survivor to store the static impulses intact indefinitely. These metaphorical containers often appear geometrical in form – "ovals, triangles, lines, rectangles, lumps, knots, holes, needles, bands, weights, etc." These detailed metaphors, as memory fragments, can be used to effectively backtrack to their source, to the originating trauma. Commonly they take their form from actual physical objects or impressions within the perceptual field at the moment of traumatization. For example, Lorraine's "triangle" and "vise" could well have been objects actually present within the garage at the moment of her encoding. Though frequently "physical" in origin, these metaphors become pregnant with the emotional power of the moment. Subsequently, they are employed by the mind to manage the overwhelming pain. Lorraine's "hot, metallic triangle" was composed from the combined sense of weight, heat (shame feelings), density, and specific somatic locations in her mouth, throat, and chest – an area corresponding to the shape of a triangle. These metaphors are comprehensive at the moment of encoding and carry a capacity for storage that is remarkable in complexity. Lorraine's metaphor was perfect for freezing and encoding her traumatic experience until she was resourceful enough and safe enough to release it. Similarly, the "vise" in her head clearly represented an intense effort on her part to grasp the blockage and to remove it. Because she did not know how to resolve these metaphors herself from within holographic space, she needed a facilitator to initially demonstrate the means to access and utilize her personal resources to heal herself. Metaphorically, the solution (vise) had been present in her nervous system for years – actually, from merely a few months after the original trauma, when she first suffered a migraine.

Learning from Lorraine's self-directed healing that the resources for our healing are present and active, we are challenged to develop them and to consciously apply them to our individual and collective evolution. We must augment our understanding of the principles of healing within holographic space. By engaging our metaphors, we see specific opportunities emerge for healing. From the case of Lorraine, we learn that metaphors are simply the gateways into holographic space. Like Lorraine, we may find ourselves unexpectedly in touch with our own scenes, preserved intact from the past. From these experiences we learn that the mind does, indeed, have the capacity to preserve and store these overwhelming scenes holographically. This freezing process is a protective measure and is the first step toward healing an intrusive and overwhelming experience. We will examine the trauma induction process in more detail in Chapter Five.

♦ *Definition of a "trauma" is relative to the sensitivity and perception of the individual.*

Trauma is, indeed, relative to the perception of the individual. Quantum physics teaches us that our perception creates our reality. An experience that is traumatic to one individual may not be so to another. Repeatedly we see this within our family histories: we may witness the same event together, but we feel and remember it quite differently from our siblings' recall. Lorraine's trauma would not be considered traumatic in the eyes of many adults. Lorraine herself commented that she had remembered the fact that the event happened, but she had not realized the emotional impact that the event had produced in her life. This memory that once seemed so insignificant to her had dominated her relational, occupational, and recovery options for the majority of her life. She had never married, feeling inadequate when speaking around males; she had chosen her occupation to help speech-impaired children learn to express themselves (which she was actually trying to accomplish for herself since age seven); and she had been unable to utilize support programs like A.A. due to the nature of her trauma, which inhibited her ability to express herself without triggering profound feelings of shame. Trauma, therefore, must be defined with respect for the sensitivity of the person at the relative age and stage of his development. The younger or less secure the individual, the more vulnerable to traumatization he is. A young child, for instance, can be traumatized by overhearing for the first time Mom and Dad fighting. In addition, I fear that we have gravely underestimated the sensitivity and sophistication of the nervous system and its ability to experience and store all of our memories. When we see the emergence of ourselves from one complete DNA pattern – from one cell, and then multiply this incredibly complex pattern times the trillions of cells which we possess, we begin to get a true sense of our capacity for memory storage. As we shall see later in this work, much more is stored in our minds and bodies than we deemed possible. From Lorraine's experience, I learned that it does not take much to traumatize a child, and that many events that we, as adults, discount in a child's world actually leave life-shaping imprints.

♦ *Trauma is a pre-moral phenomenon.*

Oftentimes traumas are induced before the age of moral decision-making at ages seven to eight, or when moral insight is only partially developed. The case of Lorraine raises a very important question: How does childhood trauma impact moral development and adult decision-making? Even when occurring later in life, trauma induction is an automatic, largely subconscious process, not a matter of morality. When traumas are induced in early childhood, for instance, blockages and triggers are placed within the subconscious of the child which influence and limit the child's choices from that moment forward. Routinely the trauma survivor will allude to her sense of increased restriction in making choices following painful experiences. (It is important to understand, therefore, that this "trauma before the age of moral decision-making" undermines a child's normal developmental stages, reduces her choices, and sets her on a path which will eventually cause this stored pain to manifest, somehow, within her life experience.) The blockage induced earlier in life can manifest on many levels in the effort of the subconscious mind to heal itself, to restore equilibrium. Understanding the pre-morality of trauma is most important if we are to allow acceptance of ourselves with all of our metaphors and triggers without feeling threatened or being self-judging. Moral self-judgment or fear of moral judgment and rejection from others is often the primary resistance to healing. The trauma that so impacted little Lorraine's life choices occurred just as she was reaching the "age of moral reasoning" at ages seven to eight. How long had the adult Lorraine identified the feeling of being defective – the "hot, metallic triangle of shame," as something totally unacceptable or "wrong" within herself, rather than understanding that this was about something done to her and not about her own goodness or worth? We will examine the pre-morality of trauma and its implications in more detail later in this account, particularly with respect to ways the various social systems responsible for nurturing us have responded to our traumas.

♦ *Trauma induction often involves a protective or memory-repressive function which, in severe cases, can result in "traumatic amnesia."*
Frequently a trauma is an experience involving amnesia; that is, the entirety of the event may be unrecalled, or, as is more common, the individual may recall the fact that the event occurred, but the emotional content may be stored in the subconscious and, thus,

more difficult to access. Lorraine stated that she had known that Dad had lost his job and that his depression had impacted her family. She was stunned by the intensity of her recollection which resurrected such profound feelings of rejection, abandonment, and defectiveness. The amnesial character of trauma has long been studied. Milton Erickson (1902-1980) demonstrated that amnesia caused by psychological shocks and traumatic events are psycho-neuro-physiological "dissociations" that can be resolved by reintegrating the frozen ego (I) state through hypnotherapy.[7] We will examine this remarkable, protective function of the mind in more detail later in this work.

◆ *The trauma induction process is facilitated by the "limbic-hypothalamic" system; there is a remarkable physiological containment process at work in all our traumatic experiences.*

The trauma containment process is facilitated by the "limbic-hypothalamic-pituitary-adrenal axis" in the brain, which regulates the functioning of the autonomic nervous system, the endocrine system, and the immune system. Lorraine found herself with a racing heartbeat, an adrenaline "rush" – unable to swallow or speak, and, momentarily, unable to catch her breath as these responses from the original memory surfaced. It is not uncommon to find trembling, tightness in the nerve centers, even momentary paralysis and pain, depending upon the nature of the trauma; chronic pain can result from these unresolved memory fragments as well. Ernest Rossi, in his work, <u>The Psychobiology of Mind-Body Healing</u>, carefully documented the research advances in understanding the manifestation of trauma in the bodymind.[8] Rossi acknowledged that the concept of "information transduction" is the basic problem of psychobiology and mind-body healing: how energy moves from, for example, a father's verbal abuse to become a ringing in the ears or a physical pain in the chest of his child. Understanding the manner in which abusive communication is encoded by the nervous system greatly enhances our ability to resolve these somatic (body) memories more quickly. By understanding the dynamics of trauma induction, we can also accelerate progress in resolving disease that presents in the body as a result of trauma.

A most recent case involved Janine, a forty-two year old woman who accessed and resolved five successive trauma memories encoded in her throat plexus. Much of her dysfunction in life centered on her inability to express her feelings, particularly during physical and verbal abuse in her relationships with her father and her current husband. After reframing all five memories, she asked me whether these recurrent traumas to her throat could be connected to her other health problems: namely, a tumor that appeared on her thyroid. Not an isolated occurrence, this case of cancer, along with others presented in this work, will illustrate the profound connection between trauma memories and disease. This is not surprising, for, as Rossi points out, the mind moves, not only our emotions and our blood pressure, but also the genes and molecules that are generated within the cells of the body.[9] He states:

> *Well, if you push any endocrinologist hard enough, he/she will admit that, "Yes, it really is true!" Under mental stress, the limbic-hypothalamic system in the brain converts the neural messages of mind into the neurohormonal 'messenger molecules' of the body. These, in turn, can direct the endocrine system to produce the steroid hormones that can reach into the nucleus of different cells of the body to modulate the expression of genes. These genes then direct the cells to produce the various molecules that will regulate metabolism, growth, activity level, sexuality, and the immune response in sickness and health. There really is a mind-gene connection! Mind ultimately does modulate the creation and expression of the molecules of life.[10]*

Rossi posits that mind-body communication involves a real process that can be seen and measured – a knowledge allowing us to utilize natural processes of mind-body communication to expedite healing. Rossi also observed that the processes of mind-body communication usually function autonomously – that is, on an unconscious level.[11] Trauma, however, profoundly impacts these processes. Trauma interrupts the natural flow of mind-body communication, resulting in illness and unwelcome symptoms.

Within this account we examine resources that allow expedient measurement and intervention in the processes of mind-body communication. Lacking rudimentary understanding of the concepts presented here, Lorraine was able, nevertheless, to access and resolve issues within a few minutes – issues that had led to multiple alcohol related relapses and inpatient hospitalizations as well as other life-changing decisions. Such is the hope we are offered by our emergent understanding of "trauma."

Chapter Four

*I know I'm not seeing things as they are, I'm
seeing things as I am.*

Laurel Lee

Trauma Metaphors
The Keys To Healing

In the last chapter we reported that many scientists now believe that "reality" for each of us is created through holographic perception – a three-dimensional imaging process that utilizes our ability to shift our consciousness and to encode it in the form of "metaphors." Similarly, our ability to move fluidly through holographic space offers us surprising options for self-healing, for it is the energy and power of these trauma-induced holograms that underlie much of our pain and illness. To grasp the mechanism by which the nervous system perceives and encodes trauma is a critical step toward healing our pain. Traumatic experiences are moments when the conscious mind becomes overwhelmed and the ability for holographic encoding is subconsciously used to stop the pain, to contain it in some manageable form, until we are better able to release or heal it. The trauma metaphors created at these critical moments of our lives are the keys to healing these powerful experiences. If we possess the remarkable ability to "pause" and encode whole experiences through the power of our multidimensional minds, do we not also possess the ability to resolve such metaphors as well? Today we are learning how easily we can alter our states of consciousness and methods of extending this ability to holographic metaphors to heal ourselves. In the cases that we shall examine in this chapter, you will glimpse the power of these metaphors and the hope we find in resolving them.

The power to use holographic perception for healing was demonstrated for me while participating in a workshop preparing me for my role as a counselor. A delightful woman named Nancy Myer facilitated the workshop. At the beginning of one of the sessions, several of us indicated that we had headaches. Immediately she suggested we visualize our headaches as we saw them inside our heads. After accessing and describing the containers of our pain, she guided us to visualize a new container – a crystal pitcher, which we filled with a "soothing, healing water" of the color of our own choosing. After doing so, we were instructed to picture an opening in the object or metaphor that contained our headache. Taking all the time that we needed to accomplish this, we proceeded to pour the beautiful, cool, healing, crystalline water into the painful headache. After pouring the water, we visualized ourselves setting the pitcher and the metaphors down; we then scanned our bodies to check the status of our headaches. They were all gone! I was amazed at how simply this persistent pain had been resolved. My first experience of the power of metaphor to resolve pain! This simple headache resolution technique contains many of the same steps that I have found involved in the resolution and healing of trauma and illness; these include:

1. Identifying the existence of a pain or distortion in the nervous system;
2. Accessing the metaphor that contains the pain;
3. Defining the metaphor in holographic space;
4. Changing the metaphor from a container of pain to a container of healing;
5. Moving the solution through the parts of the body that are in pain.

Over the next few years, my ongoing work with trauma survivors taught me to adapt and expand this simple principle to change the frozen scenes of trauma into scenes of safety, self-nurturing and calm. My initial work with trauma survivors generated profound feelings of frustration and sadness. I repeatedly faced survivors who, despite their best efforts at communicating and releasing pain, continued to experience the same painful emotions when they accessed the memory. Although they disclosed heart-rending and detailed recountings, they reexperienced exactly the same feelings, memories, and "stuck points" in their recovery. Obviously I was missing something vital about the power and nature of trauma and the way that it is encoded in the nervous system. Occasionally the survivors were amnesial and completely unaware of the actual origin of the blockage in their recovery process. Over time I came to respect the manner in which such metaphors rule the psyche.

Part of the explanation for why we are dominated by such metaphors is the concept of "state-bound" or "state-dependent" memory. David Cheek, MD, a student of Milton Erickson (a great psychotherapist who relied on hypnotic suggestion to resolve trauma memories), had posited from a twenty-five-year study of emotional trauma, stress, and psychosomatic symptoms, that severe stress produces an altered state, identifiable as a form of spontaneous hypnosis which encodes problems and symptoms in a manner which binds them to this altered state. Our pain, at a moment of trauma, becomes locked into the cells and fields of our bodies via our own self-hypnosis! In the late 1800's, Freud (1896) was already concerned with investigating the conditions for reversing such amnesia and dissociation.[2] In his paper on "The Aetiology of Hysteria," Freud discussed the role of trauma, stating that tracing a symptom back to a traumatic scene assists our understanding if the scene fulfills two conditions: "If it possesses the required determining quality and if we can credit it with the necessary traumatic power."[3] Studying the impact of trauma since the time of Freud, we are beginning to understand the specific dynamics of trauma induction which explain the ability of such experiences to determine behaviors and responses, with such power as to routinely override the defenses of the conscious mind. Some of the cases presented in this chapter will illustrate this point.

One of the first clues to the unraveling of the fixed condition of victims of trauma came from the notion of the flashback. In the same way that the study of alcoholism opened the doors to the treatment of addictions, so too, our war veterans with flashbacks and Post-Traumatic Stress Disorder (i.e., the condition created by the encoding of the pain associated with a traumatic event in such a manner that it precipitates a recurrence of the original symptoms in the form of nightmares, flashbacks, phobic responses, "startle response," hypervigilance, hypersensitivity, somatic discomfort, insomnia, "phantom pain," and marked agitation when the original stimuli are "triggered") reopened the doors to the treatment of dissociative disorders and the study of trauma induction. Three factors became apparent from my work with trauma (PTSD) survivors:

1. Among those who had flashbacks, many of the survivors had no conscious memory of the most intense moment of the trauma – they were, indeed, amnesial.

2. Trauma victims reported specific sensory data such as smells, sounds, touch sensitivities, tastes (or cravings), behaviors, and visual images that were not explicable in present time and which arose when they were triggered.

3. When asked about the location and source of the feelings accompanying the flashback, they often provided real and elaborate descriptions of objects and sensations that they visualized internally, encoded holographically at specific sites in their bodies.

Initially these observations emerged from my work with the chemically dependent population. Very early in my practice with addicts I realized that the removal of the encoded memory fragments or "triggers" contributed profoundly to the outcome of their recovery programs. I understood the traditional insistence and emphasis upon first stabilizing the addict from his dependency on drugs, but it also became evident that the failure to resolve the underlying pain and the memory triggers emerging once the detoxification was complete could result in relapse. The unresolved feelings stored during trauma could surface immediately after or even during detoxification, depending upon the nature of the trauma. The fact remains that the removal of either a healthy or unhealthy coping mechanism can result in the emergence of a stored trauma.

Illustrating this, I recall a patient whose behaviors and symptoms were actually discounted because staff assumed that the vivid somatic symptoms and emotional outbursts he experienced were ongoing reactions to the withdrawal from alcohol. In reality, he was experiencing the recall of a trauma which began, not by a visual flashback, but with an emotional one – with overwhelming feelings of anger and powerlessness which had accompanied the original traumatic experience which he had not yet consciously remembered. When I decided to suspend my judgment and simply attended to his pain, I could see that he was extremely agitated and overwhelmed by anger. I began by focusing on the evident rage.

"John, when you feel angry like this, where do you feel this in your physical body?" I asked calmly.

"It's in my chest," he quickly replied.

"And when it's in your chest like that, is it on the inside or the outside?" I inquired.

"It's on the outside," he stated abruptly.

"And when it's on the outside, does it have a shape or a size?"

"It's a green button!" he declared.

"And is there anything else about a green button like that that you would like to describe?" I gently asked.

"It hurts!" he retorted.

"And how young might you be when you first feel a 'green button on the outside' of your chest that hurts like that?" I asked.

"I'm fifteen," he answered.

"And can you see where you are when you're fifteen and there is a green button on the outside of your chest that hurts like that?" I supported him.

"I'm working at the Louisiana State Legislature as a page."

"And what happens then when you're fifteen years old and working at the Louisiana State Legislature as a page?" I mirrored back to him, using his own language.

"I'm working for one of the Representatives, and he asks me to vote for him while he's talking to some men," he described.

"And what happens next when he asks you to do that?" I inquired.

"I push the wrong button – I pushed the green button instead of the red one," he answered, with a look of fear and pain on his face.

"And what happens then, when you press the wrong button?"

"He has two of the guards take me outside, and they hurt me," he stated, beginning to cry and hold his head in his hands.

"And what needs to happen with this memory?" I questioned. "If you could go back and help a fifteen year old boy who's being hurt like that, what would you like to do first … if you could change that memory?" (pause) "Can you see where he is right now?" I continued.

"Yeah – he's being taken outside by the bodyguards, and he's terrified; I need to protect him and not let him be injured," he responded, now tapping into his unresolved anger.

"So take all the time that you need to go into that scene and do whatever you need to do to protect him," I advanced.

"OK, I've done it – I shoved the bodyguards away from him and told the representative off – that he just made a mistake and didn't deserve to be treated that way; then, I took him away from there to a safe place," John stated with less agitation.

"And how does he look now?" I asked.

After moments of contemplation: "He looks happy now – he trusts me now 'cause I protected him."

"So let's take a picture of the two of you together – the way you'd like to remember it," I suggested, "and let me know when you have the picture the way you want it."

"OK, I have it," John quickly responded.

"Now let's put a beautiful frame around it of the color or colors that you would like," I added.

Concentrating intently with his eyes closed: "All right … I have it; the frame is purple!" he stated.

"Now let's move the picture – particularly the color of the frame, through your whole nervous system, especially through your chest area where you first felt that green button on the outside; and let me know when you've done that," I directed.

John's facial muscles relaxed, and in the quiet moments of his journey with the color purple, his body progressively softened. "All right; I've done it!" he stated assuredly.

"And how do your chest and body feel now?" I questioned.

"Wow!" "It feels peaceful and calm – the button is gone!" he replied with a tone of surprise.

In contrast to his original state of distress, John was noticeably more relaxed and focused – a welcome change during his sojourn in treatment. Through this process he discovered his ability to access his memory easily, although it had been eluding conscious analysis for some time. His feelings about having done something wrong and about having been jailed prior to seeking treatment had triggered unresolved feelings about the earlier constraint and shame originating from the trauma at age fifteen. Later he shared with me that he cried for the first time in many years after this work, and thanked me for listening to him. Only after this catharsis was he able to be present for treatment without the fear, anger, shame, and self-blame that had been triggered by his recent experiences, but which originated in his trauma history. Experiences such as this caused me to become more sensitive to the cues that the conscious and subconscious mind provide to facilitate healing. Many people broadcast their traumas as a subconscious cry for help, without knowing the origin of their out of control behaviors and emotions. Particularly when the emotional reactions are disproportionate to events in present time – when there is no evident or proportionate cause for a particular emotional reaction, we are usually dealing with manifesting trauma. This was John's case.

The earliest and most outstanding demonstration of the sophistication of our memory system occurred during my work with Claire. Claire came to me stating that she was "going crazy." She had recently been informed by her husband that he wanted a divorce. Within a few days of this disclosure, she found herself "craving and eating raw flour." I informed her that my knowledge of trauma survivors indicated that nearly all behaviors originated in actual experiences from our past, but that a significant percentage of these experiences were not available to our conscious minds. Even our most irrational coping mechanisms begin to make sense when we explore our past experiences and memories. I suggested that we take a look at the origin of these feelings that had her coping with this crisis by "eating raw flour." As I listened to her, a story of abuse during her childhood unfolded. Claire had a growth within her urinary tract as a child that resulted in enuresis ("bed-wetting"). Her mother was unaware that the origin of the problem was physiological. As a result, her bed-wetting was taken as a moral failure, and Claire was punished. The punishment often involved food and was reinforced by severe verbal abuse. When Claire behaved herself and did not wet the bed, she was rewarded with her favorite foods: fried chicken and baked goods, especially pies. When she wet the bed, her mother would give her siblings her favorite foods, threaten to leave Claire hungry, or tell her that she was going to give her something repulsive (her mother's language was deemed unfit for print). Her fear of wetting the bed increased, along with fear of abandonment and rejection by her mother. Over time, the punishment and deprivation from food increased. By the age of five, still two years before the "age of moral decision-making," Claire developed her own solution to survive. When she was afraid to go to sleep at night for fear of wetting the bed and losing her mother's love, she would sneak into the kitchen, and, because there were no fried foods or baked goods available, she would eat the raw flour left on the counter. As little Claire scooped up the flour, she would repeat to herself that her mother did love her. The flour, you see, was the only concrete reminder of her mother's love for her, and, as importantly, it was something that she could control! The raw flour provided a concrete substitute for the actual love that she could not get from Mom. Hence, when Claire experienced feelings of panic and abandonment regarding her husband divorcing her, she returned to the coping mechanism that had enabled her to survive emotional abandonment and rejection as a child. Same dilemma; different players. Claire's mother finally took her to the doctor at age thirteen when she was still wetting the bed, and, in a half-hour outpatient procedure, the doctor removed the growth that had caused the bed-wetting and the subsequent emotional dilemma she had felt throughout those years.

The adult Claire's behaviors returned to normal when she allowed herself to access the memory and nurture the panicked, wounded child within her (the "ego-state" and nerve cells which held this memory) whose feelings of abandonment were perfectly preserved into adulthood. Claire "had forgotten" those ten years of abuse – evidencing traumatic amnesia or delayed recall. Upon resolving "Little Claire's" panic, her adult anxieties about the divorce became infinitely more manageable, and she was able to leave her marriage which had reflected the abuse of childhood. An abandonment trigger with such power as Claire's can leave us in a threatening living situation with little or no conscious awareness about why we experience terror when we contemplate changing our situation or leaving the relationship. Such paralyzing memory triggers can foster ongoing abuse and retraumatization. This is the power of holographic metaphors. Resolving the divorce issues, therefore, served as an occasion for her to access and resolve her unmet childhood dependency needs, to resolve her abandonment issues, to understand the dynamics of the abusive relationship, and to discover resources for completing her own self-parenting while healing the abuse of her childhood. In Claire's case, the feelings of abandonment created by her husband's announcement of his intent to divorce her triggered a "dark, black, empty feeling, like a hole" in her stomach and abdominal region. When traced back to its point of origin in her childhood, we discovered that Claire had accessed an immense body of unresolved feelings of abandonment which had triggered her original, automatic (subconscious) coping mechanism. The power of this stored memory was so great that, when it was "tapped," it overpowered her adult, rational thinking and resulted in "acting out" the script of the original trauma scenario – that of a little girl. Note that Claire was compulsive with flour before the age of "moral" decision-making (7-8 years old). (Such cases indicate that addictive behaviors and compulsivity can be in place long before the age of moral choice.) This is an excellent example of how memory triggers function. The trigger was emotional abandonment by the most significant person in her life – her mother. Psychologists and hypnotherapists (National Guild of Hypnotists) now posit that the conscious mind constitutes only seven percent of our total knowledge and awareness, while the subconscious mind comprises the remaining ninety-three percent. This ratio explains the dominance of the subconsciously stored and emotionally potent trauma patterns over the rational choices of the conscious mind. The dominating power of

Claire's subconscious memories to override her rational thinking and cause the adult to eat something as unpleasant as raw flour suggests that the subconscious mind can, indeed, seize control of our intentionality and cause us to act in ways that, at first glance, may appear irrational. Upon further investigation, they are found to be intelligently conceived, creative coping strategies.

From Claire's case and others, it becomes clear that a child's way of coping with trauma often takes a very concrete physical form. This is the natural "primary process" thinking of a child. If I feel empty in my stomach, I eat. If I feel dirty on the outside, I bathe. If I feel dirty inside my stomach, I may try to throw it up (purging as with bulimia); if I feel pain, I use whatever makes it go away; if I feel threatened or in danger, I hide. A child, for example, interprets the empty hole in the stomach as hunger, as the need for something physical to fill it. This hungry feeling is the most similar concept (metaphor) available to him for describing the pain – the emptiness, within his limited repertoire of experience. Attempts at filling the stomach with a material substance such as food (the earliest chemicals we have available to medicate with) or other mood altering chemicals will produce, at best, a temporary alleviation if the issue is trauma-based.

One of the most obvious examples of this substitution occurs when a sexual trauma memory begins to surface. Frequently the abused individual will feel a "dirty" feeling which may be accompanied by conscious recall of the trauma or by traumatic amnesia. I have never encountered a rape survivor who did not experience, on some level, this feeling of dirtiness and contamination. The actual hygiene issue has long been resolved, but as the memories of the abuse surface more clearly, the urge to bathe increases. Since the emotional trauma is actually encoded in the cells and the more subtle electromagnetic fields of the body, efforts to wash it away physically, fail. Such graphic solutions to emotional trauma can be expected from these desperate, wounded children within us. Physical, mechanical solutions to profoundly imprinted emotional traumas do little to resolve the core affect. They may enable survival, but these inappropriate solutions begin to backfire and may, themselves, begin to harm. Recent studies indicate that as many as eighty-seven percent of women alcoholics have histories of sexual abuse. The alcohol served to medicate the pain for many years, but now the alcohol itself has become a killer. Many addictions and compulsive behaviors develop as early attempts to alleviate a perceived pain or trauma. We also learn to use other experiences such as exercise, work, sex, risk-taking, and activities limited only by the imagination to produce an adrenaline reaction or a release of the body's natural opiates – the "endorphins" and "encephalins," for the purpose of medicating our pain. It is also true that we often choose our drug(s) on the basis of our traumas – that is, based on the fact that this drug or experience medicates a particular trauma pain most effectively. I have seen countless teenagers who began to smoke marijuana daily, finding that when they smoked enough of it, they no longer remembered the nightmares resultant from their trauma histories. In addition, numerous adults are addicted to prescription medications like xanax, clonopin, and valium – drugs which do, in fact, resolve anxiety for many because they work as memory-suppressants. That is, they disconnect the survivor from the agonizing emotional pain of the stored memories; the difficulty is that they create this biochemical dissociation without healing the memory, thereby fostering further dependency on the drug. Attention Deficit Disorder (ADD) (appearing as a restlessness which leaves the individual unable to remain focused on a task or project) populations provide a common illustration of dependency and the psycho-biological attraction to a specific drug or group of drugs. Feeling calm and relaxed for the first time when ingesting a stimulant such as cocaine, it is understandable that an Attention Deficit diagnosed individual would seek this new-found sense of well-being. The substance increases the flow of information to the Reticular Activating System in the brain leaving the trauma survivor feeling "normal." The response serves as a heavy reinforcement, thus leading to addiction. Initially, rather than appearing drug-influenced to their families, they may, in fact, look better than they have in years. However, the normal appearance soon becomes something nightmarish. The normalcy is brief because the cocaine becomes debilitating in its addictive progression. In a similar vein, many trauma survivors use heroin, reporting that this powerful drug enables them to feel like they are asleep although they are terrified to sleep because of their memories that surface as nightmares. Reliance on such an addictive drug gives the illusion of rest but can only sustain the state briefly, leading, ultimately, to dire consequences. From these few examples we begin to see the profound link between our trauma experiences and the coping mechanisms we choose.

Not long ago I worked with an adolescent who had experienced severe, recurring emotional abandonment, including, at age two, the death of his mother, rejection and abandonment by Dad at age three, the death of his grandmother at age five, and subsequent physical abuse by his stepmother at age ten. He was remanded to treatment for his behavioral problems and his rageful outbursts. As we looked at his abandonment pain, he accessed intense feelings of rage and anger resonating in his stomach and chest areas. He described his pain, metaphorically, as "a great big ball of fire that just wants to come out and explode." Prior to group therapy, I had not reviewed his case. As he shared his history, it became clear that his behavioral outbursts, and one particular acting out behavior made sense. He was placed in treatment because he set fire to things in his backyard and throughout his neighborhood. His language reflected desperate attempts to externalize what he described as a "fireball" of anger consuming him. His reckless behaviors equated with the desire to have someone notice it within him. Instead, his living situation simply fueled the fire. The solution was, clearly, to help him diffuse the anger that had accumulated and to provide a nurturing living environment to prevent further internalization or inappropriate expression of his anger; this is what we focused on in his treatment and family counseling.

The concrete or mechanical thinking of the wounded children within us, created by our traumas, easily carries over into adolescence and adulthood, despite our best efforts at rational control. Later in this text we will examine the consequences of this mechanical view of self and reality which impacts all areas of our lives. The cases described above suggest that our predominant approach to health and healing may be stuck in such mechanical thinking, thereby missing the true origins of our illnesses – origins in trauma. There are also larger, societal consequences to having harbored primary process or mechanical thinking about ourselves, our bodies, our attempts at finding solutions. These consequences have long limited us and our ability to successfully treat many illnesses. They have limited the medical profession as well and are, finally, with the advent of psychoneuroimmunology, being acknowledged. More needs to be done, however. The case below will illustrate my point.

A main source of inspiration for this account was the case of Diedra. I was practicing in the mental health services department of a chemical dependency outpatient program, focusing primarily on Adult Children of Alcoholics (ACOA's) and clients damaged by emotionally repressive systems. Often my concern centered on resolving childhood traumas which were causing impairment in the adult's current life. When Diedra came in for her initial assessment, she provided a narrative of her life experiences, accurate to the best of her knowledge. In sharing her history, she identified "no major traumas." A considerable portion of the assessment was, however, devoted to the details of her recent medical history. An alarm sounded in my mind, and I felt somewhat overwhelmed by the possible implications. The details of her medical history were published in the American Journal of Kidney Diseases, Vol. XX, No.2 (August), 1992: pp.180-184. With her permission, I have chosen to include certain details of the case to facilitate your understanding of 1) the extreme measures employed to treat her pain, 2) the failure at medical intervention due to an inadequate grasp of the bodymind connection between her symptoms and their origin, and 3) the permanent and life-changing results of the approaches used.

During the previous two years, Diedra had undergone four surgeries in an attempt to stop "severe left flank pain" – that is, an intense chronic pain on the left side of her kidney region.[4] At age twenty-nine, she first developed seven to fourteen-day episodes of severe left flank pain in 1986; these bouts of pain occurred at three to six-month intervals.[5] In the interim, she was treated with acetaminophen and codeine; she also received, but without significant pain relief, a course of acupuncture.[6] In 1989, the left flank pain became more severe and unrelenting, and, for two months, she required multiple doses of oxycodone for pain relief, but the use of narcotics interfered with her ability to fulfill her professional responsibilities.[7] Extensive efforts to diagnose her condition led the specialists to a diagnosis of "Loin Pain-Hematuria Syndrome" – a "poorly understood disorder in which the patients, mainly young women, experience severe unilateral (on one side) or bilateral (two sides) flank pain."[8] After ruling out all of the known possibilities to account for her chronic pain, and after efforts which resulted in disappointing short-term pain relief, the specialists decided upon an attempt to "induce permanent denervation of the kidney" via a technique called "renal autotransplantation."[9] Because of the need for daily narcotic medications, which severely interfered with her professional duties, Diedra agreed to undergo left renal autotransplantation; this was performed in November of 1989.[10] Following the surgery, she noted the pain from the left flank incision, but the deep penetrating left flank pain associated with LPHS, had disappeared.[11] Following this surgery, Diedra moved to Baton Rouge, where she continued her health care and resumed her normal activities. In July of 1990, seven and one half months after the renal transplant, her left flank pain returned with the same severity that she had experienced originally; a detailed evaluation disclosed no known cause for the recurrent pain.

It was at this point in Diedra's history that she entered my care. Early into the assessment I became aware of some type of trauma in her affect and presentation. She manifest no conscious awareness of any severe trauma at this time. Gently I processed with Diedra the information concerning current research regarding trauma induction and the medical profession's growing involvement with psychoneuroim-munology. I shared with her my research and understanding of the concept of trauma which had evolved through my interaction with survivors. I presented several case studies and explained our findings regarding the possible origins of such physical pain. I included in our discussion the research data that many "physical" pains prove to be fragments of unresolved memories surfacing for resolution. Neurophysiological research has taught us that memory is holographic, with each fragment bearing the capacity to recreate the whole – including the degree of pain present during the original experience. I shared with her how this phenomenon has demystified the previously inexplicable "phantom pain" of many trauma survivors. Recurrent, inexplicable pain frequently surfaces as the first stage of recall for an encoded memory. Professionally, it was my desire to provide her with the new "scientific" options arising from trauma research should her traditional medical interventions prove ineffective. I was, nonetheless, as surprised as she at the final outcome. At that time in my own research, I was gaining insight into the mind-body and mind-gene links which manifest through the workings of the limbic-hypothalamic system (See pages 45-46). Trauma could certainly be a plausible explanation for the repressed affect and sexuality that was evident in her speech and presentation. At this point in the development of my own trauma resolution techniques and skills, I was attentive to the functioning of the nervous system during times of trauma and its cues for the identification and access of trauma. These cues, referred to as body memories or somatic memories, were familiar to me and easily identifiable during work with survivors. These somatic memories typically appeared as "pain, pressure, aches, tightness, burning, sharp stabbing pains, lumps, knots, and trembling feelings" in the physical body. It was not until years later that a group of physicians indicated to me that they had seen sexual trauma manifest in somatic pain ranging from chronic left or right flank pain to urinary tract infections along with a variety of other ailments.

Diedra's inclination was to pursue the recommendations of the specialists in the field of kidney medicine. She was trained in the traditional medical model. At the physicians' recommendations, she underwent "epidural and lumbar sympathetic nerve blocks and received bupivicaine;" these treatments, however, only provided temporary pain relief.[12] Despite this and additional medical interventions, the severe pain persisted. After being unable to control the pain with these measures, Diedra agreed to an additional surgical intervention. In December of 1990 she underwent a "T10-L1 dorsal rhizotomy," involving the severing of certain nerves along the spinal column, which resulted in complete resolution of the pain.[13] This intervention also resulted in a permanent, significant loss of sensation in the left side of her abdominal region. Severe left flank pain recurred in April 1991, three and a half months following the rhizotomy.[14] In June 1991, a dorsal column spinal cord stimulator system was implanted, with electrode stimulation points adjacent to the fifth and sixth thoracic vertebral bodies; even this did not provide total pain relief without the need for analgesics.[15] How could the discomfort remain even when the nerves were severed? The doctors had no explanation.

Following these final efforts to medically alleviate the pain in her left abdominal region, Diedra returned to see me. At this time we investigated the readiness of her bodymind to disclose to us, at its own pace, any possible traumas that could precipitate such pain. Within a week of the first therapy session, Diedra began experiencing flashbacks of sexual abuse. From the actual memories, she came to understand that her pain was the body memory of the trauma manifesting within the left flank region of her body. The pain returned with specific memories in which physical pain was inflicted in and around her kidney region. Her pain was part of the state-bound memory – the trance that had, somehow, been accessed and which was now surfacing for resolution. I explained to her that unresolved memories begin to manifest by recreating in our bodies the symptoms of the original trance. This is simply the way in which our body-mind begins to cue us to the specific memory which needs healing. In this manner, our bodies remind us of what happened so that we may access the memory and resolve it and the accompanying pain. The left flank pain, not at all uncommon in sexual trauma survivors, was the first of many memories of trauma that she had repressed. This type of amnesia is common with sexual abuse. Even Freud himself used a type of body-work or massage to facilitate his clients' access to their memories in the effort to reverse their amnesia. The body often proves the most effective agency for getting our attention and cueing us to the locations of these encoded traumas. With such physical cues, however, we are, as an addicted society, far more accustomed to merely medicating the pain than we are to trying to trace it back to its point of origin in our memories. From working with numerous clients who experienced a persistent or recurrent pain similar to Diedra's, I have come to reverse my thinking: rather than assume most pain to originate in the physical body from a biochemical source, I acknowledge the probability that its origin is traumatic memory, and I respond accordingly. I consider medicating pain symptoms only if the pain endures after the employment of memory resolution techniques.) In the overwhelming majority of the cases I see, the pain has its roots in a specific memory or group of memories.

As Diedra acted to resolve and reframe her memories, the pain began to subside, finally. Although I did not have the opportunity to work with Diedra outside of group therapy, she continued counseling with her referring therapist who provided information about her progress. Her information confirmed my own observation that Diedra's pain was the somatic memory stored from childhood abuse. Since my initial work with Diedra, I have had numerous opportunities to witness ways unresolved memories of sexual abuse manifest in the abdominal region resulting in kidney problems, urinary tract infections, chronic unilateral or bilateral pain, irritable bowel syndrome, colitis, a variety of cancers, and an incredibly wide variety of sexual dysfunction. At a regional conference for physicians responsible for state programs designed to support fellow physicians evidencing chemical dependency or other impairments, I lectured on the impact of trauma manifestation in the physical body. I opened by asking the physicians if they had noticed any patterns of illness, pain, or other somatic phenomena common to the trauma survivors with whom they worked. Several of the physicians confirmed that they recognized patterns such as a "chronic left or right flank pain, irritable bowel syndrome, colitis, spastic colon, and urinary tract infections," in the sexual trauma survivors whom they had treated.

Although we will examine this issue in more detail later in this work, it is important to recognize that, when trauma remains unresolved in our bodies and minds over long periods of time, it will begin to manifest in our lives in successive attempts to reach our consciousness. The symptoms may begin as a feeling of discomfort or a message that "something is wrong with me." This is the classic statement of those individuals who have come to me for help and are aware that something is wrong, yet are unable to identify it precisely. When neither the emotional nor the mental warnings or messages are heard, the body will speak louder and louder, again and again, in an effort to call attention to the anomaly. The source of these messages is the trauma metaphor and its powerful content. As in Diedra's case, the pain persisted until she was able to access the trauma and commit to the process of resolution. In the midst of the pain and frustration of the circuitous path her recovery had taken, she realized that the real message was about empowerment and the healing of inhibitory patterns that had been present since she was very young. Such disclosures about trauma bring transformation. Diedra's pain was an invitation to understand behaviors, fears, anxieties, and triggers that had plagued her throughout her life without explanation. Though it was painful to face the realization that someone central in her life had abused her in a terrible way, there was tremendous energy released when the constraints imposed by the trauma and the accompanying amnesia were lifted. She was able to make decisions more freely, from a place of strength, rather than from a position of avoidance and fear. Diedra was able to be more open in relationships and, once free of the pain associated with the trauma, was again able to use her gifts and strengths to advance her personal goals and career. The growth that she has made since this time is a tribute to her openness and willingness to resolve pain, at whatever cost. In reality, the empowerment that came from facing these traumas that had debilitated her physically, emotionally, mentally, and spiritually, proved to be worth the price. Unfortunately, the lesson also included the traditional dependence on medical solutions without more timely access to the therapeutic options and new alternatives that could have identified the trauma-induced cause more readily. There remains a hiatus between the medical profession's approach to the treatment of the symptoms in the body and the new science of the bodymind that is emerging from contemporary data about trauma induction. The gap grows smaller, and, it is my hope, that the scientific process introduced by this work will contribute to the bridging of our disciplines with the common goal of providing the highest quality of care and the most expedient healing.

Through cases like Diedra, we deepen our understanding of the interrelationship between those aspects of the self that we have called body, mind, and spirit, which we often separate and compartmentalize. From the study of trauma we learn the profundity of the link of mind and body. We also learn to respect the power of these emotions which seem so indelibly imprinted in our bodymind at these traumatic moments. They connect and bind us to persons, places, situations, objects, and specific sensory experiences, though these events are long past, submerged in cellular memory. Emotions, as we shall see, form the principal bridge to relationality and, therefore, to our spiritual selves as well. Ultimately we witness the emergence of "the physics of the soul." Recognizing the power and healing potential already manifest though this new physics, we will examine by means of this writing, the implications of this development for both science and spirituality. These disciplines are much more closely joined than once thought. It has been stated for many centuries that "God is Truth." Truth is the common pursuit of science and spirituality and it is on this level that the convergence of the spiritual journey and the scientific journey occurs; it is in the common pursuit of healing that our disciplines unite.

The reality of the trauma metaphors that we have seen in this chapter was all too apparent for John, Claire, and Diedra, whose lives were profoundly affected by them – on all levels. By learning to trust their internal perceptions, they were able to draw upon, for purposes of healing, resources that they did not know that they possessed. These containers were created by the bodymind to facilitate a healing process that we are learning to employ consciously. Experiences such as these reveal to us the importance of being open to the lessons of trauma, open to our loss of energy and our pain. Our enlightened understanding of the manner in which trauma is encoded promises more expedient diagnosis and resolution of trauma-induced somatic pain without risk to the nervous system. Diedra's experience challenged both her own and her physicians' traditional understanding of disease and necessitated her exploration of alternatives for healing. Must we cling to such narrow, one-dimensional primary process understanding of pain as "physical" at the cost of our health and at the risk of permanent injury? The anomalous pain in Diedra's body was her bodymind presenting a distortion for healing. I feel great sadness when I look upon the power structures that rule our medical professions and see the limitations imposed that leave the entire realm of holographic space virtually untouched. Classically, the holographic realm has been termed "psychosomatic" and, thereby, discounted, as though trauma induced from human emotions is something less than real "scientifically" and unworthy of the attentions of the medical profession. The greatest weakness of our medical sciences is the lack of attention to and the undervaluing of the power of affect. Emotions are incredibly complex biochemical, electrical, multidimensional forms of memory. They are bridges that form the foundations of human relationship and easily transcend space and time.

As a child it was quite apparent to me that emotions are e powerful and are not to be underestimated. My mother could feel in her own body, simultaneous with the event, any accident that befell my siblings and me. There was little separation between body, mind, and spirit for her in these moments. She felt these events as a physical pain in her own body. She would note the time on the clock and spend time in prayer and meditation for us until she was "officially" notified of the accident or event. When my brother was domiciled at the veteran's home in Gulfport, Mississippi, acting upon "a feeling," she called and asked of my brother's whereabouts just as the ambulance arrived to take him to the hospital due to an injury from a fall. To this day, there is a social worker on staff who believes that my mother was called prematurely by another employee. The administration wanted to reprimand "the employee who breached protocol." My mother knew and trusted the holographic statements of her bodymind; their verity was dependable. Simple examples as these provided my introduction to the "physics of the soul" and provided the pathway for my own journey, my legacy into the exploration of holographic space.

Emotions are the content of trauma-induced metaphors and carry immense power. When stored during a moment of trauma, these biochemical reactions are encoded or stored intact and do not complete their dynamic processing cycle (See Chapter Five). If left unresolved over time, these frozen feelings of trauma will become evident in successive efforts to reach the bearer's consciousness. This is part of our innate capacity to heal. When left unattended, these emotions will speak with increasing volume on the spiritual, mental, emotional, and, ultimately, on the physical level. As Chris Griscom states: "If we are not listening, the body, as cosmic teacher, will start talking louder ... the dissonance is called disease."[16] Supporting this concept is the work of Louise Hay who, from her own experience with cancer, indicates the consequences of holding the unresolved energy of trauma within our nervous system.[17] She provided specific correlations between specific fossilized emotions and certain illnesses. Just as we are coming to appreciate the link between the mind and the body, so, too, are we learning to recognize the advantages of collaboration between the psychotherapeutic and medical disciplines. Whatever our venue of care for others, the mechanical thinking of the child within each of us and the influence of the old Newtonian physics has left us with a diminished and limited understanding of healing. This mechanical view of the individual has left us with a reductionistic philosophy, such that we have often come to see healing as the successful treatment of the immediate symptoms in the body, and have remained ignorant or inattentive to the actual origin of most of our illnesses in the memory capacity of our bodymind. We are in discovery and exploration of the "neurotransmitters" that mediate the functioning of our immune system. We are in the initial stages of grasping the intricacy of the nervous system and its ability to protect us from the devastating effects of trauma, whether emotional, physical, mental, or spiritual. Research in this area has given birth to the new field of "psychoneuroimmunology," which is a fancy medical term acknowledging that health and well-being are dependent upon the close interrelationship between our minds and our bodies. The case of Diedra, and many others like her, propels us into this new field with an urgency and a purpose. Let us not abuse out of ignorance. The power of the metaphors of trauma and their impact on the bodymind will emerge more clearly as we explore these remarkable containers of the overwhelming experiences of our lives.

Chapter Five

> *Just as our immune system protects us against infections from bacteria, our psychospiritual immune system is activated when attacked by the malevolent intentions of others.*
>
> Larry Dossey, 1997

The Dynamics of Trauma Induction

A most exciting breakthrough in the healing sciences has occurred through our growing understanding of the dynamics involved in trauma induction. At last we are coming to appreciate the remarkable power of our nervous system to shield us from the traumatic events of our lives. Furthermore, we are recognizing that each of us has induced or encoded experiences that would have overwhelmed us if not for the assistance of this self-protective system. None of us is without trauma. In addition, our past traumas, we are now learning, are nothing to fear. They are part of an extremely sophisticated healing resource that has always been in place within our bodymind. Rather than avoid the pain of our memories for fear of retraumatization, we are discovering that our systems are designed to provide access and resolution to stored memories without the need to fully re-experience or relive them. Let us examine the explanation for this phenomenon.

Among the most important therapeutic insights of this century is the understanding of the profound dynamics of trauma induction. Countless cases of Post-Traumatic Stress Disorder (PTSD) have come to our attention as a result of war traumas. To our credit we have developed a heightened awareness and greater disclosure of sexual, ritual, physical, and emotional abuse. Study of these cases has led to a greater understanding of the induction of trauma and ways it is stored. In reality, much more than what we have traditionally categorized as feelings is preserved in body memory.

Previously I stated that trauma is relative to the perspective of the perceiver. By this I intend that certain painful experiences which you and I might easily discount as an insignificant event could be extremely traumatic for a child or a person of different disposition or for someone with a different life experience history. Many therapists and authors indicate that chemically dependent persons, for example, evidence a high sensitivity level which sets them up to feel more pain and, consequently, predisposes them for trauma.[1] Regardless of this sensitivity factor, however, a trauma is induced by a sense of: "I feel like I'm going to die." Such induction occurs through physical, mental, emotional, sexual, or spiritual stimuli. The mind seems to work automatically in such a moment to protect its victim by stopping the threat. This is achieved by arresting and containing all incoming data: sensory information – sight, smell, sound, touch, taste, body perceptions, emotions, thoughts – literally, everything experienced at the moment when the pain becomes overwhelming. In addition, in order to survive, the mind "freeze-frames" and encodes this data in a fraction of time just prior to when the experience becomes absolutely overpowering. David Grove, a psychologist from New Zealand, who researched the dynamics of trauma encoding, referred to this as "T minus one" (T-1), indicating one millisecond prior to the trauma itself.[2] I shall employ his terminology, as it is accurate and descriptive when discussing the nature of trauma. "T-1" is a most important concept. Most of us avoid accessing memories for fear of fully reexperiencing the original pain. We now understand that: 1) the inherent design and function of our nervous system helps us to avoid retraumatization, and 2) it is not necessary to relive the entire emotional experience in order to heal. We do not encode the whole experience; we encode only the peak (T-1) moments. Therefore, we do not have to relive the entire experience to obtain resolution. This phenomenon was noted when studying Vietnam veterans and discovering that their flashbacks were not their worst moment or "T" itself, but were an incredibly vivid experience of T-1.

At T-1, the mind and nervous system, through the functioning of the limbic-hypothalamic system of the brain, consolidate all the incoming data and encode this information in holographic form – as metaphor. This metaphor (as referenced earlier) is simply the fragment of the larger holographic scene. In an incredibly powerful and expedient manner, the holographic metaphor serves to contain the event and also halts the damaging effects that would have been caused to the psyche of the victim. The easiest way to grasp the power of this process is to understand that the entire event, as perceived, is paused like on a video recorder and held in stasis in the nervous system. Time and space perceptions are halted and contained in the metaphor. This creates the altered state, the spontaneously induced hypnotic state referred to previously as "state-bound memory."

Recently I worked with a client, Sylvia, who indicated that she wanted to resolve the intense feelings of loneliness that had surfaced over the past few days. When asked about where in her body she felt this loneliness, she stated that it was "just under the surface" in her chest area. After focusing on the sensation, she described it as a "white circle about the size of a golf ball." When asked if there were further distinctions about the circle, she stated, "Yes, it has red dots!"

"And how old might you be when you first feel a circle with red dots and a lonely feeling in your chest like that?" I asked.

"I'm five, and I can see myself in the kitchen," she responded with surprise.

"And what happens next when you're five, and you're in the kitchen like that?" I asked.

"I go up to Mom and tug on her dress to get her attention," she stated.

"And what occurs then, when you do that?" I inquired.

Sylvia responded: "She turns to me and says, 'Get the hell out from under my feet; I don't want you in here right now!'"

"And what follows next when she says that to you?" I continued.

"I feel so rejected and heartbroken ... I just start crying and wander into the living room by myself," she indicated, becoming tearful as she accessed the child's feelings. "She never yelled at me that way before. Mom had started drinking again at that time," she added.

"And so what needs to happen for a little girl who's being treated that way by her own mother? (pause) ... if the adult you could go and help her, what would you like to do first?" I asked, highlighting the opportunity which stood before her to heal her unresolved abandonment and loneliness due to mother's alcoholism.

Sylvia bowed her head without speaking, pondering her options. "I'd like to take her out of there and let her know that it wasn't about her," Sylvia affirmed. "It was about Mom's drinking; I was a good little girl."

"So, take all of the time you need to do that – to make her safe and let her know that it wasn't about her at all, and let me know when you've done that," I added.

After a quiet pause – "OK, she's fine now; I have her in the safe place with me," she stated with a sigh.

"Let's take a picture of this scene – the way you want it, and let's put a frame around it of the color or colors of your choosing. Can you see the color of the frame?" I asked.

"It's silver and blue," she said, smiling.

"Then let's move the silver and blue color through your whole body, especially in your chest where the white ball with the red dots was located," I directed.

"OK," she stated, "I've done that!"

"And how does your chest feel now?" I inquired.

"It's fine now," she reported.

"Sylvia, do you know the origin of the white ball with the red dots that you felt in your chest?" I asked.

"Oh, yes, now that you mention it. It was what my mother was wearing that day – her white dress with the red dots," she replied with a new appreciation for the "white circle" that initially appeared in her chest when she began to think about the pain of her loneliness.

This is one of many examples that demonstrates the power and function of holographic metaphors. These simple geometric forms serve to contain and encode experiences that prove overwhelming to us. Our minds focus on these simple, geometric patterns to gain control of the scene, holographically, using a shape or sensation that they recognize and can manage, thereby reducing the whole to a manageable fragment. Subsequently, these fragments become the triggers that, with incredible power, draw us back into our memories. The process by which the metaphor is derived from the trauma scene is apparent in many cases – as in the case of "mother's dress," above. These holographic fragments, as containers of the whole conscious experience, carry immense power. By willingly focusing our attention on these metaphors, we return to the age, sensations, emotions, body, clothing, etc. that we possessed at T-l. This is our inherent, natural capacity to enter into holographic space – the multidimensional locus of healing.

In my practice it has rarely been necessary for a client to relive the entire trauma experience in order to resolve it. The fact remains that we have all lived through our traumas once already and did not find emotional resolution. The key to resolution is in addressing our consciousness at the correct moment in space and time when the altered state (trance) was created – the exact moment when the memory fragment was encoded. At that place and time, the portion of the experience that we could not effectively process was preserved perfectly intact in the metaphor. Unless this specific metaphor is accessed and resolved, the fragment of the trauma scene and its contents will continue to present themselves to the psyche for healing. This means that the survivor may suffer for years with a feeling like "there is something wrong with me" or that "something inside me doesn't belong there." This is the feeling often presented by the metaphor's presence in the nervous system – identifying itself to the psyche for healing. Lacking knowledge about the trauma induction process, the survivor may assume that there is something wrong with him, instead of understanding that he is carrying unresolved trauma — something that was done to him, something that was stored within his bodymind when he became overwhelmed by the experience. This confusion is even more pronounced if traumatic amnesia is involved as part of the encoding. In cases of amnesia, the client, while remaining anchored in present time, may be assisted in viewing, without emotionally reliving the new memory, by observing the entire (previously repressed) event before enacting the solution.

Once the event is conscious, the client can return safely to T-1 armed with adult ego-state resources and enact the appropriate solution. The memory still need not be fully relived with all its emotional distress in order to be resolved.

There are several important points to be noted about the trauma induction process:

♦ **Metaphors (holographic memory fragments) are encoded and manifest in the location(s) of the body where the pain was most intense at T-1.**

The nerve centers of the body and the surrounding muscles react promptly to perceived threat. For example, a five year old boy watching his intoxicated father choke his mother feels a tightening in his throat and encodes the trauma in his throat plexus as he watches Mom gasping for air. A young child slapped in the face encodes the trauma in the nerve centers on the side of the face where the blow was taken. A sexually abused child, knowing little about sex, will often encode the fear and betrayal in the stomach plexus, where it manifests as nausea or emptiness. The death or sudden loss of a loved one typically is perceived as a sharp pain or emptiness in the heart, where emotional absences are so keenly felt. Traumas, therefore, may appear in forms such as a lump in the throat, a weight on the chest, a black and bottomless empty hole in the stomach, a chronic stabbing pain in the heart or abdominal region, a vise around the head, etc. When these metaphors present themselves for healing, they are called "body" or "somatic memories" (from the Greek word, soma meaning "body"). Body memories are the initial indicators of the location of stored memory. Sometimes these hints are not subtle, and they may be accompanied by flashbacks of visual, olfactory, auditory, or other sensory experiences of T-1 memory fragments. Remember, these experiences are the mind's cues and maps to healing. As the facilitator of the survivor's own process, I simply follow the cues and maps that he provides to heal himself. We will examine the specific dynamics of the emotional encoding later in this work.

♦ **When a metaphor is created at the moment of trauma, it may not appear in the conscious short-term or long-term memory.**

It does appear, however, to be encoded as a physical sensation in the nerve cells and electromagnetic fields where it was felt at T-1. This process often leaves the individual amnesial without any conscious memory that the event occurred. (This mechanism, called "traumatic amnesia" or "delayed recall" has successfully been proved in courts of law; now there have been many such cases.) The containment function of the metaphor also includes this protective option (amnesia) which is easily understood when we see how the individual's own sense of security and identity would have been compromised. This is often necessary, as seen in the case of incest, where the child cannot reconcile such betrayal by the very person(s) that she turns to for life, love, and nurturing on a daily basis. The amnesia magnificently saves the life of the child or adult by preventing a trauma of such magnitude from reaching the conscious level – a rupture which could close the door to any option for further nurturing from her own parent or loved one. Such an experience would precipitate a relational break of indescribable proportions to the psyche of the vulnerable child who has few, if any other, options for nurturing.

♦ **The painful symptoms of trauma, encoded within the nervous system of the survivor, particularly when accompanied by amnesia, precipitate profound feelings of defectiveness which can be mistakenly attributed to the self.** *low self-esteem*

Over time the survivor may become accustomed to living with the feeling that "there is something inside me that doesn't belong" and may come to believe in profound, personal defectiveness. When the survivor has no conscious awareness of the trauma's origin, and, since he is unaware that it was induced from the outside by a perpetrator or external event, he might very well conclude that "it's all about me ... I'm bad ... there's something wrong with me ... there's something evil inside me ... I'm a mistake ... I'm the cause of all the pain." With no knowledge or memory to explain his negative self-talk, he may conclude that he is its source. The wounded ego-states within us support such negative thinking: "if there is a bad feeling inside me, I must have done something to cause it." A survivor could live the entirety of his life acting out this falsehood, basing his decisions on erroneous self-perceptions. Frequently the memories precipitating these feelings and their locations (as metaphors) are hinted at throughout life. Other survivors begin accessing their trauma memories between the ages of twenty-eight and forty-five due to stabilization and enhanced safety which allow the memories to surface. Some individuals are forced to address their traumas as a result of a crisis which triggers their encoded pain. Irrespective of the precipitating cause, most of us learn, quite early, to medicate our surfacing metaphors with drugs, alcohol, food, relationships, religion, sex, work, exercise, etc. As you see, we have both conscious and subconscious mechanisms at work to foster survival. Having traumas encoded in our nervous systems with no recognition of their external origin, we claim the metaphors and their contents as our own and come to identify with them. It's really quite simple: "Because this feeling (metaphor) is in my nervous system in my body, it must be about me." Between the coping mechanisms of denial and amnesia, the self appears to be the obvious culprit. This tendency toward "self-attribution" has its origins in early childhood development. As children we self-reference everything – i.e., if a bad thing happens, "it must be about me." Additionally, a child will self-blame in order to maintain the image of a loving Mommy or Daddy: "I must just be bad – that's why Daddy does this to me." As abuse victims we are encouraged by our perpetrators to "forget about it," to keep the secret, or to face dire consequences. The repression of memories is one of our earliest and most effective survival mechanisms; it is largely subconscious and automatic. These defenses can keep us alive until we are old enough, safe enough to begin dealing with these powerful metaphors which contain our very consciousness. Now we must begin to examine what this containment of consciousness means for us.

♦ The holographic containment process includes the internalization and freezing of all perceptions, including the image of the abuser and all associated emotional exchanges occurring at that moment.

If quantum physics is correct – that we create our reality through our act of perception, then something powerful occurs when we utilize that same ability to freeze our perceptions. What, exactly, is internalized when such an altered state is created – when our consciousness itself, in that instant, is put on hold? Is there a physics to this transaction? Let us consider the following case:

Michael came to me stating that he needed to address feelings of "shame." When asked where he felt the shame in his body, he observed: "I feel it over my head and shoulders on the outside like a wet towel."

"And how young might you be when you first feel a wet towel of shame over your head and shoulders like that?" I asked.

"I'm five," he replied.

"And where are you when you're five, and you're feeling shame like that?" I inquired.

"I'm in my bedroom," he reported.

"And what happens then, when you're in your bedroom, and you're five years old?"

"My Dad bursts through the door and this wave of anger hits me," he whispered, instantly reverting to a quiet, frightened, child-like voice.

"And what happens next, after the wave of anger hits you?" I encouraged.

"I pull the blanket over my head and hide 'cause I'm terrified," he responded, beginning to reflect a cowering posture in his chair.

"And would a feeling of shame like a wet towel over your head and shoulders have anything to do with a five year old boy, a blanket, and a wave of anger?" I inquired.

"Yes, it's the same thing!" he stated with surprise. "It wasn't a towel, it was a blanket!"

In an instant, Michael realized that he was carrying his father's abusive rage in his body as anger and shame, in the holographic form of the "wet blanket" over his head and shoulders. At this point the adult Michael became angry that he had been carrying his father's abusive anger around as his own all these years, preventing him from expressing his anger appropriately as an adult. He was then able to enter the memory and remove this five year old from the abusive anger and presence of his father, bringing him to a safe place. He wrapped him in a warm, dry blanket and provided love, safety, and nurturing. At the close of the process, there was no evidence of the "wet blanket of shame" in his body.

The study of this transaction reveals that, when a metaphor is created, when time and space perceptions are arrested at the moment of trauma, all awareness on the physical, mental, and emotional planes is imprinted and stored within the cells and electromagnetic fields of the body. The child's outgoing emotional impulse to protect himself collided with the perceived "wave of anger" – the incoming emotional impulses of his father, and froze. These sensations were encoded somatically at the nerve centers in his body where the threat was perceived. This is not simply a matter of internal psychological perception, for this transaction manifests in an external, physical manner in the nerve cells and fields of the body and can be measured by instrumentation. Scientists have known for some time that states of stress from trauma remain in the body from the moment of traumatization onward. Quantum physics shows us that our consciousness – our act of perception, indeed, creates our reality. This includes the physics of our bodies, minds, and spirits.

The distinctions between mind, body, emotion, or spirit begin to blur when we recognize the sheer power of consciousness and the perceptual act. The physiological sciences and psychology affirm that emotions and thoughts are biochemical-electrical impulses. Trauma induction, therefore, suggests a capacity to store these impulses in some form of stasis over indefinite periods of time. The metaphors which accomplish the storing contain, not only the perceived impulses of the survivor's own nervous system, but also the perceived intrusive impulses of the abuser/perpetrator. Michael froze, not only his own emotional impulses, but also those which he felt projected by his raging father. Understanding these dynamics is most important, for they also provide clues to better understand how destructive patterns are communicated intergenerationally. Long have we sought to understand the means by which family secrets and other undisclosed experiences of shame and trauma are transmitted intact, allowing them to be repeated generation after generation. Comprehending the nature of these metaphors and their powerful programs is crucial in this endeavor. Great freedom and healing are found when we discover that we internalize and carry the reality of others within these arrested states of consciousness. Once we access the memory and realize that the perceptions we carry are not exclusively our own, we can eliminate the confusion created in the trauma scene – the confusion consisting of two opposing emotional realities which, at that moment (T-1), could not be separated or resolved. The product of trauma induction, therefore, is not merely an "altered state," but, based upon the theory of quantum physics, is a confusion of two opposing realities. Such a condition will, of course, impact reality and self-perception profoundly. When we acknowledge our capacity to internalize the reality of others through trauma induction, we can individuate from them.

♦ **Trauma results, not only in the internalization of the reality of others, but also in an emotional splitting within the self.**

If, at a moment of near trauma we had been able to access and utilize our anger to prevent the violation of our boundaries, traumatization might have been prevented. In every case of actual trauma, however, there is a "peak" moment when a sense of powerlessness is reached – a moment when even our best resources cannot seem to halt what is about to happen to us. As a result, there is necessary emotional splitting that occurs: there is sadness, pain, and hurt felt on the one hand, and an anger that is instilled on the other. Quite often, the "wounded child self" bears the sadness, pain, and hurt, and the "adult-parent self" inherits the anger. In the case of Michael, he became terrified and overwhelmed by his father's anger and had to put his own anger aside. From the trauma, he stored both his father's anger and his own. The adult Michael developed a "temper" over the years and went to extreme measures in his life to avoid venting his anger inappropriately on others. He lived in terror that he would become his rageful father, which remained a very real possibility as long as his anger was suppressed. Expending such effort to avoid his anger, however, he also missed a key ingredient for his own healing. That very emotion that he was avoiding was to eventually become the vehicle for his healing. The power to resolve such conflicting realities often comes from the direction that we least expect: without sufficient anger to provide us with the strength to confront a rageful perpetrator, we might never enter the scene to rescue our wounded self. Anger gives us the gift of energy. The anger of having carried around another person's unresolved feelings of anger, guilt, and shame is often the very energy which allows us to filter our realities from those of another. The amount of anger that we carry from our past is, in fact, a measure of the amount of unresolved trauma that we carry. This anger is most useful in providing the strength needed to enter the scenes to liberate the wounded inner selves imprisoned since the moment of the trauma. Does the existence and power of such frozen ego-states surprise you?

As young children, especially between the ages of zero and five, we imitate and encode what we see, hear, smell, taste, and touch; this is how we learn language so quickly. From my experience, I know that, by age four, I had already internalized much of my father's shame, fear, avoidance, and shyness. He was a child of trauma who never overtly addressed his personal issues. Once I realized that the shame I carried was not my own, it became considerably easier to release. Nor did I find it necessary to blame my father for the patterns I carried, for neither were they original to him. He, in fact, improved his coping strategies over those he inherited from the previous generation. After I began to release the family trauma patterns, I was shocked to discover, for instance, that I was actually more extroverted than introverted. How many years I had lived out that early emotional programming leading me to think, feel, and believe that I was so much less than I am?

Trauma induction imprisons consciousness, spirit itself, with messages, perceptions, and emotions which are not our own, and it often alienates us from those emotions which are ours. Over the years we come to identify with those containers of trauma as well as their contents – coming to believe that we are powerless, shameful, immutable, and unable to change the past. Trauma "blurs" our boundaries, merging our realities with those of others. As we will see in the ensuing chapters, the solution for trauma induction must involve an individuation or separation, initially, from the false, confused messages of the wounded ego-state. Those of us who have suffered trauma have lived with internal messages of defectiveness and shame, and we have never been able to trust that, just perhaps, this is not about us "being bad." To further complicate our healing efforts, most of us were taught to follow a "moral model" and, thus, find it easy to judge ourselves and others. Trauma is not about morality. It is about "survival" and is automatic and subconscious in its induction. It is "pre-moral." In the instance of sexual abuse, for example, the abused child often acts out promiscuously in light of the premature sexual awakening and the sexual shaming that arrests her with a preoccupation with sexuality and with a subconscious message that sex is love. The powerful subconscious mind implodes with the assertion that I am an object for the gratification of others. The acting out which then follows is the subconscious attempt to release her own shame – often in the same manner that it was programmed during the perpetration. Such acting out, however, does not heal the original scene. In addition, such trauma-induced programs are often much stronger on an emotional level than any mental or moral precepts that may have been taught to guide moral decision-making. This incredible emotional power which defies rational control and diminishes moral guidance underlies the cases reported here. As we saw earlier, traumas induced before the age of seven or eight developmentally precede the ability to make moral decisions, negating potential moral reasoning. Irrespective of the age of its encoding, the effects of the trauma create an intense need to "undo" the wrong felt inside. Sometimes we have tried to release these emotional imprints by medicating or suppressing the pain, but, with trauma, the only permanent solution involves converting our specific trauma from a destructive to a constructive experience. This requires accessing the original scene at T- I. Repressing it will only cause it to manifest more obstinately somewhere else in our body or life, for the psyche demands the solution that will make us whole, nothing less. Michael was able to release the shame over his head and shoulders by saving his five year-old self who was fixed in space and time while his father raged. Using the anger as a resource for his own healing, he transformed his fear of anger into an energy which was utilized to love himself, free himself, and release the shame that had followed him around like a "wet towel" every day since he was five years old. This is the challenge and the power that we have to heal and liberate ourselves.

Studying the dynamics of trauma, we see this process as a part of an emotional immune system that preserves and contains, with great efficiency, the overwhelming experiences of our lives until we are ready to address and resolve them. By freezing these perceptions at a pre-overwhelm instant, the nervous system indicates that it does not want to re-live the experience in question. Our minds work in magnificent cooperation with our bodies to provide containment until resolution is possible. Our lives are filled with opportunities for accessing and resolving these unfinished scenes from our past. Just as our bodies, minds, and spirits worked together to contain these overwhelming experiences, so do they work to illumine these memories that we might integrate them and, in so doing, advance our personal and collective evolution.

Chapter Six

A crisis event often explodes the illusions that anchor our lives.

Robert Veninga

"Triggers" – The First Glimpse of Trauma

Research on the manner in which memories are encoded indicates that the capacity of the mind to store memory – no, to store more than what we traditionally thought of as memory – to store consciousness itself, is remarkable. This ability is a function of the holographic nature of the mind. If, for instance, I wish to think of my favorite food, because my mind and my senses operate holographically, I may access this food in a number of ways: I may simply recall who cooked it, its smell, the sound of its preparation, or the kitchen in which it was prepared. There are innumerable possibilities for accessing holographically encoded memories. Any one of these memory fragments can be used to provide access to our stored experiences. In the course of a day we make contact with hundreds of such memory triggers. Our tastes, our choices, our likes and dislikes are shaped significantly by our memories. But how is it that a mere thought, a face, an image, a smell can possess power sufficient to propel our conscious minds backward in time into the stored emotions of a past experience or event? And, with respect to trauma, how can it be that such events, once triggered in our memories, can influence us to act in contradiction to our rational thought and moral judgment? We are well acquainted with the emotional potency of such memories. How frequently, for instance, we hold unresolved anger about an injustice done to ourselves or someone we love; we need only think of the one who inflicted the harm to resurrect in mere seconds the unresolved pain we hold. Furthermore, this pain maintains us in relationship to those persons who inflicted it, keeping us connected on the powerful subconscious level. Frequently we chide ourselves for holding such resentments and not forgiving our offenders when, in fact, it is more likely that these scenes and their potent emotions are restraining us from the subconscious. Few of us would choose to consciously retain our negative memory triggers – the phobias and fears, the uncontrollable impulses and reactions. The persistence of these triggers is based, not so much in our rationality, as in the domineering emotional content of our memories. It was their overpowering emotional nature that originally led to their encoding as trauma; let us examine this nature.

Some years ago at a seminary library book sale, I acquired a collection of texts entitled, <u>The Literature of All Nations</u>, edited by Julian Hawthorne. This ten volume collection of literature was published in 1901. In the introduction, Justin McCarthy states the following:

> *The root and origin of human speech is emotion. The distinction between emotion and thought was artificial and comparatively recent. They were originally one; and if we penetrate beneath the surface, we shall find that they are so still. Thought, in its basis, is the contemplation of emotional impressions. Though such contemplation may, in the abstract, be considered apart from the impression, in reality, it is never so separated. The two make one as do substance and form. We may abstractly consider the form of a thing apart from the thing itself but if we take away from a thing its constitutive substance, obviously there will be nothing left. We can only say that form is a universal property of substance; and in the same way we say that thought is an inalienable property of emotion. Without emotion, the mind is and must remain an inoperative, a blank.[1]*

The profound connection between emotion and thought, referred to by McCarthy a century ago, has clearly emerged as we study the dynamics of trauma induction; and, indeed, we find that emotion and thought remain as one. In fact, recent studies of the brain indicate that emotion is central to the process of rational thought; it is a crucial element for learning and decision-making. But how does emotion support our cognitive processes? Emotion potentiates or empowers thought. Items or concepts to be remembered are assigned a subjective attribute via emotion, ensuring that the brain "captures" the specific item and sets it apart from other less meaningful data. What types of life decisions would one make based solely on rationality? Archaeological and anthropological studies of ancient man confirm the need to make sudden, lucid decisions in order to survive. Survival continues to depend on the combined effort of emotionality and rationality.

Thoughts and emotions are similar; both are identified as biochemical-electrical impulses or movements. The trauma induction process involves the arresting of these movements. This freezing is indiscriminate, meaning that all incoming impulses are preserved, whether they are emotions, thoughts, or sensory perceptions. This explains the process by which a given trauma, captured in its complex metaphorical form, may be elevated to consciousness by such stimuli as a thought, a feeling similar to the emotion of the original scene, or sensory perceptions resembling those of the first experience. Such triggers, as holographic fragments of the original scene, carry immense power, for they are able to access the whole event, the entire trauma scene and, in an instant, to recreate this state of consciousness within our contemporary nervous system. These metaphorical containers carry the power to transport us instantaneously to the past place and time when we were violated and our boundaries were penetrated. These metaphors resurrect the intensity and level of psychic distress that was present in the frozen scene. An understanding of these triggers is essential. Otherwise we may be overwhelmed by the metaphors when they arise.

Among some of the most common types of experiences that serve to ignite memory triggers are the following:

♦ **Stabilization and Safety:** Periods of stabilization as are experienced during recovery from addictions, from stressful periods of life, or from financial insecurity, may leave a victim of trauma with the opportunity to give himself permission to feel. When the survivor is not distracted or medicating his feelings, this stability may allow his feelings and his memories to surface unprompted. Periods of safety provide the opportunity to deal with those issues that have been buried since the moment of traumatization. A "safe" person like a partner or significant other may provide the level of security needed to release the original subconscious barrier and allow oneself to face memories of sexual abuse, for instance. If amnesia is involved, the survivor may not understand, at first, that it is actually the sense of safety derived from the partnership that enabled the memory recall, rather than a deep-seated aversion or incompatibility that is in evidence. One's significant other may provide the occasion for a memory to surface, but need not be its source. In working with trauma survivors, it is important to include the partner who may have been responded to or treated like an abuser when the source of the marital conflict was the original trauma.

Tony and Bridget's story demonstrates the profound effects of stabilization and safety and the role they play in recalling trauma memories. Having been married to Bridget for twenty-one years, Tony was successfully completing outpatient chemical dependency treatment for alcoholism. Bridget came to me in tears stating that she could not "figure out" what was happening to her. Now that Tony was doing so well, she found his touch and romantic overtures "disgusting." She could not be near him or accept any sexual overtures without feeling ill. She identified this "disgust" feeling as a "black box in my abdomen." Focusing on this metaphorical container, she began to access a memory. As she recalled the scene, she identified her age as twenty, and the location, as a black truck she and Tony had owned. She proceeded to describe how Tony, while in a blackout from drinking, had beaten and raped her. They had been married for only a few months when this occurred. Bridget experienced traumatic amnesia and had no conscious memory of the experience for the next twenty-one years. In fact, she described their sexual relationship as "good" over those years. It was only when Tony stopped drinking and entered recovery that she subconsciously felt safe enough to remember. He was in a "blackout," and she had traumatic amnesia; neither knew that this had occurred between them. After accessing and resolving her memory, we invited Tony to join us in a counseling session to process the experience and to enable them both to heal from the trauma. After she resolved the memory, she feared that the "disgust" feeling would return to sabotage her marriage. Much to her delight, once the somatic memory was resolved, she experienced no recurrence of the "disgust" feeling, despite her knowledge and fear of "self-fulfilling prophecies." Stabilization experienced in recovery from alcoholism and other addictions often allows unresolved traumas and feelings to rise to the surface, to the conscious level. The removal of alcohol from her marriage was the trigger – a spark of stabilization and safety – which ignited the "disgust" feelings which provided access and healing of the trauma.

♦ <u>**Somatic Memory Triggers:**</u> A sensory response – a touch, smell, taste, sound, or sight that is identical or similar to the encoded memory will immediately access the stored metaphor. A gesture or body perception that duplicates any portion of the original memory can easily access the subconscious scene which, then, picks up at that moment in past time – suddenly sending the individual to a different place and time. We believe the holographic memory principle (where each memory fragment contains the whole) to be accurate. Therefore, one sensory fragment can replicate or trigger the whole of a stored memory. The validity and value of this principle is to be found in the effectiveness of the memory resolution techniques and the exemplary cases presented in this work.

Among the most frequent trigger experiences that I have encountered are those of touch, smell, and sight. To be touched in a manner similar to the original abuse experience frequently produces instantaneous recall; tactile triggers are very powerful. Recently I worked with a client, Jan, who, at the outset of the process, nearly jumped out of the chair exclaiming: "It's hot! It's hot ... on my back." I had begun with the traditional process, simply placing my hand on the dorsal point of her back. The heat sensation generated by my light contact roused a memory of Jan and hers siblings dyeing

Easter eggs. Her brother, who was abusive with her, threw the hot water from the boiling eggs on her back. Immediately she was able to reframe the scene and resolve the body memory from the original trauma. Oftentimes the extremes of our discomfort with certain forms of touch give us our first warning of the presence of an unresolved memory.

Olfactory (smell) triggers are among the most powerful fuses for igniting encoded memory. The smell of whiskey, for instance, on someone's breath often resurrects countless memories for those abused by alcoholics. One client reported how a "musty" smell in a cedar chest always brought back memories of her grandfather's home in which she was abused. A recent client, Stephanie, as a child of seven, witnessed the explosion of an airplane flying over her family's corn field. While she was too terrified to watch the experience, a "horrible smell" pervaded the air as she fled for safety. It was this smell that haunted her long afterward.

Visual triggers may be the most common. Persons resembling the abuser, symbols, objects, or scenery from early trauma are readily accessible to us in our everyday lives. It is impossible to detail the number of memories that were accessed by simply seeing the image of the bleeding, wounded child broadcast on television screens throughout the world within hours of the Oklahoma City bombing. Most of you know the image to which I refer – a picture that was chosen to elicit an emotional response. My clients, my friends, and I discovered that we accessed memories of traumas involving childhood accidents and injuries which contained the sight of a bleeding, wounded child. I responded by recalling the incident when my childhood friend Keena accidentally hit me in the head with a golf club, creating a particularly bloody and terrifying scene. Fortunately, I possessed a "hard head" and didn't require stitches, though I still carry the "knot." Keena, however, thought that he had killed me and hid behind a couch for three hours before anyone could find him. I wonder what he felt when he saw the televised image? Such images carry power because of the remnants of traumas we hold within us. Some media folk know, quite well, how to stimulate visual triggers. Innocently, we tend to refer to their work simply as news, journalism, or advertising rather than abuse.

Auditory triggers are among the most tenacious. Among the most frequent of the early childhood traumas that surface in my work with survivors is the first time a child hears Mom and Dad fighting – particularly if the fighting escalates to violence. "How can Mommy and Daddy be fighting and still love each other ? ... And what's going to happen to me?" The child's world is "black and white"; conflict creates confusion – a dilemma in her mind. Along with abandonment trauma, this experience of domestic violence is the most recurrent trauma I see in resolution work. Many survivors who lived in households punctuated with screaming, fighting, and violence find themselves agitated around loud, chaotic situations. They are easily triggered in such settings and may even react in protective, isolative, or aggressive ways to perceived provocation, or situations that even remotely resemble the aggression displayed in their past.

An unforgettable case is that of Todd, a very muscular male client. He would inexplicably strike out with violence at anyone near him when he heard a loud noise. He admitted that he had even "knocked out" his wife when he was startled by a rock hitting the bottom of the truck in which they were traveling. On another occasion he nearly killed someone in a bar when he heard a loud noise while holding a glass. He had no conscious explanation for his behavior. When I asked him where in his body he felt the impulse to strike out, he explained: upon hearing a loud noise, he would feel an instant pain on the outside of his right ear. During our session, while focusing on the pain sensation outside his right ear, he immediately reverted to a scene of himself at age four seated at the kitchen table eating breakfast. Dad came home, entering the kitchen smiling, although he was actually drunk that morning. Suddenly, catching Todd completely by surprise, Dad struck him full force on the right side of his head "with a bag of frozen candy" (as the child's mind perceived it at the time), knocking him to the floor. In a spontaneous reaction to the shock (the adrenaline "fight or flight" response of the endocrine system), he "came up swinging," fighting for his life. His self-defense reaction was bound to the (T-1) scene at the same moment as the blow to the right side of his head. This event created a powerful imprint that negated any conscious control when it was auditorily triggered. This is the power which trauma imprints on the nervous system. Todd had never recalled this incident. He was able to reframe the memory to create safety for the wounded child, and to resolve all the associated triggers. As we saw earlier in the case of Claire and the "raw flour," the subconscious coping mechanisms can easily override conscious control, abandoning logic and leading to the reenactment of the original scene. The "acting out" of our old subconscious coping strategies reveals the power of trauma memory.

◆ **Affective Memory Triggers**: Feelings and emotions similar to those of the original trauma are frequent provocative triggers. With a wide variety of emotional experiences available in a given day, it is easy to see the potential for encountering events which readily spiral us into memories where, in an earlier episode, we felt the same or similar sensations. The mind has a magnificent capacity for drawing together memories in a non-linear (i.e., non-chronological) fashion. Intense affect such as anger or panic, once induced and stored, can be incited by like feelings, even of lesser intensity. This gives rise to the familiar shame, fear, anger, and depression spirals to which we are susceptible. Claire's sense of fear, panic, and abandonment, activated by her husband's announcement of his intention to divorce her, sparked the need for an immediate coping mechanism; hence, her old childhood strategy of "eating raw flour" was relied upon when the adult felt overwhelmed. Such can be the power of affective triggers.

◆ **Transference**: A person bearing the traits, profile, emotional characteristics or features similar to those contained in the memory can easily provoke the unresolved feelings. Innumerable times, I have been the object of someone's ire by simply walking into the room and "looking like" the client's ex-husband or ex-partner. Similarly, in my work with hundreds of sexual trauma survivors, the coincidence of my dark hair, light colored eyes, and olive complexion have roused survivors' memories because their perpetrator bore these traits.

♦ <u>**Reenactment or Retraumatization:**</u> Even though there may be amnesia after a trauma, <u>a reenactment of the original event</u> often <u>provides rapid access to the original</u> memory. This explains why "psycho-drama" (a therapeutic re-creation of the experience using substitutes to represent the characters and symbolic representations of the abuse environment) is effective in summoning the affect buried in an unresolved memory. To recreate the scene certainly provides a powerful bridge for the encoded memory to surface, if the subconscious mind allows access. A retraumatization or actual re-experiencing of the same type of trauma will also resurrect these frozen feelings. It is important to remember that unresolved traumas from the past often repeat themselves and, in so doing, serve to provide another opportunity for healing the original, painful event. We are magnetic to the patterns we bear. This is never more evident than when we subconsciously recreate the relationship of our parents – the first who demonstrated and defined for us "love" and intimacy. Subconsciously bound by this early definition of love, we repeat the same patterns until we become conscious of the need to change. We frequently become angry upon realizing that we have "retraumatized" ourselves, not realizing the powerful impact of the underlying, subconscious, family programming.

♦ <u>**Intensification of Stored Memory:**</u> The intensification of feelings of shame, fear, anger, and guilt may <u>result in an eventual inability</u> <u>to contain the increasing number of similar emotional experiences,</u> <u>and give rise to a breakdown in defens</u>es. This is particularly evident in the case of the addict where the use of the mood altering drugs, relationships, or behaviors actually produces more shame, thereby intensifying the very feelings that the individual is trying to mask or medicate. This commonly leads to "hitting bottom," where the unhealthy defenses and denial break down. Intensification is one of the main tools of our subconscious for raising the real problem to consciousness for purposes of healing. The deeper we try to push the ball of emotion under the water, the more the pressure increases, forcing it to the surface. Try stuffing a little angry air into it every now and then and see what eventually emerges!

Identifying these categories of trigger events provides valuable clues to trauma survivor behavior and response. The list is not exhaustive, but rather open-ended and fluid as I continue my observations. Nearly all of us have awakened such stored responses in our everyday events. A temper, for instance, is created by a body of unresolved emotions stored in our nervous system to the degree that a very small stimulus, not even necessarily pertaining to the original anger, causes the entire body of anger to surface. Our emotions are stored holographically, for a fragment will cause us to spiral or access the whole. One small memory fragment can stimulate an unresolved feeling of depression, fear, shame, or worthlessness and, by association with other similar traumas stored in the subconscious, cause us to spiral faster and faster into a feeling of utter worthlessness and despair. This is the shadow-side of our holographic nature surfacing for healing. I have shared an extraordinary number of cases where individuals were triggered by a particular touch, song, color, type of clothing, smell, food, person, etc., and found themselves overwhelmed by a flood of perceptions belonging to a different place and time. This is the power of the metaphor – the holographic containers that hold our trauma memories.

A metaphor, as I use the term here, is a multidimensional container. Within the consciousness of the individual, it serves to embody the overwhelming experience in a comprehensive fashion that allows the subject suffering great pain to survive. The metaphor encompasses the entirety of the experience as it was perceived by the individual at the moment of preservation, and each metaphorical container is unique. Seven subjects, in fact, encode seven different perceptions of the same event. In light of what quantum physics teaches us – that my perceptive act creates my reality, we begin to see the inestimable value of honoring our memories, our perceived reality.

During a workshop that I provided for one hundred and twelve sexual trauma therapists, we investigated the accuracy of memory. One portion of the discussion centered on the issue of the existence of objective or "real" memory. I raised the point that, to one child in a family, an act might be a very traumatic experience, whereas it might go unnoticed by another. This introduces the issue of perception. Why, for instance, did I think that my childhood was so good, when my younger sister predominantly remembered the conflicts between herself and my mother? When comparing our memories, it was evident that we each had constructed different frames of reference from which we perceived and judged our experiences. It was also clear that these perspectives had been under construction since our earliest development and were, in part, roles assigned by our family dynamics and a product of the internalized perceptions from our parents. Family Systems Theory teaches us that such role assignment often leaves one child in the role of the "hero" of the family while designating another the "black sheep/scapegoat," "lost child," or "mascot." My sister and I concluded that our different frames of reference did not invalidate our individual experiences nor our memories. Neither of us found it necessary to convince the other that our personal perception of the event was the sole one. We both now understand and are learning valuable lessons from each others' apperceptions. The differences that emerged are quite comprehensible in light of what we now know about family systems theory, role assignments, personality types, and birth order.

Respect for our personal perceptions becomes crucial for healing. Accepting our perceptions as real and viable truths facilitates our openness to the healing process. It is my reality that is encoded in holographic form at the moment of trauma: my sensitivity, emotionality, and vulnerability will determine the instant that I become overwhelmed. It is neither the therapist's, nor any of my family members' perceptions that will be found encoded so intricately in my nervous system. Because it contains a frozen moment in time and space, a frozen experience, it holds all of the aspects and dimensions involved in the containment of consciousness. This process is infinitely more sophisticated than simply pushing the pause button on a video recorder, for smells, sounds, tastes, feelings, thoughts, environmental details, body image, other persons or realities, emotions – all are encoded in this holographic metaphor. In light of the hologram's sophistication, it is no surprise that it can be accessed through the wide variety of triggers already outlined. It also teaches us that physical sensations, thoughts, and emotions are simply different facets of the same crystallized experience. Indeed, they are one. This is readily seen in the metaphors we access within ourselves. It was Einstein's Theory of Relativity that revealed to us that matter is simply slowed or crystallized energy. The body is energy; thoughts are energy; and feelings are energy. Our memories are complex forms of energy. Traumatization adds to the crystallization process by slowing our energy and arresting a profound level of human experience in metaphorical or holographic form.

Dr. Karl Pribram, a well known brain researcher, indicates that the brain's most profound structuring is essentially holographic, and that the brain structures hearing, sight, taste, touch, and smell holographically.[2] Since, as physics confirms, each fragment of a hologram contains the picture of the whole, one can understand how a single triggered sensory perception could, therefore, access the whole encoded experience, resulting in a spontaneous regression or re-experiencing (abreaction) of the original event.

The healing of trauma does not require a comprehensive understanding of the metaphor itself, but, rather, sufficient, authentic access to allow its release and transformation. I may not know why my abandonment fear appears as a baseball-sized black hole in my stomach plexus, but, by focusing on this metaphor, I can, nonetheless, return to the event which caused it and resolve it. Since our subconscious mind contains the complete knowledge of the metaphor, it can also provide a solution which is complete. Given the metaphor's complex nature, only my own subconscious mind, in cooperation with my conscious efforts to heal, possesses the wherewithal to make such a perfect change in my holographic world. The accomplishment of this transformation within my mind reveals to me the power I possess to heal myself. But, what is the role of the therapist or facilitator, you might ask? As a facilitator I simply mirror and help to create the bridge between the conscious and subconscious mind of the survivor. He gradually becomes aware of his own inner access to the unlimited resources within him through the questions that I ask – which are based on his subconscious cues. Once this bridge is recognized and internalized, the survivor can often accomplish further memory resolution on his own. Our subconscious minds are, in fact, our own best experts and know exactly what needs to happen for us to reach wholeness.

Metaphors, as fragments of the overwhelming experiences of our lives, are the vehicles through which we survive and contain these traumatic events, preventing them from completely paralyzing our lives. In protecting us, they maintain our healing potential until we learn to activate and utilize it. From this purview, they possess a profoundly spiritual nature and function. It has long been said that the language of healing is the language of metaphor. This has proved true in the mythologies and spiritual writings of all nations. These bodies of wisdom express, via metaphors, truths that transcend space and time. Such is the power of metaphor – to bridge the collective conscious and subconscious minds. The Bible is one recognized example of this type of literature. There is a timelessness to its metaphorical language which allows us to transcend space and time in order to invoke its healing message in the present. I have personally experienced it. Similarly, the metaphors within us containing our past are the magnificent vehicles to wholeness and transcendence. They are the instruments for the growth and expansion of consciousness. As we evolve, we move into higher and higher metaphorical expressions and understandings of ourselves and all that surrounds us. As we evolve, our metaphors converge and resolve toward singularity. We are energy; we are light. Our consciousness manifests at any given moment as this slowed or crystallized energy. In metaphorical language, Jesus cautioned us of the importance of "not hiding our light under a bushel-basket" (Mark 4:21).

Advancing our metaphorical implications a step, we can state that: we are the metaphors of a higher consciousness to which we are evolving, and, as such, are containers of that consciousness manifest in space and time. Like all the holographic metaphors or fragments that we have studied, we ourselves are more – and we reflect that total reality. The great mystics of all ages knew this. At times we recognize this – when we glimpse ourselves in the right light. Every metaphor is, in varying degrees, an expression of the one light. As such, each metaphor promises access to something which clearly transcends our bodies, intellects, and emotions. This is the spiritual nature of metaphor. The triggers in our everyday experience broadcast to us these truths – that we are holographic in a holographic universe; and even these bothersome emotions seem to be fragments pointing us toward a greater consciousness. Our most severe traumas, therefore, in their holographic nature, hold the promise of a grand disclosure – a creative, healing power calling us to wholeness.

Chapter Seven

Forge thy tongue on an anvil of truth.
And what flies up, though it be but a spark,
Shall have weight.

Pendar (518 - 438 B.C.)

The Language of Healing

Among the many gifts that I have gained from my work with trauma survivors is a new respect for the power of words and their tone of delivery. I quickly learned that a voice raised in anger could become a pain in the heart and ears of a young listener, imprinting itself for years to come and setting up triggers of fear and insecurity. This phenomenon has been referred to as the notion of "energy transduction" – how one form of energy such as the frequency, pitch, or tone of a voice is picked up auditorily, interpreted within the brain of the listener, and translated to a physical sensation or pain in the body. I was reminded of the childhood taunt: "Sticks and stones will break my bones, but words will never hurt me." Surely this was an erroneous assumption. Within the confines of Newtonian physics we were able to remain in the illusion that when we were separated physically, the hurtful words of others would not impact us, or at least not so deeply. Through the limitations of the five senses and our scientific restriction to "observable" phenomenon, we were safe and separate, you and I. Our "illusions of separation" protected us from thinking that we could harm one another by the mere tone of our voice raised in anger. Through the insights of quantum physics, we began dissolving these illusions and opening our understanding of perception to embrace a much greater reality. In the process, we became aware that each articulation carries immense power – a creative power. Where we focus our intention and speech, we create!

Speech, for instance, can be used to shame a child, creating a split within the psyche and causing the child to devote her attention to figuring out which of the conflicting messages is "true." Words of affirmation, encouragement, and validation, on the other hand, can build a bond of love which transcends time and space and creates an everlasting relational bridge. Recognizing the power of our words, we become more attentive to what we say, to where we invest our creative energies – becoming more sensitive and aware of our creations. Listening, then, becomes a profound act of love, honoring the creations of another from moment to moment. We awaken to realize that each word is a declaration of our current creative process, our intentions, our self-understanding, and our status of relationship to others. Our words mirror our internal states, whether traumatic or euphoric. When our words are accurate reflections of our emotional states, they carry even greater force.

Working through my personal trauma memories, I recognized that I used speech, on some occasions, as an attempt to heal my traumas and, on other occasions, as a means for avoiding or detaching from my pain. Later, as the memory resolution techniques evolved, I discovered that speech can be used to keep others from spiraling into a memory and becoming lost in the feelings. It can also be employed for leading them safely through the resolution process. At one time I believed that by simply verbalizing traumas, the traumas would be expunged. We must now admit, without undervaluing the importance of breaking the spell of secrecy surrounding our abuse experiences, that simply reporting our traumas aloud does not necessarily guarantee any release of the core emotional content. In a number of instances I found myself able to articulate aloud the specific traumatic experiences within my family, educational, and religious systems, but I remained conveniently dissociated from the feelings to avoid the actual pain. Verbalization, consequently, did little to release the negative power of the memory.

Originally, I was attracted to the trauma resolution field by the immense, life-changing shift of power that occurred in my own life and in the lives of others when the core feelings from an original trauma scene were accessed and released. In my early years as a therapist, I encountered countless survivors who, often at my encouragement, spent many sessions verbalizing their recollections, only to find themselves returning to exactly the same feelings when the memory was triggered. I had been given the impression in my training as a therapist that the sufficient requirement for release was verbalization. I later encountered other schools of thought which promulgated reliving the event as the only way for releasing the trauma. However, being much more aware as adults than we were as children, many of us were more traumatized by re-living the experience from our "matured" awareness than we were by the original episode; and, again, we found little release from the original pain. In the worst cases, many of us were encouraged by our therapists to do "deep processing" which led to a vicious cycle which included an uncontrollable abreactive experience – a re-living of the worst part of the traumatic event ("T"). This often led to a weakening of the adult resource state – the survivor-self who was essential to achieve effective trauma resolution. My frustration with the inability to resolve traumas of my own and those of my clients, using the traditional methods that I had been taught, inspired my search for answers as to the origin of these stuck and fixed feelings. If full re-live of the event at "T" (i.e., the worst part of the memory, involving a complete emotional re-experiencing of the trauma sequence with the original sensory and emotional data fully present) did not provide resolution, what would?

The realization that the nervous system actually tries to protect us from overwhelming phenomena by freezing our pain and perceptions at "T-1" was the key to finding authentic resolution. The principal encoding of the affect occurred at T-1, not at T. This T-1 concept created a "paradigm shift" in my thinking, for trauma induction no longer was a matter of having to re-live the entire event in order to release the life-threatening feelings, but a matter of simply continuing the healing process that actually began when my nervous system took control of the scene. At T-1 my nervous system acted to protect me by transfixing the overwhelming feelings, scene, and circumstance until I developed sufficient resources and maturity to intervene. I survived my traumas! I had already arrived at "T+1," the post-trauma moment! The only problem was that my subconscious mind which stored most of these trauma memories had never been notified that time had progressed, that circumstances had changed, and that a solution was now available. None of us were taught how to notify those parts of our minds trapped at T-1 – that we were going to be safe and that the threat was ended. In addition, as we saw in the case of Bridget, until her husband entered treatment for his alcoholism, she did not feel safe enough to recall the rape that had occurred during one of his blackouts. No one had assisted Bridget in shifting her awareness frozen at T-1 (subconsciously) to the T+1 (conscious) realization that she had survived the trauma and that her painful "disgust" feeling was not about her own defectiveness, but the residue of "frozen feelings" indicating a perpetration. The resolution of the memory, therefore, involved completing the process begun by her nervous system – notifying her bodymind that the threat had passed, that she had survived. This allowed the healing of her marriage from the devastating impact of alcoholism, creating for Bridget a new respect for her emotions, which, she realized, were the cues for healing herself and her relationships. She eventually shared with me that she was grateful that she had not pursued her original reaction to her sudden "disgust" with her husband and "gone out and had an affair" or acted out her feelings of aversion when they arose, but, instead, had pursued her feeling to discover its true origin and worked toward its healthy resolution.

The resolution of memory requires that we maintain focus on our feelings long enough to return to the metaphor which contains the preserved pain. Because we have survived our traumas, the mature, survivor self can now provide the wounded part of our consciousness with the perfect solution needed to resolve this stored, troublesome scene. We can notify the nervous system that the perception of overwhelm is no longer accurate with respect to our current self or our present life. To most survivors, this is actually the case. An exception to this exists when the state of trauma has been remanifest in current relationships. The principal focus for resolution is to notify the subconscious that the threat has ended. Until the subconscious, which is ninety-three percent of the mind, is notified, the original scene remains potent and close to the surface. In fact, within the subconscious, there is no distinction between the past, present, or future: all is present. By the standards of the subconscious, all trauma memories were encoded only a fraction of a second ago – all of them encoded at T-1. Our memories hold such power over us because they are not ended; they are unresolved and, to put it bluntly, raw! The varied threats remain intact in the unresolved scenes of our subconscious minds. The difficulties that we have with our pasts are due to these unresolved masses of intense emotion which we hold intact in captured scenes. If, therefore, we could resolve the affective or emotional component of our trauma memories, we could recall these incidents without feeling the pain or accessing the emotional triggers that make our lives dysfunctional.

A few years ago I read an esoteric spiritual work by Jane Roberts entitled, The Nature of Personal Reality (New York: Bantam, 1974). From her intuitive perception she gleaned that the therapies of the future would allow us to resolve the affective component of memory without having to relive an entire event and without affecting the historical recollection of the memory. The memory resolution process which we explore in this work does precisely that. In other words, Holographic Memory Resolution does not tamper with our historical memory, but simply allows the release and resolution of the feelings associated with the original experience. This, then, allows us to integrate the experience as wisdom and to be released emotionally from the event. Resolution does not require traditional "depth hypnosis." In fact, entering too deeply into the trance state of the trauma memory can impede the healing process by removing the connection with the adult nurturing self (at T+1) needed for the resolution. In addition, completely re-living an episode using depth hypnosis can prove more traumatizing than the first time we withstood it, given our heightened adult sensitivities and awareness. Resolution involves integration – using our natural ability to nurture and heal ourselves and to create singularity of consciousness, eliminating paradox and conflict. As you will see, this is one of the natural capacities of the holographic mind.

In the previous chapters we examined some of the principles underlying trauma and its resolution: the holographic model and its use as the mechanism for memory storage and neurophysiological functioning, the origin and power of holographic metaphors as containers of memory, and the nature of the trauma induction experience – the recording of emotions, sensations, time and space perceptions, and all energies contained within the scene of trauma. Several of the cases presented have given an overview of the resolution process. The essential stages include: 1) identifying the presence of an unresolved trauma memory; 2) accessing the metaphor which contains the memory; 3) defining the metaphor; 4) moving from the metaphor to the original scene; 5) correcting or healing the scene; and 6) securing the new scene in the relevant cells and fields of the body, thereby replacing emotional content of the old scene with the healthy essence of the new.

A most noteworthy consideration that I wish to share with you is the ease and simplicity of the technique. My friend Rosemary observed this technique twice, whereupon she was able to use the verbal technique over the telephone with a friend in crisis who was overwhelmed with hurtful feelings from her past. I have received reports from therapists who had "heard about" the process and, upon employing the principles they comprehended, achieved immediate, though limited relief. This technique, is non-threatening and natural. Adolescents can learn it easily, and, with modifications, it can be taught to children. I observed an adolescent employing this process to help his younger brother after the resolution he experienced with me in a single session. After a one-day training for therapists, I have received reports of successful integration of the technique into their practices. Perhaps the greatest testimony to its simplicity and effectiveness has come from the survivors themselves who, upon experiencing the technique once or twice, used it effectively to access and resolve their own traumas – without outside facilitation. This is not always possible with more intense memories and histories of trauma, where the mind seems to need a facilitator to guarantee safety during the process. Yet nearly all of my clients have been able to use the process themselves, to varying degrees of satisfaction. The ease with which so many survivors have been able to employ the verbal process tells me that its dynamics are built upon a clear understanding of the workings of the mind at moments of trauma and upon our natural ability to heal ourselves.

Moving into the dynamics of self-healing, I remind you of the markers that indicate the presence of an unresolved trauma within the nervous system. Access to a trauma can occur through verbal, non-verbal, or experiential cues. Among the cues which I have witnessed are: 1) flashbacks, 2) conscious memory of the event, 3) dreams, 4) physical injuries or accidents, 5) experiences of near death, 6) sudden losses – particularly the loss of loved ones, 7) sudden or radical changes in lifestyle, 8) breakdown of early defense mechanisms, 9) recovery from drug use or other medicating experiences, 10) subconscious verbal cues, 11) consciously "scanning" the body for pain and trauma, 12) somatic (body) complaints, 13) irrational fears, 14) idiosyncratic behaviors, and 15) unconscious triggers that have little or no explanation in present awareness. (For a more detailed presentation of the unconscious triggers, see Chapter Six).

Reflecting upon my interactions with trauma survivors, I realize that many of them gave me an initial clue to the presence and nature of their trauma in their very first sentence. Trauma victims frequently send subtle subconscious messages to others asking for help — sometimes continuously. We can also deduce the presence of trauma by observing our emotional responses to life experiences. Overly intense reactions to "minor" situations are frequent indicators of a pre-history. I developed a new understanding and respect for our aversions to certain people, colors, sounds, decor, environment, habits, and lifestyles. Many of these reactions are borne in the wake of trauma or other memory imprints. By examining our tastes, responses, and daily triggers, we can backtrack to their point of origin and gain a measure of resolution. By becoming attentive to our triggers we become capable of resolving them.

Once we have the indication or suggestion of an unresolved issue from the past – a stored memory, the trauma resolution process can be initiated. If there is actually no memory nor trauma to be accessed, or, if the subconscious mind is not ready to begin resolution of this memory, the metaphor will be inaccessible (there will be neither picture nor details). In a significant number of cases, particularly with children and adolescents, the metaphors (containers of the trauma) simply can be removed and replaced for resolution to occur. Younger survivors often seem to be able to locate the "container" and remove it, thereby releasing the trigger and removing all negative emotional associations from the trauma. Due to their psychological and emotional development, adolescents and children are more "suggestible;" this would appear to be particularly true when it comes to inducing and resolving trauma. Their vulnerability works both ways: just as they are more easily traumatized due to weaker boundaries, so, too, are these containers of pain more easily released due to boundary permeability. I have witnessed an adolescent remove and replace eight metaphors in twenty minutes without needing to access a single memory, resolving all the somatic pain that was associated with each of the experiences, and without any subsequent return of symptoms or pain. Children and adolescents most readily employ the dynamics of trauma resolution laid out within this work and seem to naturally employ the process with minimal facilitation; holographic perception and movement are "second nature" to them.

Let us now review the Holographic Memory Resolution process in more detail. We will see this simple verbal technique through my verbatim dialogue with a survivor. As we review this particular case, notice that the metaphor providing access to the trauma is actually the pain from her appendicitis, although the organ was removed years ago and, therefore, could not be producing such pain in actuality (I refer to this pain as "cellular" or "holographic memory," though the medical profession refers to it as "phantom pain" and, very often, discounts it.) Dorothea Hover, a psychologist who also teaches "Healing Touch" and who published one of the first training manuals on the subject, concurs that trauma is stored in both the cells and the electromagnetic fields of the body. This type of pain, commonly classified as body memory or somatic memory, is the mind's way of letting us know that some part of the original experience remains unresolved. It is fundamental to understand that it was not the physical pain from the appendectomy but the emotional pain of abandonment that locked this sensation in the right side of her physical body. With holographic perception, an unresolved fragment of an experience can resurrect the whole; hence, if we treat the physical body but leave the emotional pain untreated, the pain complex can and often does return to give warning that the healing or resolution is incomplete. The returning pain is a declaration by the bodymind that we cannot successfully resolve it while viewing it myopically. The medical profession has often addressed the physiology, leaving the emotional and spiritual self untreated. This approach will not resolve the actual trauma because the body and mind are in unity. We can not simply alleviate the symptoms and leave the trauma trance unattended. We must treat the whole person, not the body alone, and this means addressing the matter of mind and consciousness.

Here we examine the case of Loretta. Unlike the cases we reviewed previously, we will examine the dialogue in detail and offer commentary in order to provide a clearer understanding of the process and the reasons for the language employed. The words are "repetitive" in order to allow the mind to make the link between the known (conscious) and unknown (subconscious) bodies of information available relating to the memory. It is a type of "mirroring" process which allows the client to produce the next piece of information and to make the necessary disclosures at his own pace. This process will become more familiar as we share Loretta's story.

Loretta is a thirty-seven year old married woman who came to me expressing a desire to resolve some of the memories and feelings underlying her depression. She was aware that her childhood had involved considerable abuse – living with her alcoholic dad and emotionally absent mom. Loretta began to tell her story declaring that she wanted to " focus on my feelings of loneliness." "This," she explained, "seems to be the source of most of my adult problems today { no one in my life seems to be able to take away the emptiness or meet my needs satisfactorily.")

I first identifed the key emotion that was emerging: "loneliness." "And when you feel this loneliness, where do you feel this, physically, in your body?" I asked. (This question directs us to find the storage site of the memory fragment - the metaphor.)

"In my right side!" she answered. At this point she actually grabbed her right side and bent over in pain. (While it is usually easy for most people to identify the location of the feeling in the body, it does not always occur with such intensity when given attention. The pain, however, is confirmation that the original trance or altered state which encoded the trauma is being accessed.)

(2)   I continued: "And is it on the inside or the outside of your right side?" (This question helps us to utilize holographic awareness to locate, access and define the metaphor. Trauma metaphors, when encoded, may have been perceived to be more to the inside, outside, "just under the surface," or both inside and outside of the physical body at the time of storage. This question intensifies conscious awareness of the metaphor and invites us to employ our natural holographic ability to scan our bodies in seconds, using our multi-sensory awareness. Each of us has a natural ability to do this. Utilizing trillions of nerve cells within our nervous system to collect this data, we can usually respond within seconds, and, often, in considerable detail.)

    "Mostly inside, but it extends to the outside too!" she reported with ease.

(3)   "And what's it like on the inside and outside – a pain like that?" I inquired.

    "It's a terrible stabbing pain!" she declared. She then doubled over, bending deeper to the right. (Her degree of physical pain was proportionate to the discomfort she experienced during the encoding of the original trance. It would appear that the subconscious mind uses physical pain to cue the conscious mind as to the identity and location of the memory fragment.)

(4)   Concerned by her increasing discomfort, I proceeded quickly: "And is there anything else about this sharp stabbing pain on the inside and outside of your right side that you would like to describe?" (This question – "Is there anything else about it?" is normally asked several times before the description is complete.)

    "No, but it hurts!" she declared. (This feeling statement tells us that she is at T-l and is ready to move from the metaphor to the actual scene, having enough data to complete identification of the memory scene – the source of the pain.)

(5)   "And how young might you be when you first feel a sharp stabbing pain in your right side that hurts like that?" I asked. (This question allows us to return to the moment of the trauma's induction. We enter the body and feelings at T-1, the moment of encoding in space and time immediately prior to T. Oftentimes, if the memory is very early, we only get "very young" or "little" as the mind's response.)

"I'm twenty years old," she replied.

6.   "And <u>where might you be</u> when you're twenty years old and you're feeling a sharp pain like that in your right side?" I inquired. (This question allows us to return to the place of the trauma's induction, further accessing the scene.)

"I'm just beginning college," she indicated.

7.   Her response was not yet a specific location, so I continued this line of questioning: "And <u>where are you in college</u> when you first feel a pain like this?"

"I'm in English literature class," she stated.

8.   "And what happens then when you're in English literature class?" (This question, "What happens then/next?" initiates the process of defining the event until we reach T-l where some intense emotion caused her to become overwhelmed; it is repeated <u>until the peak emotion is disclosed.</u>)

"I double over in pain," she answered, still clutching her side.

"And what happens next when you double over in pain?" I asked.

"They take me to the emergency room at the hospital," she responded.

"And what happens then, when they take you to the emergency room?"

"They take out my appendix – they told me I had appendicitis," she indicated.

In this process, the verbal cues of the survivor are followed until the key emotional pain is identified and/or verbalized, indicating the source of the encoding. Loretta, while describing profound physical discomfort, had not identified any feeling suggesting the specific origins of the loneliness that she had originally described. I assumed, therefore, that there was some other emotional pain affiliated with the appendicitis and followed her direction: "And what happens next, when they take out your appendix?" I asked.

"I wake up in the hospital room all by myself," she answered.

"And what happened then, when you wake up in the hospital room all by yourself?" I questioned. (The questions mirrors each of Loretta's last statements and provides an opening, a bridge to the next piece of information.)

"I feel so sad and abandoned – my family doesn't even come to see me in the hospital; I feel so hurt!" she responded, becoming tearful. (This feeling statement defines the emotional response that caused the scene to freeze. This is T-l! This statement identifies the emotional pain upon which the trauma is based and designates the nature of the conflict or pain that led to the encoding at this precise moment.)

Next, I allowed her time to acknowledge her feelings about the event, and proceeded: "And what needs to happen for a twenty year old girl who's in a hospital all alone and is feeling so sad and abandoned? (pause) If you could go to her and help her, what would you like to do to assist her when she feels that way?" (This double question introduces the identification of a solution which is provided by her survivor self in present time. It creates a bridge between the adult self who is safe in present time and who possesses perfect knowledge of the needs of the younger self, and the wounded self who is still trapped in the scene of past time with no help available.)

She responded: "I'd like to sit next to her and comfort her ... tell her that she's going to be all right and that I'll never leave her," she stated. (This response is her own internal solution to the crisis and, as such, allows her to heal herself using her perfect empathy for this wounded ego fragment; such complete solutions are possible when we realize that we share the same nervous system as the wounded self.)

"So take all the time that you need to go back and do that," I encouraged. (This statement allows the actualization of the integration by changing the original scene – the original trance. Loretta, in her own self-hypnotic state enters the scene and reconstructs it using her creative adult resources, thereby producing a different emotional experience. This statement assures her of the support and permission to heal herself within this frozen scene of pain. She is invited to comfort the wounded, arrested part of herself stuck with feelings of loneliness, sadness, hurt, and abandonment.) After a significant pause, I added: "And let me know when you've done that."

"She's OK now," she reported of the twenty year old Loretta.

"And does anything else need to happen for her in that scene?"

I inquired. (This question determines whether the new scene is complete – if the original trance is corrected and if the scene feels finished.)

"No, she looks all right now," she answered.

13.   "Is she safe in that place?" I asked. (This question determines if the original, threatening trauma scene is now changed sufficiently to become a "safe scene.")

"No, (pause) I want to take her away from there," she stated.

14.   "Do you have a safe, nurturing place where you'd like to take her... either in present or past time, or do we need to create one?" I asked.

"I don't think there was a 'safe place' back then; I think we need to create one," she replied.

15.   "If you could create a perfect safe place for you and her, what would it be? … The beach, the ocean, the mountains, a lake, by a stream or river, in a field of wild flowers, flying in the clouds, in a forest or a park, in a garden … what would you like?"

"We'll go to a butterfly garden," she decided.

16.   "Then take all the time that you need for the two of you to go to the butterfly garden, and let me know when you're there."

A bit later – "We're there," she confirmed.

17.   "And is there anything else that you need to do for her or to tell her in that scene?" I encouraged.

"I need to let her know that it's nineteen ninety-six, and that she'll never be left alone like that again … that I'll always be here with her … that she's going to be fine now."

18.   "So take all the time that you need to let her know that," I supported, waiting for a sign from Loretta that she was prepared to continue.

"OK, she's fine now," she said.

19.   "When you're ready, I want you to take a picture of the scene the way that you'd like to remember it," I said. (This photographing of the new scene establishes the "emotional corrections" of the new scene within the nervous system.) "And let me know when you see the scene the way you want it," I added.

"OK, I have it," she reported.

20. "Now let's put a frame around it of the color or colors you would like ... and let me know when you have it framed the way you want it." (This framing process helps to secure the memory within the nervous system.)

"All right; it's framed," she said.

21. "What color is the frame?" I asked.

"It's green and gold," she shared.

22. "Now I'd like for you to move the green and gold colors through your right side where you felt the appendicitis and any other place in your body where you felt the lonely feeling. Move the colors all the way through your body at least once, and let me know when you've done that," I stated. (Color is frequency; the colors of the frame carry the emotional corrections needed in the nervous system. Moving the colors through the nerve centers where the memory was felt replaces the old emotional message of the trauma scene with that of the corrected scene. There is a measurable displacement of energy from the nerve plexus during this release process. We will examine this phenomenon in the next chapter.)

"I've moved them through," she confirmed.

23. "And how does your body feel now?" I asked.

"The pain's all gone!" "I feel lighter," she described with some surprise.

24. "I'd like for you to think of the old scene and to see what comes to mind," I continued.

"I can remember the old scene, but all I can feel are the feelings of the new scene," she confirmed.

Afterward, I spent some time with Loretta processing the implications of this scene for her life. I encouraged her to continue moving the colors of the frame, green and gold, through her whole body during the next few days to ensure permanent placement in the nerve cells and electromagnetic fields of her body.

This case demonstrates the essential stages of the verbal process of Holographic Memory Resolution. While many components of this simple verbal process are familiar to those of you who have experienced "inner child" work or techniques similar, H.M.R. offers refinements. The photographing of the scene is based on the understanding that a trauma is a "frozen holographic scene." Resolution, therefore, requires the creation of a new, corrected scene. If the corrected scene cannot be photographed, something is incomplete in the resolution process, and further work is needed. The inability to secure the final scene sometimes occurs if stored anger needs to be released. The ability to photograph the scene can be used as an indicator to determine if the subconscious mind has accepted the proposed change(s) to the original scene. The color(s) of the frame, similarly, corresponds to the content of the picture and will change as the scene changes. On occasion, for instance, the final frame is reported to be red; while this can be a positive color, it often denotes unresolved anger. In such cases, it is helpful to ask if there is residual anger about the event that still needs to be released. A black frame denotes the need for additional resolution work; trauma remains. I have also noted that some very "spiritual" closing scenes are unable to accept a frame – e.g., as with Higher Power (God), angels, certain nature scenes, and a variety of others. To move the picture or its dominant color(s) through the body is usually sufficient to replace the negative encoding. This is most easily accomplished by picturing the color(s) as water flowing throughout the body, or as a beam of light (flashlight or horizontal beam) penetrating inside and outside the body, much like an X-ray or CAT scan.

Colors are manifestations of frequency. The framing of the final scene is actually a clever way of obtaining the frequency correction needed to "reprogram" the nerve plexus(es) with the updated, corrected perception of self. I observed that the colors often ascend in frequency during the resolution of multiple memories. The appropriate color frequencies are spontaneously provided by the subconscious mind. This is logical when we remember that trauma induction is an automatic, subconscious process. Just as the induction of the trauma by the subconscious was an automatic process to stop the pain and allow for healing, so too will the subconscious, when given opportunity, provide the precise frequency corrections. Facilitating memory resolution with adolescents, I have witnessed their progression through the order of the colors of the electromagnetic spectrum: black, red, orange, yellow, green, blue, indigo, violet, and white – the colors increasing in frequency with the resolution of each metaphor or memory. Most were unaware of the existence of the electromagnetic spectrum.

Colors, texture, materials utilized during framing all bear significant meaning for the resolution process. Similarly, difficulties which arise with respect to framing do not indicate failure. Oftentimes a second memory, related to the first, will surface needing resolution; this is indicated by the inability to acquire or maintain the frame. The color of the frame may indicate the need for additional resolution work, as with red, black, or gray. Secondary memories commonly arise pertaining to the same time period or theme as the first memory. Both memories must be resolved and both "wounded selves" must be present in the safe scene for the final framing to be possible. There are also occasions when groups of memories with a common theme emerge, and all of the relative ego fragments or wounded selves must be included in the final picture.

In summary, the Holographic Memory Resolution process involves the use of the creative powers of the mind to move within holographic space. This transformational healing process includes the displacement from the nervous system of the "old scene" and its accompanying negative affect, and replacement with the "new scene" and its positive affect, without impacting historical memory. The ability to convert the scene indicates that we possess the capacity to change our emotional perceptions of the past, as quantum physics supports. This creates a significant shift in our reality. The power of the past to cause difficulty springs from the manner in which the memories were stored or encoded within our nervous system. If the holograms which contain the past can be changed, then those events of the past which trigger our emotional distress can be released of their pain content; without such pain, we can remember these experiences without eliciting the baggage that went unresolved in the original event. In other words, **if the holograms which contain the past can be changed, the past, as far as its emotional power over us and our perception of it, can be changed.** It is precisely this emotional baggage which makes the past problematic and destines us to relive it until it is resolved. If the emotional content can be released, the memory can then be integrated as a learning experience and can be appreciated for the wisdom gained from it.

In the case of Loretta, the trauma that was evidenced was not the physical trauma of the appendicitis, but the emotional pain of abandonment, occasioned by the appendicitis. When the trauma scene was frozen and encoded, physical pain was part of her abandonment experience. Her somatic pain during the resolution process was the physical manifestation of her unresolved trauma, not the recurrence of her diseased appendix! Such cases increase our awareness of the potential to interpret as "physiological" in origin these holographic manifestations which present in order to draw our attention to spiritual, emotional, and mental traumas that left us with distorted beliefs about ourselves. (We have reached a point in our evolution where we are beginning to respect emotional reality in the same manner that we were forced to respect our physical needs.)

The process that I have presented in this chapter is scientifically grounded and precise in its form; it is also easily applied. This verbal process, while useful itself, can be accelerated by additional dynamics which foster (safety) and the release of memory from the cells and electromagnetic fields of the body. We will examine these dynamics in the next chapter.

MEMORY RESOLUTION EXERCISE: (Phrased for Self-Application)

(Precautionary Note: If, at any point in this process you begin to feel overwhelmed by the intensity of the feelings, return to the safe scene (see exercise p. 30) and proceed only with the aid of a facilitator or therapist. It is necessary to remain safe in your nurturing parent-adult self for the resolution process to be completed. If you tend to "lose yourself" in the feelings of the wounded, younger self, this process needs to be facilitated by a trained professional.)

1. Identify the key feeling surfacing for resolution: "How do I feel about _____?"
2. Ask the location(s) of the feeling in your physical body: "When I feel this feeling, where do I feel it in my body? And is it on the inside or the outside?"
3. Define the metaphorical form of the feeling in as much detail as possible: "What's it like – does it have a shape, size, color, temperature, texture, etc.?" (Sometimes more than one feeling or metaphor may need to be accessed before the specific memory can be identified.)
4. Define the age: "How young might I be when I first feel _____ _____ (as defined by #2) _____?"

5. Define the location: "Where might I be when I'm _____ years old and I feel _____?"

6. Define the scene: "And what's happening when I'm in a place like that?"

7. Continue defining the scene until you access the "peak" feeling which defines T-1. This is usually recognized by a feeling statement such as: "I'm scared ... he's going to hurt me!"

8. Identifying the solution: "And what would the adult-me in present time like to do if I could go back and change that scene, helping the younger part of me in that experience? What would I like to do first?" (Some possible solutions include: now that I'm an adult, provide the nurturing for myself that I needed; remove myself [and any others in danger] from the scene before the event happens; picture the event happening the way I would have liked for it to have occurred; bring in the support personnel needed – for example, the ideal or nurturing parent that I really needed, "Child Protection Services," a SWAT team, a guardian angel; speak to the "spirit" of the person who died; say "goodbye" to the individual from whom I need to detach, heal the disease [via color] causing the pain, etc.)

9. Actualizing the solution: "Now I shall take all the time that I need to do that." Change the scene to meet the specific needs of your frightened or wounded self. A child often needs to be held, comforted, and made to feel emotionally safe. Ask yourself: "Is there anything else I need to do for the younger me?"

10. Assess the location for safety. "Is this new scene now safe for us?" A change in location to a "safe place" may be required. Create one as needed: at the beach, ocean, by a river, in a garden, forest, on a mountain, in the clouds, etc. This place may be in past, present, or future time, actual or created.

11. Photograph the new, living scene. Any difficulty with this step means that something about the final scene is incomplete. Check to see if there is an additional feeling such as anger that needs to be released from the original scene. On occasion, a second, related wounded self in another memory must be included for the picture to be complete. Remember, the mind controls space and time perceptions. The removal of many wounded ego-selves can occur in only a few minutes if the mind gives permission; this means that multiple, repeated trauma need not, necessarily, be resolved scene by scene. Repeated abuse often causes a "blurring"

of boundaries between individual scenes, allowing a type of group memory resolution. The picture can be photographed when all of the necessary ego-selves and components are present.

12. Framing the scene. Frame the "safe scene" in the color or colors of your mind's own choosing. Your subconscious will readily choose these. If the frame begins to fade – again, there is something incomplete that needs to be addressed. If the color red surfaces during the framing, you may need to return to the scene to check and see if any anger needs to be released from the event. While red can be a positive color for some, it often indicates unresolved anger; if this is so, when the anger is released, the color of the frame will be a more soothing color of a higher frequency. Profoundly spiritual scenes often do not require a frame. The "radiant colors" associated with "Higher Power" (God) or angel, for instance, preempt the need for a colored frame. Their own natural colors are the frame, and the light within this scene can be moved through the system instead.

13. Move the color or colors of the frame (final scene) through your nervous system, particularly in the areas where the trauma was felt most intensely – the location of the metaphor(s). Using the image of colored water, a flashlight beam, a scanner beam, an appropriate feeling or sound can facilitate the anchoring of the solution in the nervous system.

14. Check your body for any additional pain. If pain remains, it will often be a different metaphor, suggesting another memory; begin the process anew, unless you require rest.

15. You may wish to write or "journal" your memories as a way of processing them. The details have a tendency to fade once the memory is resolved. In your notations, describe the color or colors that were used to resolve the issue. Use these colors for temporary respite in the future if similar feelings or issues arise. These colors are very powerful, as we will see in the next chapter, for they are your conscious choice to alter your brain wave frequency.

Chapter Eight

Our separation from each other is an optical illusion of consciousness.

Albert Einstein (1879 - 1955)

The Electromagnetic Key

The most powerful tool discovered in facilitating the healing of trauma evolved from observing the role of electromagnetic fields. This resource involves the applied use of electromagnetic energy to facilitate the access and resolution of trauma. This discovery revealed crucial information about our ability to protect ourselves from overwhelming experiences – a virtually unlimited capacity to store information, and the power to utilize these resources to heal ourselves. Understanding that consciousness manifests in the cells and in the electromagnetic fields of the body, improved the early, cumbersome resolution process I relied upon.

I have gained the greatest insights into our multidimensional nature from studying the electromagnetic form of our emotions and traumas. Today I have the ability to feel and confirm the release from the nervous system of the painful biochemical electrical transmissions stored in the cells during a traumatic event. Optimally, I am able to experience this release through my hands both in immediate contact with the body of my client and at a distance of a few inches away from the physical body. If anyone had told me six years ago that I would develop this degree of sensitivity, I would have diagnosed that individual as delusional. Nevertheless, over time I have learned to use this ability to establish an electromagnetic rapport with the nervous systems of my clients. Over the past three years I have taught this process to others, demonstrating our natural ability to focus and direct electromagnetic energy for purposes of healing. Let us begin our examination with the events that led to this revelation.

The concept of feeling the emotional pain of another as a physical sensation in one's own body was not original to me. My mother was able to do it. I witnessed this as a child. When my sister and I were in car accidents, when my brother fell and broke his ankle, when my oldest sister suffered a miscarriage, my mother felt these events as physical sensations in her own body – an "icy, cold feeling" - she described it. As children, my siblings and I became familiar with this phenomenon. I spent most of my life in educational institutions studying various disciplines, particularly spirituality, in an attempt to grasp the key to my mother's curious ability to simultaneously feel the pain of others. Even separation over great distances did little to deter her capacity. I still remember my experience of being involved in a car accident. When I finally got around to calling home and informing my parents of the accident, my mother said: "I knew something had happened – my body went cold; I noted the time on the clock, wrote it down, and started praying when I felt it. It happened at 3:23 p.m. didn't it?" The time that she had written down was the moment of the accident. Years later I discoverd that each of my siblings had experienced a similar incident with her. She was a very "intuitive" woman.

The next stage in learning to feel subtle distortions in electromagnetic fields occurred innocently and without my conscious awareness. I spent over thirteen years as an archaeologist in Israel. During my training for ministry, I regressed into my childhood love for archaeology and spent summers digging with the Lahav Research Project, centered out of Mississippi State University. I began my work with them in 1979 as a volunteer, while I was completing my post-graduate work in Rome. I was trained in field archaeology, and, among the first skills I developed was the ability to feel differences in soil density and texture using a "patish," a small hammer-like tool with a slightly curved end. Little did I know that I was receiving initial training in the ability to feel differences in density and vibration through my hands as they interacted with the earth. I developed a reputation for the ability to track elusive midden or living surfaces over seemingly impossible terrain. This seemed easy as I simply trusted the vibrational sensitivity in my hands.

The initial realization that this sensitivity involved some type of healing capacity occurred rather humorously. I developed a case of "warts" – eight of them on one hand. One day, I noticed that, after regularly touching one of them rather absentmindedly, it simply went away. I touched another one over the next week and it, too, "magically" disappeared within a few days. Bewildered by this change, I decided to make a more deliberate effort as a means of confirming my suspicion. I chose a specific order and intentionally touched each of the "sites." Each wart disappeared as I focused on it, in the order that I selected. I thought the whole experience quite bizarre and never mentioned it to anyone. Some months later, my friend Ted turned to me as we were on our way to a movie and asked: "Did you know that you can heal warts?" I was totally shocked and, I must admit, somewhat embarrassed. I had been quite "shy" about my unsightly virus and had certainly never drawn attention to the issue. "Well, yes," I responded, "but how do you know?" I inquired, feeling perplexed. "Last week," he stated, "when we traded 'bodywork', you pushed on my foot with your hand, and I felt a tremendous wave of heat go through my body; six of the 'planter's warts' on the bottom of my foot went away within twenty-four hours, and the one that had been the source of the others – the one that had been surgically removed and then grew back, went away within seventy-two hours." I was speechless. It is one thing to have peculiar experiences privately, but to have these strange suspicions confirmed by a friend was another matter, indeed. The issue suddenly became more "real." "Great!" I thought. "Now I could make a living as a 'wart-off' like in Russian folk-lore." I minimized the whole experience and, at the same time, thought it ironic that I should stumble across any awareness about healing capacities subsequent to leaving ministry. There I had been anointed to heal and told that I possessed the faculty to heal, but had never "felt" anything of a healing nature, nor been given any impression that I ever would.

These experiences, on a more subtle level, raised questions as to whether there could be a more scientific or direct explanation for this "energy" phenomenon. The next step occurred spontaneously. I noticed, in my work with trauma survivors that when I asked about the physical location of the principal feeling(s) associated with the traumas, my clients consistently described detailed objects or metaphors that were located along a central axis running parallel to the spinal cord. The blockages causing the pain were consistent in location, including: the lower back or base of the spine, the abdomen or stomach, the solar plexus, the heart, the throat, the eyes and forehead, and the crown of the head. These seven locations in the body, I knew from my study of Eastern spirituality, corresponded to the locations of the major nerve plexes, called "chakras." They were the intersections and largest groupings of nerves along the spine; hence, they were also the locations where pain was felt most intensely at moments of trauma.

In research literature and ancient spiritual tradition, it was acknowledged that these intersecting electrical nerve pathways produced electromagnetic fields, as occurs when electricity runs through coils of copper wire. In my work with trauma survivors, many of them actually reported seeing a "tornado-like vortex," a "circular spinning sensation," or a "swirling black hole." Subsequently, it also became evident that my clients utilized some type of holographic perceptual process, closely tied to these electromagnetic processing centers, that was providing them with the detailed information. They were able to see how the nerve centers were impacted at the moment of trauma. Over time, I concluded that these vortices of electromagnetic energy were clearly affected by the increase or decrease in impulse caused by emotional reactions at a moment of trauma. Finally, I asked, were the detailed metaphors – the lumps in the throat, the knots in the stomach, etc., that my clients described in such detail, fragments of the original trauma scene that were "caught" or encoded in the nerve plexus where the pain became overwhelming? Was this plainly an effort to stop or contain the unspeakable pain that occurred at the moment of traumatization?

After observing this phenomenon over time, the conclusions were indisputable. Consistently, the locations of the pain corresponded to these vortices created by the nerve pathways. Through ongoing observation, it became apparent that some of the traumas were encoded at sites of minor or lesser vortices. The sensitivity of these processing centers confirmed that it was possible for feelings to become "stuck" or holographically imprinted at these locations when the nervous system was overwhelmed. Even when the feelings appeared in the extremities, the metaphors were located at nerve plexes where electrons were flowing through the perineural cells, thereby creating electromagnetic fields.[1] I found, for the first time, a plausible explanation for the origins of holographic metaphors which were evidenced in my clients' bodies and which were associated with extreme pain. While this insight was helpful, it was not until I confronted a series of additional trauma cases that the practical nature of this information emerged.

Tricia first drew my attention to the constructive role of electromagnetic fields. A sexual trauma survivor, Tricia was terrified of accessing any feelings or memories associated with her abuse. She had a tendency to spontaneously regress or "lose herself" in the feelings of the wounded child-self when those feelings began to surface. As a result, when I observed an increase in feelings of desperation, I sat immediately adjacent to her to better anchor her in present time. She became calmer and was able to proceed. At one point in the process, my pen, with which I was detailing her account, ran out of ink. I rose to acquire another pen and, upon returning, and without realizing it, sat one seat farther away from her. She immediately interrupted the process and announced that the "violet light" that had previously been surrounding her was no longer present and asked me to resume my former position so that she "could feel safe enough to continue." I was surprised both by her ability to note my position change with her eyes closed and by the violet light phenomenon.

Through my continuing work with trauma survivors, I found that the perception of an "indigo-violet" light was common during the process when I sat next to them. My familiarity with the electromagnetic spectrum suggested that a very high frequency of light was in evidence which fostered a feeling of calm and thereby enhanced the resolution process. The color-frequency of violet is the second highest frequency in the visible spectrum – second only to white light itself. After working with Tricia, I knew to sit immediately adjacent to my client in order to foster an enhanced sense of safety. I learned from Tricia the importance of proximity. Particularly with clients who tended to dissociate during trauma resolution work, adjacent positioning is necessary. Because safety is the number one prerequisite for effective trauma resolution, the "violet light phenomenon" was a welcome lesson.

After my experience with Tricia, I began a personal search for understanding the mysterious nature of electromagnetic fields. After describing the violet light experience to a friend, he introduced me to the text, Hands of Light, written by the physicist and psychotherapist Barbara Ann Brennan. Brennan not only provided a clear and scientifically grounded explanation for the violet light phenomenon, but also suggested that electromagnetic fields could be felt and used for purposes of healing. I was skeptical; and I did not foresee how such a practice could have relevance for trauma memories stored on an emotional level. Nonetheless, I continued studying Brennan's claims and discussed the findings with colleagues. Somewhere in the midst of this personal journey I confirmed that I could "move my headaches around" and often resolve them using the electromagnetic fields in my hands. I wondered if this was not, in fact, the same phenomenon that had helped me free myself from my unsightly virus. Within a short time I found that I could actually feel the headache pain most precisely at a distance of two to five inches away from my head. As I continued to practice on myself, my hands seemed to become increasingly sensitive. Over time, I gained awareness and sensitivity allowing me to monitor and distinguish a variety of distinct types of pain sensations experienced by my clients. I developed the ability to read the vibrational frequencies through my hands. According to Brennan, and as I have come to believe, we all possess this inherent ability within our bodies, our hands. Brennan observed that we each carry a surplus of electromagnetic energy in our hands, a result of their constant interaction with the energy fields all around us – from sunlight, nature, and the magnetic fields of the planet. Again, I mused, how ironic it was that I discovered this natural ability to heal after I had left formal ministry in the Catholic church where I had been anointed and authorized to heal through the "laying on of hands." Why had I been given no information about these simple scientific principles that could have enhanced and empowered my ministry? Was associating the "metaphysical" movement's involvement with electromagnetic fields exploration preventing established religious systems from accepting and integrating this simple scientific data? Despite the mysterious reasons and agencies through which this information was entering my life, I felt profoundly grateful!

Now that I had this information, what was its practical value? Never did I imagine that this increasingly powerful journey into self-healing would so profoundly impact my nicely defined, quasi-traditional therapeutic practice. Though I had formally left ministry, I continued to operate within fairly traditional parameters and belief systems. Interestingly, it was another of my clients that brought me to the next stage of growth.

Barbara was an incest survivor. Her "body memories" were very intense as her recollections erupted to the surface. In casual conversation on the topic of "alternative healing techniques" before our session one evening, I shared with Barbara my personal success at alleviating my headaches using the electromagnetic fields in my hands. I look back at the irony of this event because Barbara, with a strong Catholic background, knew that I had served as a Catholic priest. In her mind, the laying on of hands was a natural concept, and she also, logically, thought it natural to me. Little did she know that I had met very few priests who had ever noted any sensations whatsoever during the laying on of hands process. This was not to say that healing did not occur; it was merely that no conscious control of it had ever been implied in our training. In the middle of one of our group therapy sessions, she disclosed that she continued to have intense physical side effects accompanying the trauma work – like a "three day long" headache. Would I use my hands to "dissolve" her headache as I do my own, she asked. I was startled at her request and said that I would talk with her privately about this during the break.

At Barbara's request, and, given that I did not have another opportunity to see her for individual therapy for another week, I agreed, during our brief break, to try the electromagnetic field technique on her headache, as I had done on myself. This was my first attempt to use this ability on another. As soon as I placed my hands two to five inches away from her head, I felt the most intense pulsation – as though my hands were being waved back and forth by a stinging, invisible electromagnetic force. In less than five minutes, the disturbing wave-pulse subsided and, in an unparalleled move which left me standing in my office in open-mouthed shock, Barbara suddenly stood and announced: "Thanks, it's all gone now... I think I'll go have some popcorn and juice in the cafeteria." After confirming that there was no pain left whatsoever, she smiled, gave me a hug, and walked away with a nonchalance conveying that it was nothing more than she had expected. It took me some time to integrate the lesson she had just taught me – a gift.

Increasingly I came to realize that this was not merely a subjective phenomenon, nor simply a matter of some "faith healing." These electromagnetic blockages produced by trauma had an objective reality – that is, they could be felt by an outside observer. Emotions had substance! I knew this because I could now feel them through my hands, and I was alerted to the fact that I could also feel these pains in the bodies of others.

The next step in the integration of electromagnetic field principles into the trauma resolution process came through Linda. I had worked with her in an outpatient setting for longer than a year. We discovered that she had a number of distinct types of migraines. The headaches were distinguished by their location, their intensity, and their particular metaphorical presentation – that is, the "stabbing-pain-in-the-right-temple" type contrasted with the "cold-throbbing-gnawing-at-the-base-of-my-skull" type. Linda actually came into my office and showed me a diagram of the work that we had been doing over the previous year. Included in one diagram were depictions of specific traumas that had generated each designated category of migraine. On another diagram she illustrated emotions which had allowed us to identify the traumas as well as the verbally abusive messages from her mother which had precipitated the migraines. Finally, she represented each of the compulsive behaviors that had been generated in response to the abuse. Comparing her diagrams with my notes, it became clear that, as each of these particular traumas was resolved, the specific migraine ceased and she became less compulsive in her behavior.

At the beginning of one particular group therapy session, Linda's face appeared haggard, and she disclosed that she had a "terrible migraine." "It hurts so bad," she shared, "that I haven't been able to even visualize and employ the headache resolution technique you showed us." Having worked with all of the group members teaching and practicing the verbal technique, I made a therapeutic decision to ask them to move their holographic thinking into the external world. I provided them with a brief explanation of the electromagnetic field technique (non-contact), and checked their comfort level with this new application. They were willing to support Linda's effort. As Linda closed her eyes I placed my hands near her head. I felt a dense electromagnetic field, an intense pulsation accompanied by a "tickling" feeling in the palms of my hands. After a few minutes this sensation diminished, and I moved my hands to the spot where I felt a type of electromagnetic pain ridge. Each time I moved my hands, Linda, whose eyes remained closed, described a swirling motion on that part of her head. The group members were somewhat startled that she was able to correctly identify the location of my hands at a distance of two to five inches away from her head. After about five minutes I sensed a decrease in the pain in my hands. I asked her about her migraine. She stated: "Oh, that went away after the first minute." Her face was noticeably brighter, and feedback from the group was very positive. As the group session proceeded as usual, I noted this was the first incidence that I consciously utilized an electromagnetic field technique during a group process.

At this time in my work with trauma survivors, however, I had little indication of the function of this electromagnetic resource in the resolution of trauma memories. I assumed the verbal and electromagnetic techniques to be separate and independent therapeutic modalities, never imagining their profound rapport. I continued to use the verbal technique (See Chapter Seven) and to employ the electromagnetic field component only when headaches or other secondary symptoms were interfering with the verbal process. The next step in the integration of the electromagnetic field techniques occurred when I started working with Paulette.

Paulette was extremely sensitive, intelligent, and intuitive. She could not enter holographic memory via a voice or sound-facilitated bridge because it threw her back into present time. She was a trauma survivor whose sensitivity to sound, frequency, and vocal tone caused her to reorient to present time whenever she heard any sound, including my voice. What emerged was the fact that only by holding her hand during the process was she able to enter the memory to achieve resolution. The physical contact grounded her sufficiently, allowing her to remain in holographic space to access and resolve her memories. She insisted that I needed to use more physical contact to better ground my clients, to foster safety, and to facilitate the bridging needed to access the wounded ego-states within. Indeed, as I continued to work with Paulette, she was able to feel more comfortable entering and resolving her memories, relying on holding my hand to keep her "safe." She also reported seeing the "indigo-violet-colored light" each time we worked.

The most significant leap in the process of learning effective ways of utilizing my sensitivity to electromagnetic fields came when my clients and I were uncertain whether a presenting headache or symptom was due to current stress, trauma, or a physiological problem. In the effort to make this determination, it was logical to approach diagnosis using the simplest solution available – the color replacement technique for resolving stress. If the complaint remained unaffected by the stress reduction effort, an unresolved memory fragment was most likely the cause, and the verbal trauma resolution technique was employed. On the infrequent occasions when these two approaches proved ineffectual, and the pain remained, the discomfort was found to be physiological or spiritual in origin (in the case of the latter, serving a higher purpose). In approaching new cases, I came to discover that most suffering labeled as physiological actually originated in encoded memory; specific cases repeatedly validated the need for this diagnostic shift in expectation.

A client, Andrea, described very frightening memories of incest and physical abuse that she had never addressed in a therapeutic setting. She was experiencing extreme physical discomfort from intense body memories in the form of frequent headaches. At the beginning of a session she looked particularly frightened. She asked me to use the electromagnetic field technique to ease her headache pain and to help her relax. When I placed my hands near her head, I felt the pain ridges, and, while they briefly decreased in intensity, they returned with full force. She noted that the pain was not subsiding. At this point, I suspected that the issue was memory related and that she needed to consciously face this memory if the pain were to be resolved. I told her what I was "sensing," and she responded with a reluctant acknowledgment that this was her belief also. With support she was able to enter a specific memory of physical abuse involving trauma to her head. Through this process she resolved the headache pain completely. More surprisingly, when she first recalled the scene, I felt a sudden pain in my hands. When she later accessed the scene of the trauma, the pain in my hands increased even more, and when she created the "safe scene" with the corrections and began moving it through her body, the pain in my hands disappeared completely. Over time, I practiced leaving my hands in place near the sites of the metaphors and found consistent patterns of pain-increase when the memory was accessed, and dissolution of the pain in my hands when the memory was resolved. I added this manual scanning of my clients' electromagnetic fields as a tool to help them locate their memory fragments and to gauge the effectiveness of the resolution process. This adjunct proved a powerful tool for facilitating healing and led to an even greater application.

Though naturally cautious in the early exploration of my sensitivity, I became obligated to use this skill when I discovered its ability to accelerate and enhance the access and visualization of memory. The sensitivity in my hands increased through practice, and I became aware of a consistent "hot spot" on the dorsal point of the spine in the majority of my clients. This "hot spot" shifted from the dorsal point only when the pain was located exclusively in the regions of the head or in the extreme lower body. I began to notice that when one hand was placed over this spot on the back of the body and the other hand positioned over the metaphorical memory fragment stored in the nerve plexus in the front of the body – for example, over the "lump" in the throat, my clients could suddenly see the trauma scene as it was transfixed at T-1. In addition, many of them claimed that they had never been able to visualize their memories prior to this experience. With enhanced visualization, we were able to proceed at an accelerated pace. Eventually I came to explain this phenomenon, comparing the process to a sophisticated, multidimensional video-recorder. The focused use of the electromagnetic fields in my hands appeared to work somewhat akin to accessing the VCR and pressing the "play" button. From the instant of the original trauma, the recorder had been on "pause," producing only a static, obscure image – a fragment of the original scene, preserved at T-1 in the nerve cells and electromagnetic fields of the body. Once this static state was stimulated by higher frequency energy, access to the stored memory was nearly instantaneous. The entire holographic memory resolution process proceeded more quickly.

Repeatedly, instant visual access occurred when 1) I placed my left hand on the most intense access point, which I found by scanning the back, and 2) placed my right hand over the nerve plexus containing the metaphor (memory fragment) in the front of the body. Over a period of time I realized that, just as a hologram is created by splitting light into two beams – a "reference beam" and an "object beam," which then intersect with each other at right angles to create a 3-D picture, visual access to memory was enhanced when I used my right hand to intensify the electromagnetic current running vertically along the spine (the reference beam) while I used my left hand to focus on the location of the encoded hologram (the object beam). (See Figure 1, p. 37). This made sense in light of Karl Pribram's confirmation that the mind functions holographically. Eventually I came to use the left hand to track the specific "object" – its location, progress, and resolution. With my hands in place over these sites, I could feel the whole release process. In the more severe cases, such as incest, the release of the energy would actually "sting" my hands and necessitate a pause for clearing this unpleasant energy from my own electromagnetic fields. This necessitated an enhancement of my own "self-care" practices, including meditation, proper diet, and exercises to raise my own energy levels. I found it equally important to process my experience with colleagues or supervisors while protecting the confidentiality of my clients.

With my clients I found it most important to explain to them that I was not healing them, but, rather, that I was facilitating their own self-healing ability by increasing the accessibility of their holographic perception. Herein lay the beauty and empowerment of this process, for it does not foster an external dependency upon others who "heal us." Instead, holographic memory work instructs us in the development of our skills to heal ourselves. Over time, I found that the focused use of electromagnetic energy during trauma resolution work proved beneficial in the following important ways:

♦ Creating a sense of safety which facilitates access to the stored memory;

♦ Fostering co-consciousness – helping the survivor to remain grounded in the present while simultaneously accessing the wounded ego-state;

♦ Preventing total regression into the memory when the survivor begins to be overwhelmed by the intensity of the original trauma – helping to anchor the individual in the present;

♦ Facilitating the release of the memory from the electromagnetic fields and cells of the body;

♦ Allowing the therapist to confirm and validate release of the low frequency energy from the cells and fields of the body;

♦ Supporting the anchoring of the new scene in the nerve cells and electromagnetic fields,

♦ Expediting sequencing during the resolution process – cueing the facilitator and the client to the next step required for resolution of the trauma memory(ies);

♦ Enhancing the effectiveness of the verbal technique;

♦ Fostering spiritual growth and healing by expanding awareness;

♦ Intensifying the holographic picture and facilitating access of the metaphor;

♦ Validating the survivor's own multidimensional awareness and ability to heal himself;

♦ Assisting the therapist/facilitator in discerning the absence or validity of a presumed, suspected, or reported memory.

The impact of the simultaneous implementation of the verbal and the electromagnetic field techniques is the creation of a symbiotic relationship between the trauma survivor and the facilitator. When applied in its entirety, this interconnectedness with the survivor enables me to gauge continuously the movement of the subtle memory forms which can shift to various locations in the body during the resolution process. This symbiotic relationship also allows me to determine the degree of resolution achieved and indicates any remaining memories stored in the same nerve plexus or in other parts of the nervous system. This energetic rapport provides simultaneous access to other areas of the nervous system that may not be directly related to the memory in question. (This often predisposes the survivor for the next encoded memory fragment to surface at the appropriate time.) For example, while it is quite easy to miss certain dark objects in a dimly lit room, heightened illumination dispels the darkness, eliminating any doubts as to the presence of such undesirable objects and makes the most prominent "object" visible while fostering the requisite safety. With such visibility and safety, the stages of memory resolution are greatly accelerated.

(Movement from one memory to another is readily achievable when safety is continuous and uninterrupted.)Each time a memory is resolved, a blockage removed, there is an influx of energy and an accompanying sense of empowerment in the survivor. This allows for multiple memory resolution in the majority of cases. Such a process is designated as "brief" therapy. Resolution of a single memory using the verbal technique alone originally required a lengthier period of time. Supporting the client's process with the electromagnetic field component allows for the resolution of multiple memories in less than half an hour. This is most easily achieved when the individual has a strong motivation for recovery and a strong parent-adult ego-state to intervene in the arrested scenes of trauma. At the time of this writing, I utilize a group therapy format that allows a group of five trauma survivors to resolve an average of one to three memories per person in a two and a half hour time period, providing opportunity for processing.

The feedback received from participants indicates that: 1) The survivor himself often feels the moment when the metaphor is released from the nervous system. 2) The pain associated with the original memory or trance resolves at the moment the nervous system is notified of the change, the new scene. 3) There is typically no recurrence of the original metaphor or its accompanying symptoms once resolved. 4) The survivor is empowered by the increased energy flow within the nervous system and is often "lightheaded" immediately after the release. 5) At the moment of release, the survivor often experiences an intense "tingling," even to the point of numbness in the hands, particularly in the two outermost fingers and, sometimes, in the feet. 6) Extra rest and water are needed to allow the nervous system to adjust to the changes which transpire. 7) Spiritual empowerment occurs when the survivor realizes that he possesses the capacity to locate and resolve these powerful scenes of stored pain. 8) The pervasive sense of isolation and defectiveness created by trauma is greatly diminished when the survivor realizes that there is someone else who can, quite literally, feel the pain resulting from these traumas. Realizing that others acknowledge this pain also helps to remove any denial and self-doubt that may have originally inhibited access and resolution of the traumas.

While it is normal for an individual to doubt the authenticity of a trauma memory which is very frightening and overwhelming to the nervous system, the validation of such a memory is not difficult. As we have noted, a trauma is an actual trance state that is created at a critical moment to protect us from being overwhelmed emotionally. Some clients were "led" in the past by well-intentioned though "misguided" therapists to suspect or even believe that they were sexually abused. This gave rise to the discussion of what was labeled "false memory." This is, in a true sense, a misnomer, for, since a trauma is actually an authentic trance state which is accompanied by specific and measurable changes in the nervous system, the mere idea or suspicion of a trauma does not produce supporting somatic data to validate the existence of the trance since the supposed trance does not, in fact, exist. Those clients with whom I have worked who were "led" by a therapist to believe that they were sexually abused when they were not, could not and did not produce any somatic or electromagnetic data to demonstrate or validate the existence of their "purported" memory. Simply "willing" oneself to have an abuse history will not produce such a reality somatically, neurologically, or electromagnetically, for the thought alone does not have this power. One of the advantages of the electromagnetic field technique is that the facilitator has feedback from the somatic level about the presence and intensity of the trauma involved, as well as its state of resolution (The client's own data is also more intense and vivid, rich with detail, as evidenced by the technique.)

As originally affirmed in the pioneering research of Milton Erickson and David Cheek, stress creates a spontaneous state of self-hypnosis. My research with trauma survivors indicates that we can take this observation one additional step: traumatic experiences produce such an acute state of stress (traditionally diagnosed as "Post-Traumatic

Stress Disorder") that victims naturally employ the mechanism of self-hypnosis to contain the overwhelming pain. Trauma produces a state of self-hypnosis, an altered state, which is protectively engineered by the limbic-hypothalamic system. This system regulates or "seizes control" of the autonomic nervous system, the endocrine system, and the immune system in the effort to manage the crisis. When trauma experiences arise, this remarkable system, the "limbic-hypothalamic-pituitary-adrenal axis" responds to protect us. These responses are observable and measurable and have been explored in research studies since the 1930's. Research psychologists are presently developing more precise tools for gauging these responses during access of the state-bound memory to provide means for assessing purported memories of trauma. Today's technology is producing mechanical instruments with sensitivity to detect the subtle distortions in the electromagnetic fields of the body. As we have often heard, however, the human body is more sophisticated than any computer that we could develop. The diverse capacities of my hands to locate and distinguish many types of electromagnetic anomalies exceed my ability to describe. Yet, it is this very sensitivity of my nervous system and my clients' nervous systems that enables the resolution of trauma using this process.

Seeking an explanation for "how an experience can manifest in the cells and the electromagnetic fields of the body" is not a new quest. It is an issue long under scrutiny. Ernest Rossi, in his book, The Psychobiology of Mind-Body Healing, points out that the central issue which has emerged from the study of the psychobiology of mind-body healing is the concept of "information transduction" – that is, how information is converted or transformed from one form to another.[2] Rossi uses the example of a windmill to demonstrate this:

> *A windmill transduces energy into the mechanical energy of the turning blades. If the mechanical energy of the turning blades is attached to a generator, it is transduced into electrical energy, which can in turn be transduced into light energy by an electric bulb.[3]*

Rossi also confirms that studies such as these, along with the basic concepts of information, communication, and cybernetic theories, have led to a view of all biological life as a system of information transduction.[4] In his text he provides a history of the concept and establishes the connection to the principles of hypnosis. Once we comprehend that trauma is a spontaneous state of self-hypnosis, his insights have great value for our understanding of the dynamics of trauma resolution. His research shows the history of the evolution of the concept of information transduction from the work of Bernheim (1886) to Mishkin (1982).[5] Bernheim, one of the "fathers" of therapeutic hypnosis, helped us to understand that ideosensory and ideomotor reflex convert hypnotic suggestion into body processes.[6] By the 1980's we came to appreciate the role of the limbic-hypothalamic system in the storage and transduction of sensory information.[7] The major breakthrough in mind-body research occurred, however, when Hans Selye (1936, 1982) formulated his theory of how mental or physical stress is transduced into "psychosomatic problems" by the hormones of the "hypothalamic-pituitary-adrenal axis" of the endocrine system.[8] In his "General Adaptation Syndrome," Selye provided an overview of the entire process of mind-body information transduction. The main focus of research on the information transduction issue has been to understand the process by which information received and processed at the semantic (verbal) level is converted into information that can be received and processed at a somatic level.[9]

From the trauma scenes shared with me by clients, it is clear that a five year old child, for instance, may transduce the energy from witnessing Dad strangling Mom during a drunken rage into a tightness in her own throat as she watches Mom gasp for air, or into a pain in her ears from the fighting and yelling. All of us translate the energies of our experiences continuously, but rarely have we been taught ways to use this transduction to assist the release of painful energy from the electromagnetic fields of the body. We have not been attentive to our own energetic transactions, much less those of others. Those who proved more "energetically sensitive" often were reluctant to make such contact out of fear of "taking on" the burdensome issues or energies from others. Resistance to this powerful notion of energy transduction is also comprehensible when we recall that most of us were taught that it was necessary to re-live the pain of our memories to completely release them. Depth hypnosis was often employed to accomplish this, frequently resulting in emotional retraumatization by a full reexperiencing of the entirety of the original event. The victim of trauma did not encode the entire experience with the same emotional intensity, although the whole experience may have been repressed, as in cases of amnesia. Remember that a trauma is a hypnotic state encoded at T-l, not an encoding of the whole experience. Trauma resolution can best be achieved by enhancing the client's own skills to address the T-1 moment, using her facility to focus or self-hypnotize to address the encoded pain, not to relive the whole of the original experience. Knowing what we have now affirmed from interventions at T-1, we need not induce a trance state deeper than the client employed to protect herself originally. The client is the expert who determines the necessary depth of the trance to resolve her personally encoded T-1 scene(s). With Holographic Memory Resolution, the facilitator simply uses her abilities to enhance the survivor's own self-hypnotic skills and precision. This allows the survivor's conscious mind, in cooperation with the subconscious, to safely gauge the moment of reentry and degree of entry into the original memory, using a fragment of the original scene to access it. Once the specific scene at T-1 has been identified for the conscious adult-self that has survived the trauma, the scene can be resolved from a safe, post-trauma position without having to relive the entire sequence. Memory transduction of the original trauma is achieved by allowing the conscious mind of the survivor to follow the cues of the subconscious, which holds the memory in stasis. The subconscious mind of the survivor provides the cues to the memory, the event's location in time and space, by resurrecting the body sensations encoded at the T-1 until conscious recognition occurs. The subconscious mind speaks eloquently through somatic channels. Once the memory is raised to consciousness, it can be transformed from a scene of pain to a scene of calm, and resolution is easily achieved. The gentle, non-traumatizing interplay of the semantic and somatic components of the technique are the hallmark of the Holographic Memory Resolution process. The expediency of this process is easily understood when the roles of both the verbal and the electromagnetic field techniques are considered. The effect is a doubly enhanced self-hypnosis – that is, an "energetic trance" and a verbally facilitated trance, coordinated by the bodymind of the survivor. The electromagnetic field technique rapidly induces the "energetic trance," often measurable as a "Theta" state (4 to 7 Hertz on the brain wave scale), producing a sense of safety and calm in the body which allows the conscious mind to remain more fully present than in traditional hypnosis and allows the subconscious to surrender its hold on T-1. The adult, conscious mind remains present to assist in the resolution process by utilizing the resources gained from its years of experience. This approach is considerably more flexible and empowering than traditional hypnosis because it is based upon the expert interplay between the client's conscious and subconscious awareness. Its effects are cognitive, behavioral, and affective.

One of the most valuable roles of the electromagnetic field technique arises when the verbal technique is hindered. While facilitating group therapy with inpatient adolescents some months ago, it became apparent that they were self-conscious and reluctant to acknowledge any personal experiences and accompanying emotions. I facilitated a progressive relaxation exercise and, upon completion, worked with them individually, though each denied any trauma or somatic cues. As each youngster sat in the chair, I "scanned" his body to identify any prominent trauma sites, which manifested as a pain or tightness in my hands. Once a site was identified, I called his attention to this location so that he could become aware of the presenting distortion and address it. I assisted each adolescent in 1) focusing on the nerve plexus where the pain became most intense, 2) identifying the trauma memory that surfaced in his conscious thought, and 3) in resolving the memory and its accompanying emotional pain. Each group member accessed and resolved three memories! Having denied suffering any unsettling feelings or bothersome issues whatsoever at the onset of the process, they were amazed at themselves. What a privilege it was to share their self-healing experience!

It is important to note: when resistance from the conscious or subconscious mind is engaged, the bodymind often utilizes the body or somatic resources to gently allow the memory to surface for healing. I have worked with many shy, frightened, or reluctant individuals who, when assisted by the electromagnetic field technique, were easily able to begin verbalizing their somatic cues, though they initially felt inadequate for the task. In fact, many had been unsuccessful in prior therapeutic endeavors.

I recall the case of Mike, an adolescent who, when I encountered him, was a newcomer to treatment. He denied awareness of any trauma or intense feelings at the start of our group session that day. Immediately upon placing my right hand on the "hot spot" or primary access point on his back, before I could scan the front of his body or begin the verbal technique, he loudly exclaimed: "My arms are burning! My arms are burning!"

I immediately responded with: "And how old are you when your arms are burning like that?"

"I'm thirteen!" he answered quickly.

"And where are you when you're thirteen and your arms are burning?" I asked.

"I'm at my best friend's house," he stated.

"And what happens then when you're at your best friend's house and your arms are burning?" I inquired.

"I'm shooting up heroin for the first time, and my arms start burning," he declared.

"And what happens then, when you're doing that?" I questioned.

"I think I'm going to die," he concluded.

By engaging the electromagnetic field technique, Mike's bodymind immediately took him to a very intense memory of his first heroin use when he was afraid that he would overdose, and he experienced the burning in his arms. This traumatized him both emotionally and physically, inducing profound feelings of shame and fear that became bound to his heroin use. Such shame induction accelerates the addictive cycle and binds the psyche to the shame-inducing behavior. This initial traumatic drug use accelerated the progress of his addiction and led to his need for inpatient treatment. The electromagnetic field technique accelerated the healing process by alerting him to the presence of this intense somatic pain induced from his "play" with drugs. The memory was easily identified and resolved once he "recalled" the original pain.

Those who are unfamiliar with trauma resolution work are often surprised at the clarity of their own somatic cues when they pause to listen to their bodies. They are equally surprised that another person can feel and assist them in finding and experiencing these memory cues. Emotions are not merely private or subjective realities. They are powerful interpersonal, relational bridges and messengers that are stored at moments of trauma. (We shall examine the nature of these relational bridges in the ensuing chapters.) A by-product of Newtonian influence, it was the absence of an instrument to measure these subtle electromagnetic distortions that led to our skepticism. On a scientific level, however, it is now clear that these more subtle energy forms can be precisely identified and measured – and beyond the limited capacity of our "five senses."

Upon completion of my post-graduate work in Rome, I arranged to do a six week study program with N.A.S.A.'s Earth Resources Laboratory connected with the John C. Stennis Space Center in Mississippi. My goal at the time was to see if airborne "thermal infrared multi-spectral scanners" could be used to detect archaeological remains below the surface of the earth and, thereby, accelerate our ability to do archaeological research in the Near East. (Since that time, many of these objectives have been achieved using ground-based radar.) Previously, such technology had proved effective in locating archaeological sites beneath the sands of the Sahara along the Nile through the use of "Shuttle-Imaging Radar-B" (SIR-B). Actually, this event occurred as an "accident" when the radar was left operative during a "fly-over" of Egypt. While studying these scanners, my instructor, a brilliant man who later went to work in Geneva to help develop the United Nations Global Database for Endangered Species, indicated to me that all forms of energy, including electromagnetic distortions in the environment and the human body can be detected utilizing certain calibrated scanners. I saw cases where even overgrown man-made structures could be distinguished from the surrounding vegetation that now covered them. The scanners that I was studying at the time had only been declassified from military use two years earlier in 1982. Now instruments have been developed that can detect and measure electromagnetic distortions in the human body – Magnetic Resonance Imaging (MRI), for instance, and the Superconducting Quantum Interference Device (SQUID) at New York University, among others.

Encoded holograms, which have been described here, carry an electromagnetic signature as unique and personal as our own handwriting. Recognizing that each hologram is unlike any other is pivotal to understanding this work. This information is not new to us – but is, perhaps, to the general public. One Christmas holiday spent on an Air Force base in Germany, I met an Air Force intelligence officer who, upon discovering my archaeological pursuits, asked probing questions about my interest in the applications of "remote sensing" technology. He later informed me that he worked in the military's own version of "remote sensing" technology. Employing a touch of humor, I asked him if it were true that we could now read license plates in downtown Moscow. He jokingly responded, "Only if the license plate is facing upwards." Although we are on the evolutionary and technological brink of developing the instruments needed to measure precisely the spectral signatures of the holograms of emotional trauma, we have long possessed a far more sophisticated multidimensional resource – our minds and hands – whose powers of information transduction, by far, surpass our most advanced technology.

Over the past two years, working with thirty or more trauma survivors per week, I have had ample opportunity to exercise the electromagnetic scanning technique to facilitate the identification and release of trauma from the bodyminds of my clients. With frequent practice I have noticed an increase in the sensitivity of my hands which now allows me to distinguish the trauma left from head injuries and other severe physical injuries, for instance, from other types of pain. Anger stored in the nerve centers often manifests as a "burning" sensation, whereas a nervous system injury feels "icy cold" – a total absence of energy at the trauma site. Certain emotions such as anger produce a thermal or heat reaction distinct from other emotions. I invite each of you to explore the potential for the ethical application of this inherent sensitivity. In honing these skills, there have been times when the sensitivity flows so naturally that I perceive it to be inherent to our nature – an ageless part of our minds that are remembering forgotten skills and abilities.

Through my archaeological work and research, I know that many of these techniques, such as the electromagnetic field applications, were documented in the ancient literature of Egypt and Greece and are now returning to the forefront of our search for truth – both through science and spirituality. This common pursuit is now empowered by the scientific research emerging from quantum physics, field theory, and the study of "psychoneuroimmunology." Among these "revived" techniques are those that we consider in this text. I can attest to the fact that Holographic Memory Resolution feels much more natural to me and is far more effective than the methods I was "traditionally" taught. We are beings of light and energy; we are energy transducers. We are now learning to "see" from our multidimensional awareness and to consciously interact with each other through this natural expertise.

Chapter Nine

A rock pile ceases to be a rock pile the moment a single individual contemplates it, bearing within him the image of a cathedral.

       Antoine de St. Exupery (1900 - 1944)

The Physics of the Soul

The interrelationship between science and spirituality is a recurrent theme of my personal reflection. The intrigue offered by the interconnectedness of these two fields, viewed by some as mutually exclusive, has heightened my fascination with trauma and motivated me to develop tools for healing that would never have evolved without the interplay between science and spirituality. These two disciplines, I have come to recognize, are not as separate as I once thought. It does not appear that one can study and experience the dynamics of trauma induction and resolution without exploring this rapport.

A common bond exists uniting the fields of science and spirituality: it is the pursuit of truth. A study of the process by which the mind grasps truth indicates that it is a dual process. On the one hand, the transmission of truth always involves a constant – an unchanging element that remains the same throughout and beyond time. But there is also a variable – something which changes, grows, and evolves over time. Let us look at ourselves, for example. We are told that the cells of our bodies are renewed and replaced over a seven year cycle, yet there is something about us which remains the same. I am still who I am after all the cellular changes. I am both constant and variable. There is a stability that remains despite all the changes and a growth process that is evidenced as well. Even my understanding of who I am as an individual remains stable while seeking ever more precise articulations of my "true self." Both our personal and collective histories proceed, therefore, as a "dialectic" process – one in which the "truths" we learn about ourselves are subsequently challenged by life experiences which lead us to further refinements in understanding who we truly are. We begin with the "thesis" (initial truth) which is then challenged by the "antithesis" (opposing notion); this interaction eventually gives rise to "synthesis" in which we move to a "higher" or more precise articulation of the initial truth as a result of the confrontation. Trauma is the most profound human experience where our "truth" is confronted by that of another. It is the "antithetical" human experience par excellence. From these experiences our "higher" truth can emerge.

An examination of the history of science and spirituality shows points of commonality. Much of what was once considered "science" to ancient man is viewed as "spirituality" in the assessment of modern times. The "shaman" or "medicine man" was the scientist of ancient times. But that which one generation considers scientific truth may be greatly diminished, becoming "superstition" or "myth" in the eyes of the subsequent generation. Nonetheless, there is a truth that we share with ancient man that is, has been, and ever will be constant. This constant is the experience of Truth itself. As we evolve, we seek to express our personal and collective truths more and more clearly. The truths that were communicated by ancient man in myths and stories constituted his "science." In modern times, we seek to make distinctions between these ancient "primitive" articulations of truth and "more advanced" science. Suddenly, however, we see a convergence between many of the ancient teachings, especially those of spirituality and the attributes of quantum physics. Is it possible, then, that the tension between "scientific" truth and "spiritual" truth is simply a misperception?

One of the great surprises to me was the discovery that my ability to work with electromagnetic fields and to discuss this subject scientifically immediately triggered intense reactions – from the scientists, on the one hand, and from religious advocates on the other. To the traditional Newtonian scientists, the discussion of electromagnetic fields was considered outside the purview of their "traditional" training and outside the scope of their understanding of the "measurable data" of science. Many of them viewed any discussion of "electromagnetic fields" as suspect and, quite often, unworthy of the attention of their "tried and true" methodologies. Many of them were unaware of the vast amount of data generated regarding the healing effects of applied electromagnetic energy used in the clinical setting – research long under way at New York University and in Dr. Valerie Hunt's "energy laboratory" at the University of California at Los Angeles (U.C.L.A.), for instance. They were also unfamiliar with the vast body of research literature accessible in any medical library under such titles as: "Healing Touch," "Therapeutic Touch," or "Reiki" — all variant electromagnetic field techniques. The resistance I encountered also seemed related to many of the scientists' attachments to their own belief systems.

The extreme reaction which I received in ongoing encounters with "religious" advocates came as a surprise as well. As long as I spoke of the laying on of hands from a traditional, scriptural, or biblical perspective, there was little tension. When I began to discuss the subject in terms of science, there was a sense of threat and suspicion. This issue, as I was well aware from my study of the history of science and religion, was not new. If, for example, we return to the controversy surrounding Galileo, the father of modern mechanics, we see his initial rejection by many of the powerful systems of his day (including the Roman Catholic Church) due to his contesting certain age-old "truths" regarding the nature and movement of planetary bodies. The controversy surrounding him had less to do with the validity of his observations and more to do with the politics and established systems of power of his day. His scientific research was perceived as a challenge to older philosophical principles that rested at the heart of these political systems.

During my seminary training, the dialogue between science and spirituality was explained as a natural and healthy tension between physics and metaphysics. Both were viewed as valid scientific endeavors. Nevertheless, it seemed that there was a hiatus or gap between the "truths" posited by my religious system, and the ongoing and evolving attestations of science. Scientific truths seemed to be integrated into religious systems only after long, protracted, painstaking delays and scrutiny – all justified in the name of protecting the innocent and less-informed. I understood the caution and the intention involved, but the price exacted was spiritual and emotional pain to many who saw in science the presence of evident Truth. I saw many religious systems struggling to understand and integrate the data of "evolution" and the "Big Bang theory," as well as other hypotheses. It was big news recently when Pope John Paul II gave verbal endorsement to the concept of evolution. Yes, there remains a delay in the transmission of truth in some important circles. In my efforts to resolve this personal struggle, I vowed to study the history of both science and spirituality hoping to bridge this gap within my thinking. Along the way I encountered some remarkable mentors. Their observations were provocative and surprising.

Thomas S. Kuhn, in his book, The Structure of Scientific Revolutions, speaks eloquently of the struggle with our understanding and image of science.[1] From his observations it becomes clear that the notion that science provides us with a secure, absolute knowledge or experience of truth is an illusion. He points out that science proceeds as a dialectic process in which competition arises between segments of the scientific community which results in the rejection of one previously accepted theory in favor of the adoption of another.[2] In talking about scientific revolutions, Kuhn states the following:

> *Copernicus, Newton, Lavoisier, Einstein (sic.) ... each of them necessitated the community's rejection of time-honored scientific theory in favor of another incompatible with it. Each produced a consequent shift in the problems available for scientific scrutiny and in the standards by which the profession determined what should count as an admissible problem or as a legitimate problem-solution. And each transformed the scientific imagination in ways that we shall ultimately need to describe as a transformation of the world within which scientific work was done. Such changes, together with the controversies that almost always accompany them, are the defining characteristics of scientific revolutions.[3]*

Later in his work, in a chapter entitled, "The Resolution of Revolutions," he discusses ways competing or opposing views of truth are resolved, drawing particular attention to the <u>verification process</u> – that is, the matter of determining which is "true."[4] In a statement which I found surprising and enlightening, he observed the following:

> *To the historian, at least, it makes little sense to suggest that verification is establishing the agreement of fact with theory. <u>All</u> historically significant theories have agreed with the facts, <u>but only more or less</u>. There is no more precise answer to the question whether or how well an individual theory fits the facts ... it makes a great deal of sense to ask which of the two actual and competing theories fits the facts better.[5]*

What we discover, therefore, is not that science provides an "absolute" knowledge that is incontestable, but that science itself is a growth process. In discussing the movement from one scientific paradigm to another, as from Newtonian physics to quantum physics, Kuhn states the following:

> *The transfer of allegiance from paradigm to paradigm is a conversion experience that cannot be forced ... The source of the resistance is the assurance that the older paradigm will ultimately solve all its problems, that nature can be shoved into the box the paradigm provides ... Though some scientists, particularly the older and more experienced ones, may resist indefinitely, most of them can be reached in one way or another. Conversions will occur a few at a time until, after the last holdouts have died, the whole profession will again be practicing under a single, but now different, paradigm.[6]*

What, precisely, is this emerging paradigm? The main content of this work draws attention to the paradigm shift occurring in the transition from Newtonian "mechanical" thinking to quantum, multidimensional or holographic thinking. In my interchange with scientists, therapists, ministers, and medical professionals (allopaths), there is clearly evidenced a lack of awareness of this multidimensional nature of reality. The age-old attachment to our limited five-sensory perception is quite understandable when we examine the history of scientific, educational, religious, political, and medical systems and their reliance on the old paradigm.

The mechanical thinking of the old paradigm found its origins in Newtonian physics which saw the human individual as a solid object. Isaac Newton placed his emphasis on the "observed laws of mechanics" and "physical causes" underlying the movements of "corporeal bodies."[7] The mechanistic model of Newton, which successfully detailed planetary movements, laws of motion, and gravitational phenomena also fostered a belief that the world is a closed objective system where all physical reactions have a physical cause. Time was linear; space was three-dimensional; and all was measurable by one set of systems and observers.[8] Convenient! Simple! Comfortable! Tidy! During the nineteenth century, Newtonian physics was extended to describe the universe as composed of tiny solid objects consisting of a nucleus of protons and neutrons, with electrons revolving around the nucleus. These tiny building blocks were called atoms. This overly simplified, mechanical view of the universe offered a certain false security – a convenient, closed, solid, largely unchanging, predictable system with definite rules that governed its functioning. In time, however, we were to learn that the actual picture of the atom was something quite different. For instance, the analogy has been made that, if we were to build a scale model of the atom using something the size of a ping-pong ball for the nucleus, it would be necessary to have an area the size of a football stadium to contain even the innermost orbiting electrons. And if the ping-pong ball were placed at the center of the fifty yard line, a green pea on the uppermost seat in the stands would represent the nearest electron of the atom. We begin to see, therefore, that there is very little "actual" matter in "physical" matter. We would appear to be 99.999% space! The notion that the human body is a solid object and that the various forms of matter that I observe around me are "solid" is, in fact, a carry-over from the old paradigm, from Newtonian physics. There are both scientific and spiritual restrictions created by maintaining this thinking, as I discovered for myself.

With roots in some very traditional systems, I was, nonetheless, through my commitment to support others in their healing process, mandated to move beyond the restrictions which held my clients trapped in their pain. I was forced into a much more expansive perception of the universe and its human population through my struggle to understand the dynamics of trauma. The first lesson taught to me by trauma survivors involved recognition that I could not proceed with resolution if I thought of the human body or the human person as merely a "solid object." Included among these earliest insights was the realization that the encoded trauma could be perceived to be located on the inside, the outside, or both, with respect to the "physical" body. It was simply a matter of holographic perception. In addition, once the initial location of the metaphor was established, inquiry into the size or shape of the metaphor usually resulted in very elaborate and detailed multidimensional pictures. Work with these multidimensional images immediately impressed upon me and my clients the fact that we were not working with the notion of the self as a "solid object," but with forms of consciousness which presented as subtle electromagnetic fields which readily could be felt and perceived. These metaphors or containers of memory seemed superimposed within the electromagnetic fields which extended beyond the confines of the "physical" body. Summarizing the placement of metaphors reported by my trauma clients, I noticed a proportionately higher incidence of metaphors located "on the inside" with the balance located "on the outside," "just under the surface," or "both inside and out." We all possess this ability to "scan" both inside and outside the electromagnetic fields that comprise our consciousness, for we are more than our physical bodies.

Not long ago I was asked to demonstrate the trauma resolution process during a workshop with one hundred sexual trauma therapists. The first question that I was asked was, "Why did you ask the volunteer whether the feeling was on the inside or the outside of her body?" Newtonian "mechanical" thinking has left us with residue of an outdated notion of solidity. Today we are moving beyond the belief that the "boundary" of the human person is to be equated with the physical body or that emotional metaphors are less real than that which is physical. As we are now learning, emotional metaphors are as real as "physical" reality. The invitation is to move beyond the old illusions of separateness and apparent solidity to a more accurate, fluid perception of reality. In their intent to move us past these illusions toward "truth," both science and spirituality are fully engaged, albeit on different levels.

I often, playfully, challenge my new clients' Newtonian thinking by reminding them that I am not as I appear to be – that, in reality, what they assume to be "me" is, in fact, the reflection of photons off of interference patterns caused by the confluence of the living waves and particles of energy comprising my "physical" body, which are then imprinted on the retina of the eye upside down and are reinterpreted by the brain right side up. I point out to them that the energy fields of the human "body" actually extend thirty-two to forty feet in all directions. I am much larger than I appear, and, while confined within a room, we overlap profoundly. The limitations of our "five senses," however, tend to reduce me to a much smaller perception. Our eyes, normally, only register the "densest," heaviest particles or wave patterns. In the past, those who did speak of seeing the interactions of these living energy fields around the "physical" body were often discounted, though many ancient cultures, for example, depicted the radiance of their "en-lightened" beings as extending outward from the physical body. Jesus was often depicted with a "halo" or accompanying manifestation of light or energy which revealed his grander nature and origins. While spiritual traditions comfortably discussed the phenomenon of light or energy associated with spiritual beings, science remained skeptical. The presence of electromagnetic fields was discounted until recently when machines were developed that could photograph and measure them – that is, Kirlian photography and instruments like the Superconducting Quantum Interference Device (S.Q.U.I.D.) at New York University.[9]

Irrespective of multitudinous scientific advancements, we have certainly managed to hold onto old Newtonian influences. Perhaps we are, indeed, prone to be addicted to our own beliefs. Certainly Kuhn's observations about the resistance to paradigm shifts is accurate; but, as a result of the Newtonian mechanics, have we reduced ourselves to greater trust in machines than in the infinitely subtle and sophisticated perceptions of our own minds and bodies? How do we explain the metaphysical phenomena of our experience that seems to substantiate the existence of our nature as spiritual?

Statistics, for instance, tell us that one in twenty-five persons among the standard population has undergone an "out of body" (OBE) experience. For those of us who work with the memories of trauma survivors, the "out of body" dissociative experience is familiar. My clients who have experienced this phenomenon often describe the scene in detail, observing themselves at some distance from their own bodies, while remaining blissfully removed from their emotions. They are able to accurately describe all the details of the event as detached observers. I studied this phenomenon myself in a college course entitled: "Death and Dying." I was studying for ministry at a Catholic university at the time. Such esoteric studies were usually assigned to the domain of theology (meaning "study of God" – though it, too, is considered a science). Since the "out of body experience" could not be "reproduced in a lab situation" and due to the fact that the witnesses could not be considered "reliable" (since they did not "remain dead"), it was argued that they did not provide valid proof about life outside the body or a life hereafter. It appears that when our perceptions stretch beyond established scientific parameters, they are often consigned to the realm of spirituality or discounted completely. To do what I do from the standpoint of a minister, for instance, is considered "normal," whereas, to approach my work from the perspective of science is suspect until it can be reproduced and analyzed in a lab. Acknowledging the demands of current scientific method, however, my colleagues and I, at the time of this writing, are preparing to measure with biofeedback and electroencephalogram (EEG) instrumentation, the electromagnetic shifts and brain wave changes that occur during such trauma resolution.

In studying the history of the relationship of science and spirituality, it is notable that, to ancient man, most of reality was a "mystery." Attempts to grasp these mysteries resulted in created mythologies which articulated the emergent patterns and cycles evident in life, nature, and the universe. In the mind of ancient man, there was obviously an invisible force that sustained all life. Attempts to articulate this phenomenon drew attention to the notion of "breath," "wind," and "spirit" – all manifestations of this invisible power. Studying the etymology of the concept, we trace the Latin word "spiritus" (spirit) back to the Greek work "pneuma" (breath, spirit, soul), and even earlier to the Hebrew word "ruah" (breath, wind, spirit). This mysterious power, with its animating properties, was an accepted fact for ancient man, for it was evident that when this invisible breath or spirit was present, there was life; when the breath left a being for a prolonged period of time, the corporeal life of the being ceased. The Hebrew language had no concept for "nothing." Everything was a real force, a "thing," including this invisible sustainer of life.

Articulations of "higher truth" have always involved, by necessity, the use of metaphor. This ancient notion of "breath," while now interpretable through physiology, biology, physics, and a host of other sciences, has proved a persistent metaphor for the invisible "force" which animates all. In reducing the breath to a biochemical formula, we may have missed the deeper mystery and truth that underlies its reality. This notion of breath is, itself, one of the meeting points of science and spirituality. The study of trauma contributes to the nexus of the two realms.

As recorded in ancient times, the focusing of the breath has been associated with the creation of various states of consciousness. Disciplines of breathing were found to produce altered states of consciousness. Since a trauma is also an altered state of consciousness, there is an interesting and positive correlation with this notion of breath. For many researchers in the trauma field, it is believed that the intake and holding of the breath initiates the "freezing" and encoding of the electrical impulses that comprise the survivor's perceptions at the moment of trauma. I can often determine when a survivor's approach to T-1, for there will be a sudden intake, slowing, or holding of the breath. Consider what happens when someone comes up behind you and scares you. There is a sudden, sharp sucking in of breath, a tightening of the muscles, especially in the part of the body where the intrusion is most strongly felt. This physiological response is one of the mechanisms that transforms incoming electrical impulses from a dynamic flow state to a static state and stores the impulses in the cells and fields of the body. This process is the "energy transduction" that was described earlier. The nervous system attempts to "take control" of the situation which is perceived as life-threatening on physical, mental, emotional, and/or spiritual levels. The sudden capture or holding of the breath facilitates the freezing process. An understanding of this storage mechanism contributes to our grasp of the profound connection between what we have traditionally defined as "science" or "spirituality." The effort to comprehend the mechanisms of consciousness is, by no means, new.

Millenia ago, the teachings of the Eastern religions described a subtle life-force uniting and sustaining all living things. In India, for example, this life-force was called "prana" and was, particularly, associated with the breath.[10] In all forms of yoga, for example, breathing exercises known as "pranayama" (meaning, "the regulation of prana") involved the enhancement of this life-force through focusing and balancing energy flow.[11] In the eastern religions it was recognized that the holding or storing of this prana at a moment of crisis enables the storage of the overwhelming perceptions. During the final stages of my mother's illness, I taught her a breathing technique which allowed her to remain relaxed and centered when the pain of her condition threatened to overcome her. We can learn to use our breathing to release tension and stress, rather than waiting until our nervous system becomes overburdened and "forced" to encode the feelings. It would appear from the legacy they left us, that some of our Eastern brethren were acutely attuned to their bodies and, thus, accurately observed the functioning of what we now perceive to be the Limbic-Hypothalamic system's response to crisis and trauma. They developed techniques to help heal and improve the nervous system's functioning, even without the advantage of Quantum physics. Techniques for directing and regulating breathing such as Stanislav Grof's "Holotropic Breathwork," among many others, have now been developed to help us identify and access trauma memories for resolution.

An additional point of convergence between science and spirituality relates to the "oneness" or interconnectedness of all things. Both science and spirituality have sought to address this notion in their own manner. Current scientific research, for instance, seeks comprehension of the mechanism by which universal life energy demonstrates the characteristics of a vast electromagnetic field or force field; this area of research is called "field theory."[12] The pragmatic implications of such a theory are profound. Ongoing research through N.A.S.A., for instance, and from independent scientific research suggests that we are, in fact, on the verge of a "unified field theory." Some scientists with whom I speak state that we already possess it. Currently N.A.S.A. and other government agencies sponsor symposia for scientists to discuss such themes as "alternative propulsion systems" based on the physics of an emergent unified field theory. There are, however, other practical applications.

Addressing field theory from the perspective of the "healing sciences," I can affirm that I have gained both valuable data and illumination working with the electromagnetic fields of my clients. The realization that I could feel the energetic distortions, the precise low-frequency memory forms "within" the bodies of other individuals has led to a re-defining of the concepts of intimacy and relationality. Feedback that my clients could also feel my energy transactions within their bodies occasioned further revision in my thinking. It would appear that we are capable of profound levels of intimacy and interaction with others that were not even suggested in the most advanced training for health professionals and clergy.

From the onset of my work, I found it required little effort to feel intense distortions in the electromagnetic fields within the bodies of my clients. Distortions such as those resulting from incest manifested as a sharp, stabbing pain in my hands. The energy that presented as headaches, chronic somatic pain, etc., actually "stung" my hands as it exited the client's body. Migraines suffered by my clients caused a sensation so intense that it felt as if my hands were being violently waved back and forth. When the violent wave motion in my hands subsided, my clients' headaches normally were gone. From the "five-sensory" standpoint, my hands had not moved at all. The old five-sensory awareness could not adequately explain my experience. There were clients and ministers who tried to reduce the explanation to the religio-moral sphere of "faith healing," but this was not a case of "faith healing." Faith was not required, though permission always was sought first. Let me explain.

The first session in which I used directed electromagnetic energy to resolve a migraine headache involved a nine year old boy who, I was informed, had been waiting in our reception area with an intense migraine for a few hours while his parent attended to some hospital business. The receptionist who knew my work informed me of his condition and asked if I could assist in any way. He looked agonized. I introduced myself, inquired about his migraine, and then asked if I could place my hands near his head, three to five inches away. After about three minutes, he suddenly looked up with surprise and asked:

"What did you do?"

"It's energy," I explained. "How's your head?" I asked.

"Better!" he stated with amazement.

A "gray area" now exists between our traditional "five-sensory" awareness upon which our science has been based, and all that was otherwise relegated to the field of spirituality. Traditionally, when healing occurred that was not explainable by our accepted level of science, it was called "faith healing." That is not the focus of this work. For the effective application of electromagnetic field therapies, permission is all that is required, not faith. This, of course, is a point of contention with religious systems who "claim" proprietary rights for healing from "divine will" and use those instances of healing to prove their claims. For example, in one episode with a "born-again" addict who was suffering a relapse with alcoholism, I was accused of operating from the "dark side" because I was not healing as a minister of his church and because I would not agree that all healing is simply a matter of "faith." Even quoting scripture on this matter left little impact on him. I feel sadness when I see religious rigidity or addiction blinding individuals to the offerings of spirituality. The belief that healing can occur only through "faith" is largely the product of the old "moral model." What about the healing of the child who has not yet reached the "age of reason" to possess the informed decision of "faith"? The universal energy or presence that is manifest in all healing is not limited by our moral model.

Through my work with trauma survivors, I must admit that I have developed a particular love for the atheists, pessimists, and skeptics. I recall my first work with a skeptical physician. He entered my office complaining of head, neck, and back pain. He also explained that he was "old school" and a product of "traditional medicine." Nonetheless, he indicated that he needed help and was open to exploring new avenues. Within the trauma resolution process he was able to identify and access the trauma that had caused his pain which he recognized as an incident of betrayal by peers within his own profession. After completing the trauma resolution work and reframing his specific memory, all of his somatic complaints were resolved. "I'm a believer!" he stated. His healing experience required less than twenty-five minutes.

During my work, I sense the interaction of my own electromagnetic fields with those of my clients. I feel a flash of heat through my nervous system when our fields actively engage one another; my client often experiences a similar response. Commonly, I experience a "cooling down" period when the trauma is resolved and the work is complete; my client typically feels the same coolness. With the dissolution of my old thinking that I am my physical body, comes the conclusion that my clients are, likewise, more than what my five-sensory awareness has led me to believe. If I am no longer just over here, and you are no longer just over there, there is a constant energy exchange taking place between our electromagnetic fields. My motivation to facilitate trauma resolution has deepened tremendously from the realization that we are all much more a part of each other than I had previously comprehended. It is profoundly moving both for myself and those with whom I work to realize that we can "perceive" each other's "internal" emotional states. The "illusions of separation" which we were taught and which have left us "alone in ourselves," once they dissolve, raise questions about our need to elevate our consciousness to be more sensitive to ways our thoughts, feelings, and actions influence the open energy fields around us – whether this is in concert with other persons, the global population, nature, the planet, or beyond. Research indicates that, as complex energy fields in constant interaction with our environment, we are under an illusion if we think that we can "close out" the influx of energy from around us. We are intrinsically open to surrounding energy sources. I can delude myself into thinking that I am an isolated, invulnerable entity with precise physical boundaries, but this misconception cannot be maintained. The energy fields of our nervous systems must remain open for us to live and to thrive. This openness is part of our blueprint. As much as I might like to withdraw from interaction with other systems, I am a living part of a totally unified, living energy exchange. Once I realize my connection to the whole, I have immediate access to unlimited resources and forms of energy so that my old defenses of isolation are no longer necessary, and certainly no longer serve my best interest. There is abundant energy to foster safety, protection, well-being, and health without having to withdraw or isolate to create a personal sense of security.

Under the Newtonian notion that we were "solid," physical isolation and withdrawal served to maintain an illusion of security. Such limited attempts at preserving our inner power and security did not suffice long-term, for they did not address our deeper needs or exigencies. The illusion that security can be found in the isolation of the physical body does not honor our true nature as beings of light. Physical isolation is quite different from our intrinsic need for solitude. In solitude, we may, in fact, unite more closely with others by transcending our physical limitations – as through meditation. By feeling that I am not just my physical body, but that I am light, I open to a whole new paradigm and way of perceiving reality. There is a heightened consciousness of others, of my own thoughts and feelings, of my intimate interactions with nature, food, animals, the planet, and the universe. There is much more interconnectedness than I was led to believe by the "illusions of separation." With this consciousness comes the heightened ability to respond – the gift and the responsibility. (Science is now supporting this expansion of consciousness by moving into the realm of quantum physics and beyond.) By doing so, it is also demonstrating the truth of our own power as the creators of our reality.

This expansion of our consciousness to see the interconnection of all things was anticipated through the work of physicist J. S. Bell. In 1964 he published "Bell's Theorem," a mathematical proof that supports the principle that subatomic particles are connected in some way that transcends both time and space; in other words, if anything happens to one particle, other particles are simultaneously affected.[13] The effect is instantaneous and immediate – that is, it is not time transmitted. The importance of this theorem is that effects can be "superluminal" or faster than the speed of light, contradicting Einstein's Theory of Relativity which indicates that it is impossible for particles to travel faster than the speed of light.[14] Support for Bell's Theorem has now been established by research, providing the potential for further paradigm shifts. On a more personal level, it has the potential to revolutionize all forms of communication. The implications of understanding how this instantaneous interconnection works would profoundly intensify our capacity for communication with each other. Our communication would no longer be as limited by time or space.

I was already aware from my family history that some such superluminal communication probably existed. Previously I attributed this to a mysterious "spiritual" phenomenon. It appears that science and spirituality are converging — agreeing that we have the capacity, by our very nature, to transcend space and time in our communication practices. In effect, this principle informs us that what was once considered "spiritual" power is profoundly connected to the very makeup of reality, physical existence, and the functioning of subatomic particles. This phenomenon suggests the unification of reality in ways that provide new possibilities for communication and reveal to us new options for shaping our own reality. At this level, science and spirituality are no longer distinct. While examining the remarkable implications of this interconnection, we might find ourselves asking what practical value such an understanding would provide? One implication was suggested to me through my work with a young trauma survivor, Zack.

This nineteen year old, like many teenage trauma survivors, was chemically dependent and sought treatment when his parents could no longer live with the specter that only resembled their beloved son. While in inpatient treatment, Zack joined my trauma resolution therapy group to explore the trauma he had undergone as a result of his drug addiction. When he described intense feelings of shame and remorse about the damage his addiction had caused, I asked him: "When you feel this feeling, where do you feel it in your body?"

"It's in my stomach," he stated.

"On the inside or the outside?" I asked.

"Both," he responded.

"And what's it like in your stomach?" I inquired.

"It's like a black hole the size of a baseball," he answered.

"And how old might you be when you first feel a black hole like that?"

"I'm fourteen," he replied.

"And where are you when you're fourteen, and there's a black hole like that?"

"I'm at a friend's house; we're drinking, doing 'shrooms (mushrooms) and smoking pot," he explained.

"And what happens then, when you're doing all that?" I asked with concern.

"I almost overdose 'cause I can't tell how much I'm doing," he replied.

"And what happens then, when you almost overdose?" I questioned.

"That's when I feel the black hole for the first time and get scared for myself," he answered.

"So what needs to happen with this scene?" "If you could go back and help him, what would you like to see happen?" I asked.

"I'd like to warn him about what he's about to do to himself and get him to not do it," he replied.

"So take all the time you need to go back and do that ... and if you'd like, you can show him pictures of what's going to happen to him if he continues on this path – show him pictures of his future and see if he's willing to accept your help and do it differently," I suggested. "You already know some of the painful things that are going to happen to him as a result of his drug use."

"OK," he stated. Then he paused, lowered his head, and after a minute said, "Oh yeah, I remember now when we did this!"

"What do you mean?" I asked, confused by his last statement.

"I remember when a guy that looked like you, and me – yeah, I see, it was me the way I look now; I didn't recognize me back then ... We tried to convince me to do it different ... I just thought that they were dreams or something. I was fourteen. I just blew 'em off ... I didn't think they were real. But those dreams worried me. I remember you now."

I paused in silence to assimilate the concept he was suggesting. For years I had been taught about the implications of quantum physics and the relativity of our space and time perceptions, but I had never encountered a case where the principles had been demonstrated – and certainly not in a personal context. Nor had I ever considered the implications of dialoguing within the mind from different space and time perceptions. I was unsure what to think about his disclosure and, to this day, have seen only one other case where a client reported a similar recall. He "resolved" the dilemma of the original trauma by visualizing himself dialoguing with his "addict self" at age fourteen, securing the adolescent self's cooperation, and picturing both of them safely in treatment together in present time (T+1) – the post-trauma scene. We concluded the resolution process, with his fourteen year old self accepting the factual result of his drug usage and at last with a willingness to "do it differently." I filed the information and, more lightheartedly, told myself that I was probably just having a flashback from a "Quantum Leap" episode. The implications of the experience have remained in my mind and have given me a new respect when I ask my clients to dialogue with those other injured or addicted parts of their own minds, borne in the experiences of other places and times. I have no absolute means of authenticating the internal experience of another, except to say that I know that the memory he shared possessed its own unique pain, a portion of which I felt in my hands. When he resolved the memory and secured the cooperation of his "fourteen year old wounded self," the pain dissolved. I felt this as he released the encoded trauma from the cells and fields of his body. Beyond this, I leave you to your own reflections and exploration of this phenomenon.

The intricacies of my clients' memories along with the broader implications of their trauma experiences served to challenge my understanding of the mysterious interplay of body, mind, and spirit. Quantum physics suggested that the mind is the nexus where a creative act occurs – a place where we can, for instance, freeze space and time perceptions to protect ourselves from pain, and that this act constitutes reality itself. From my family environment I was aware of some of the "higher" capacities of mind, as I watched my mother obtain information that was inaccessible according to the laws of traditional physics. These experiences stimulated my quest to grasp the implied interconnection of all these realms of reality. This interrelationship is so profoundly a part of our nature and of reality as a whole that the scientific and spiritual traditions are, themselves, converging. Bell's superluminal theorem, for instance, supports the age-old understanding of experiences that we have previously labeled spiritual or "mystical" in nature. From the perspective of spirituality, that consciousness which we associate with "the numinous" or "the divine" always possessed the ability to transcend the limits of time and space. What are the implications of science's declaration that consciousness is a creative act – that each and every act of perception is the act of a "creator" and that this is inherent to our nature?

While the new, emergent paradigm can only be limitedly anticipated, it suggests a profound leap in the direction of healing distortions in space and time. The tenets of this new paradigm hold equal promise for intrapersonal and interpersonal healing. Whether we seek to heal those frozen moments of our own consciousness held in stasis in some quiet, hidden place within ourselves, or whether we seek to resolve the social and historical conflicts that have fostered separation and schism on familial, societal, and global levels, the new paradigm offers hope by teaching us that all of the breaches are simply ruptures in consciousness – acts of perception which can be changed. The profound nature of our "interconnectedness" may allow the healing of these fractures to our natural unity by reminding us that alienation of the "other" is only an alienation from self; the traumatic perceptions we hold are dissociations from ourselves. Therefore, there is no benefit to oneself in fostering these illusions. Barbara Brennan, in her work, Hands of Light, applies the principle of "interconnectedness" to the healing dimension. She states the following:

> I suggest that since we are inseparable parts of that whole, we can enter into a holistic state of being, become the whole, and tap into creative powers of the universe to instantaneously heal anyone anywhere. Some healers can do this to a certain extent by merging and becoming one with God and the patient. Becoming a healer means moving toward this universal creative power which we experience as love by reidentifying self with and becoming universal; becoming one with God. One stepping stone to

this wholeness is to let go of our limited self definitions based
on our Newtonian past of separated parts and to identify
ourselves with being energy fields.[15]

Both science and spirituality support this understanding of ourselves as beings of light. Ancient Indian literature spoke of our sustenance by "prana," that universal life energy which permeates, constitutes, and sustains all life. The Chinese referred to "ch'i," the vital universal energy which permeates and comprises all matter. The Kabbalah, the Jewish mystical literature, speaks of these vital energies as the astral light. Christian literature indicates that "God is light" (I John 1:5) and that when God becomes incarnate, He is called the "Light of the World" (John 1:1-18; 8:12). In view of this history, are we not supported spiritually by our growing understanding of the nature of subatomic particles? Spirituality and science have become intimate indeed!

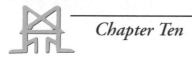

Chapter Ten

> *What makes the desert beautiful is that somewhere it hides a well.*
>
> Antoine de St. Exupery (1900 - 1944)

The Hierarchy of Healing

Once we accept, as Einstein affirmed, that all matter is simply slowed or crystallized energy, we begin to realize that we are living energy fields. As this truth dawns upon us, we begin to grasp ways that higher consciousness could be associated with higher frequency. Blockages in the electromagnetic fields of the body manifest as very low vibrational frequencies and commonly present themselves in the colors consonant with the lower end of the visible portion of the electromagnetic spectrum. We all possess an inherent understanding of these frequencies. What colors come to mind when I ask you to consider the notions of death and hatred? What colors do you associate with rage and anger? My clients routinely inform me that death, depression, and hatred appear to them holographically as "black" (the absence of light), whereas anger and rage appear as "red" (the "lowest" color in the visible portion of the spectrum). When we are angry we state that we "see red." Our emotions, our traumas, our thoughts themselves are biochemical-electrical transmissions, and these frequencies are perceived through color.

In seeking to understand the individual in terms of the interactions of these electromagnetic fields, various authors such as Barbara Brennan and Chris Griscom have identified and described the interplay of the various frequencies or states of consciousness by designating them as "bodies;" hence, we find discussion of physical, emotional, mental, and spiritual bodies.[1] For purposes of our forum, our interest in these bodies relates specifically to the impact of trauma. How does trauma impact our consciousness on the physical, emotional, mental, and spiritual planes? What occurs energetically?

Observing the dynamics of trauma induction and resolution, it becomes evident that there is a kind of hierarchy of consciousness which structures the healing process – a hierarchy which orders the flow of energy within the electromagnetic fields that comprise our reality.[2] This descending hierarchy exists as follows: 1) the spiritual body, 2) the mental body, 3) the emotional body, and 4) the physical body.

In reality, these distinctions are somewhat artificial, since consciousness is a continuum reaching from lower frequencies and lower consciousness to higher frequencies and higher consciousness. Even within the human person, the identified bodies associated with certain colors and frequencies represent an attempt to explain or grasp this infinitely smooth continuum. We can see a tendency to oversimplify observable reality in the case of the "rainbow," where we reduce the phenomenon to the predominant descriptors or "colors" when, in fact, the rainbow actually consists of the visible portion of the electromagnetic spectrum – a smooth merging transition from one color to the next, including all the colors in between. Due to our finite vocabulary, we reduce the rainbow to a few major colors to describe it. Similarly, all of the bodies are profoundly connected. The study of trauma and our capacity to freeze our perceptions instantaneously at overwhelming moments indicates that all aspects of the self are involved: the physical, emotional, mental, and spiritual. Similarly, effective trauma resolution actually relies upon this interdependency. Access to the emotions of a traumatic experience allow us to find where and how the physical body was impacted, enabling us to locate the scene and identify the hurtful or abusive mental messages that were imprinted during the trauma. Once accessed, these messages and feelings can be released of their negative content which has so deeply affected our belief system – our spirituality itself. Trauma resolution, therefore, is profoundly empowering and spiritual in nature. We begin to understand reasons for the hindrance of our emotional and spiritual growth when we seek spirituality while avoiding trauma memories. Trauma "metaphors" are the cues to the locations of our blockages in our physical, emotional, mental, and spiritual bodies. In order to understand more clearly the impact of trauma and its role in the healing process, let us reflect upon the interrelationship of these bodies. One of my favorite meditations is a reflection on these aspects of self. It is a personal adaptation of the meditation from Morton Kelsey's book, The Other Side of Silence.[3] The meditation goes as follows:

♦ **Physical Body:** I have a body, yet I am not just my body. My body is the precious vehicle of experience and action. Moreover, it is the manifestation of how I see myself consciously and subconsciously. It is my self-expression. My body may be rested or tired, but it is not my total "I." I try to treat it well and keep it in good health. It reports to me about my health and well-being on emotional, mental, and spiritual levels, and when I ignore these messages, it helps me to redirect my attention by making me aware of the problem areas through physical pain or illness. I seek to nurture and care for my physical body in its present form. Every seven years the cells of my body are renewed, but, throughout this transformation, something about me remains the same. I have a physical body, yet I am not just my physical body.

♦ **Emotional Body:** I have emotions, yet I am not just my emotions. They are infinite in number, varied, spontaneous, and powerful. Though constantly changing, I know that something about me remains the same in times of hope or discouragement, joy or pain, trauma or serenity. My emotions provide direction for wholeness and happiness, drawing my attention to unresolved events and experiences which can further my growth, attracting me to certain events, people, and situations. My emotions are a relational bridge that connects me to persons and experiences that define the very quality of my life. They direct my attention to my spiritual lessons and the work that remains to be done. I am also learning that I need not be the victim of painful emotions – that they can be resolved though long repressed or frozen in time and space. Emotions connect me with those who are forever a part of me though physically absent. They help me to explore my interconnection to all things. They are wondrous, challenging, and infinitely varied. But, amidst all the continuous emotional changes, something about me remains the same. I have emotions, yet I am not just my emotions.

♦ **Mental Body:** I have an intellect, yet I am not merely my intellect. My rational mind helps me to see clearly and to not be ruled solely by my emotions. It assists me by grounding me and anchoring me in an ever-changing world. This "logical" mind assists me in organizing my reality and in problem solving. It is the vehicle of my growing knowledge and helps me to make sense of my everyday experience. My knowledge has grown and developed over the years, helping me to increase my personal power and choices. It is a precious vehicle for the discovery and discernment of truth within my reality. My intellect enables me to express and articulate who I am and my life experiences. It allows me to bring order and comprehension to my daily life. My rational mind allows me to focus and direct my attention to persons, events, and circumstances needing my attention. I am an intelligent being, yet I am not just my intellect.

♦ **Spiritual Body:** I am a spiritual being of light, capable of infinite growth. I am more than my physical body, more than my emotions, and more than my intellect. I am one with that which is unchanging, infinite, and eternal. By my choice I embrace my physical, emotional, and mental bodies, yet I am more than all these. I am capable of moving beyond my feelings of individuality or isolation to experience my oneness with all that is. I am learning that I am more than my lessons in space and time. Time and space, I am discovering, are matters of perception and illusion which can be transcended. I, as all expressions of art, am a reflection of my creator, the one Source of all. I am a living extension of that which is eternal and undying. As I move beyond the illusions of separation, I see and experience myself as part of this much greater light. By learning to transform my physical, emotional, and mental bodies I come into my true power and discover my true nature as a creator. I discover that I can and do have the power to create my own reality consciously. I am, by my very nature, capable of extending this power to love and heal myself and my other-selves. I am returning home, to know my oneness with All That Is. Above all, I am a spiritual being. [4]

The hierarchy reflected in the meditation above, suggests more about our nature than science has been able to "prove" regarding consciousness. Speaking as one scientifically trained (as in archaeology) to rely upon my powers of observation and the necessary collaborating data, I do not draw my conclusions lightly: we are immensely powerful beings who, in simply focusing our minds, evidence a mastery of our overpowering experiences – a mastery over space and time, though it may not appear so at a moment of trauma induction. The field of trauma has taught me much about the expansive nature of consciousness. For example, I have seen trauma survivors access detailed memories which, when verified by their family members, appear to have occurred during the pregnancy; in other words, the event seems to have been witnessed from within the womb and was profoundly linked to the emotional experience of the mother. When my client Justin, whose left eye was distorted by forty degrees (always angling to the outside left) since birth, accessed the feelings associated with his condition, he first reported seeing his father standing in the kitchen in front of him. Suddenly, during his recollection, his father pulled a gun and shot himself. Justin recalled the moment of the trauma's encoding – accompanied by feelings of pain and terror, accompanied by a sharp pain in his left eye. I was much surprised when, upon resolving the scene, my client reported that he was "in the womb" when this event occurred. He then shared that his father committed suicide while standing in the kitchen in front of his mother; she was pregnant with him at the time. I am uncertain as to whether the trauma occurred during the period of development of the optic nerve of the fetus, but his father did, in fact, shoot himself in the left eye. I have learned that it is quite common for trauma to be induced visually by witnessing trauma to another, especially a loved one. Justin, while within the womb, somehow experienced his father's suicide and internalized the trauma in his own left eye. A beautiful and phenomenal conclusion to Justin's work involved a "substantial correction" and decreased light sensitivity in his left eye.

My work with this case and others like it forced me to go beyond the traditional scientific parameters of my training and to utilize the spiritual resources that had proved invaluable in my pursuit of "truth." One of the challenges that I faced in working with trauma survivors, for instance, concerned the notion that memory could not be accessed prior to the end of the first year of life due to the lack of development of the brain. If, however, we accept the existence of a spiritual consciousness, we are no longer limited to the notion of memory storage in strict dependence upon the developmental stages of the physical body, particularly the nervous system. If there is, for instance, an afterlife, then we are, indeed, more than our physical bodies or body-dependent memory. I know of countless cases where individuals have reported the conversations that occurred in the operating rooms and waiting rooms of the hospital when they "died" on the operating table, experienced an "out of body" experience, and returned to provide detailed accounts of the conversations which occurred "in the waiting room" before they were resuscitated. Reports would suggest that we do not lose our memory when we leave the physical body. We may lose the emotional pain which is closely bound to the functioning of the cells and fields of our physical bodies, but we do not lose our identities which are so intricately tied to our memories. There are tremendous implications for this concept. How differently some of us will view or treat a child when we realize the total memory capacity suggested by this more adaptable spiritual consciousness. Much abuse has occurred to children under the assumption that one so young and limited in development surely could not remember such treatment. This is not proving to be the case.

Emotional memory has repeatedly been discounted as well. Our earliest developmental messages are profoundly emotional in content. Before we are able to perceive ourselves as physically separate from our mothers, we are recording and internalizing "felt" messages through direct biochemical-electrical transmissions. Our earliest and perhaps most impacting messages are these felt messages. The power of this early memory becomes evident later on in life when we find ourselves recreating and attracted (subconsciously) to those situations that felt normal to us as children. Our earliest, operative definitions of love are not mental, but emotional. This is a result of our early imprints from the womb and from our early neonatal, infancy, and toddlerhood stages of life. Considering the fact that most of our parents assumed us to be unconscious and had no idea that our young memories could incorporate such data, we may have witnessed and imprinted some rather surprising notions about life, love, and relationships. I know that, by the age of four, I had internalized my father's trauma patterns and unhealthy ways of coping with life and relationships. The early formation of the emotional body has profound implications on our subsequent choices as well. In spite of my most elevated thoughts and ideals, later in life, I found myself magnetic to those people, situations, and relationships that resembled my childhood upbringing.

The principal consideration in grasping the impact of trauma concerns the following question: If the mental body has priority over the emotional body, why are we drawn to recreate a host of unhealthy situations when "we know better"? After our experiences of childhood trauma, how can we be attracted to those persons and relationships that we swore we would never repeat in our own lives or with our children? The explanation for this phenomenon is pivotal for resolving trauma in body, mind, and spirit. Let us explore the answer through the following principles:

1. When we say that the "mind rules the body," we mean that the mental and the emotional bodies which together comprise our "mind," dictate the functioning of the physical body.
2. Trauma empowers the emotional body, effecting dominance over the mental body. When trauma is present, the emotional body is "energized" to cope with the impending threat, overriding conscious, rational thought for purposes of safety and self-defense. Consequently, the mental body can only influence the traumatized emotional body in a limited behavioral way.
3. The emotional body and the spiritual body are profoundly connected. Resolution of trauma in the emotional body is, oftentimes, the path to spiritual awakening.

As we investigate the impact of trauma, the close connection of these four "bodies" will become apparent. It is the intimate interplay of these four aspects of self that allow the fluid movement from a body sensation to the unresolved perceptions and emotions encoded in the trauma scene. Access to these scenes, pregnant with the stored physical sensations, emotions, thoughts, perceptions and beliefs of an earlier time and place, enables us to change these outdated messages of trauma to those which reflect a more authentic sense of self. Let us examine these principles in more detail.

The body tells the truth to ego.

Principle One: The Mind Rules the Body

Deservedly, this principle has received much attention. The work of Deepak Chopra, Andrew Weil, Bernie Siegel, Ernest Rossi, Louise Hay and many others has left an indelible imprint on our self-understanding.[5] Few now contest that the "mind" rules the body. The study of trauma induction has led me, however, to the need for a further clarification of this concept. The word "mind" has a variety of meanings. Among the most common definitions for "mind" are the following:

1. The consciousness that originates in the brain and directs mental and physical behavior.
2. Memory; recollection.
3. Conscious thoughts, attention.
4. Opinion or intentions.
5. Intellect; intelligence.
6. Mental or emotional health; sanity.[6]

According to these diverse definitions, the notion that the "mind rules the body" could be interpreted in very different ways. We could interpret "mind" to be the consciousness that directs mental and physical behavior (#1), though, as we have seen, it is the repressed content stored in the subconscious through trauma that often exerts far more influence than the conscious mind; in cases of conflict between the conscious and subconscious, it is the latter which dominates. Perhaps we simply mean, therefore, that "memory" rules the body (#2). This second definition would certainly give us cause to take a closer look at the dynamics and influence of trauma memories, particularly in light of the scientific claim that the body is one hundred percent memory. Mind is also equated with conscious thought (#3) – with intellect and intelligence (#5). These two definitions of "mind," while commonly accepted, are reductionistic in their pure rationality and fail to include the important component of emotion. Both emotionality and rationality are important for healthy decision-making. The task of rendering judgments or opinions – that is, the "making up of one's mind," is alluded to in the fourth definition. This same definition speaks of "intentions;" we will examine the crucial issue of how trauma impacts our intentionality in Chapter Twelve. In the sixth definition, we see the inclusion of emotion as part of the understanding of "mind." When we use this term, therefore, what are we saying, precisely?

When I use the term "mind," I refer to the combined influence of both the intellectual and emotional bodies. This understanding involves more than thought, intellect, or intelligence, for it includes the integral component of emotion and incorporates the more expansive "consciousness" that honors the "subconscious" and its powerful intentionality. When I say, therefore, that the mind rules or controls the physical body, I am affirming the combined impact of the emotional and intellectual bodies over the physical body. The word "mental" comes from the Latin term "mens" meaning "mind."[7] This can be a source of confusion. When I speak specifically of the "mental body," I am using our more common understanding of the intellect or intelligence, as in the fifth definition, and I am not equating it with "mind." A clear grasp of this notion is essential for understanding the dynamics of trauma induction. "Mind" is that greater, combined consciousness created by the interaction of both the emotional and the mental (intellectual) bodies with their concomitant conscious and subconscious intentionality. But why is this distinction so essential?

If we are told, for instance, that health is simply a matter of "mind over body," but are not provided with the knowledge that "mind" includes the emotions and the intellect, we may be given the false impression that a thought alone has the power to heal the physical body. This can, in fact, be the case when there is no opposition or resistance from the subconscious mind. The subconscious mind is the operator through which all intentions from the conscious mind are routed on the journey to empowerment and enlightenment. When, however, our conscious intention is confronted by the subconscious, the subconscious mind routinely wins, particularly when it is empowered by trauma. While we do not want to underestimate the power of the intellect, a distortion manifesting as trauma in the emotional body cannot simply be corrected by a thought originating in the mental body. Minor distortions may dissolve with changes in our thoughts and cognition, but experiences encoded as actual trauma will not. The mental body can only be effective if it has the cooperation and support of the other bodies – the spiritual and emotional bodies. When the emotional and spiritual bodies are in alignment with and supportive of the mental body – that is, when the trauma-induced blockages are removed, thought creates without interference from the subconscious. Subsequently, healing can occur on the physical level when these "higher bodies" so influencing the physical body come into harmony. With alignment and consent of all these aspects of ourselves, illnesses can be healed.

When we state that we "create our own reality," we must, therefore, be careful to note that we are speaking of all the bodies that contribute to the creative process. The confused situations that we manifest externally in our daily lives mirror the internal conflicts within these aspects of our consciousness. Often we are unaware of the tensions between the beliefs of the spiritual body, the messages imprinted from childhood in the emotional body, and the old Newtonian thinking imprinted in our intellect. Yet, we are surprised when we cannot heal ourselves.

I believe that the key to unlocking our healing potential involves removing the constraints imposed by trauma encoded in the emotional body. The fragmentation that occurs to the emotional body via trauma results in a "splitting" of consciousness and intentionality. When "standoffs" occur due to opposing intentions, the subconscious will always win. The emotional body is the principal agent of the process of trauma induction. The instantaneous awareness of feeling "overwhelmed" to the point that the individual's traditional coping mechanisms become ineffectual, creates a trauma. At the critical moment that the individual's boundaries are violated, the limbic-hypothalamic system in the brain reacts automatically to contain and immobilize the overwhelming experience to prevent further damage or even death. When this internal "emotional warning system" is activated, an "ego-state" is immediately created. This fragment of the "ego" is a protected, contained form of "me" – preserving my "reality" as an altered state of consciousness. It is the acute emotional state that cues the system for the encoding and containment of the scene) The fragility of the moment which necessitates this protective encoding is created by intense emotional pain. Once encoded, these feelings and this aspect of consciousness will endure intact along with all the sensory data about self, the environment, the perceived threat, and the accompanying emotions –fully preserved until they are effectively resolved.

Initially, frustration motivated my research into trauma resolution approaches. I was baffled by the fact that an inordinate number of my clients returned to therapy, repeating the same stories over and over as though they refused to release them. At times I felt angry, only later realizing that my anger was at myself for my inability to better assist my clients in their pain. My traditional training failed to provide the necessary tools for this work. By continuing to observe survivors, I discovered that their refusal to release the pain was not a conscious one. Their emotional bodies continued to hold the memories of trauma intact, while their mental bodies tried to process them at a safe distance, not wanting to be retraumatized by having to re-live them. Cognitive therapies produced only minimal success, mostly by providing limited behavioral management for self-destructive impulses. The traditional "Rational-Emotive Therapy" of Albert Ellis, for example, succeeded in predisposing the conscious mind for change, particularly when the emotional body was willing to support the reasoning or thoughts, but was clearly unable to resolve the core feelings induced from the trauma. They continued to resurface. Similarly, affirmations were ineffective without the underlying support of the emotional body. They did, however, help to create a predisposition for change and often facilitated the emergence of the trauma memory by fostering safety and intrapersonal strengthening. Effective resolution of the encoded affect, however, was still needed. In order to better grasp the mysterious resistance mechanisms of my clients, I began to explore the nature and depth of the imprinting that occurred at the moment of trauma.

The encoding that occurs during trauma induction is initiated by the emotional body through the limbic-hypothalamic system. This imprint extends to the cells and electromagnetic fields of the body. Only now in our evolution are we learning ways to use our minds to reach into and to change the messages on the cellular level. "Biofeedback" has shown us that focusing our minds on any particular part of our bodies can immediately result in an increase in body temperature in that part of the body. Similarly, the imprint of trauma, occasioned by our mind sending the message to a particular nerve plexus to "stop," "freeze," or "contain" a feeling, carries immense power. Through biofeedback, many individuals have been taught to reduce the symptoms of their chronic pain, to manage stress and trauma symptoms. By learning how to alter our states of consciousness, we can produce remarkable changes in our bodies. At long last we are learning to extend the principle of "mind over body" to the cellular level.

There is a "cellular mind" which rules the cells of our bodies with incredible sophistication; it governs the functioning of the cell.[8] It would appear that the holographic principle extends to this cellular level, with these tiny units of life reflecting the consciousness of the whole. Recall that each of these cells already contains the biochemical picture of the whole self (i.e., DNA, RNA). Do we expect less on the level of consciousness? The group of cells which store a trauma are capable of arresting and storing intact the whole of an experience: sight, sounds, smell, touch, taste, body size, attire, environment, all participants, all emotions occurring within the perceptual field, all relative space and time perspectives. By focusing on the cells in our body which encode our traumas, we access the holographic fragments of our memories. Such fragments are the storage mechanisms of our experiences. We have already learned that, by focusing on specific cells in certain areas of our bodies, we can change our heart rates, blood pressure, temperature, threshold for pain, etc. Now we have discovered ways to focus on nerve centers to quickly enter encoded states of consciousness and change them. The physical body is the manifestation of mind, of consciousness. As we recognize and explore this intimate relationship between the mind and the body, the transformation and the healing of our consciousness and, subsequently, of our bodies becomes possible.

Principle Two: Trauma Empowers the Emotional Body, Effecting Dominance Over the Mental Body.

Founded in professional and personal exposure to trauma, I hold this principle to be of singular importance for the healing of body, mind, and spirit. Among my first observations upon entering work with trauma survivors was the evident "irrationality" of their behaviors and coping mechanisms. Despite every rational effort to change their behaviors, address their addictions/compulsivity and amend their lifestyles, they continued to manifest the same dysfunctional patterns. Case after case reinforced this awareness until the force empowering these behaviors emerged.

Frustration over her inability to quit smoking catapulted Myra into therapy. She provided every possible reason for quitting smoking, including a frightening bout with cancer. To her credit she had managed to alleviate the physiological craving for nicotine using nicotine "patches." She had also tried acupuncture and hypnosis. Nonetheless, she continued smoking despite all of her efforts and rational determination. Her inability to alter her behaviors indicated the possibility that her smoking was related to a deeper emotional imprint or trauma. Tenacious holding on to debilitating addictive behaviors routinely is rooted in unresolved trauma experience. The related compulsive behaviors are frequently "locked in" to the psyche by an emotional trauma which links the need to medicate with a traumatic event. When the trauma goes unresolved, the impulse to medicate remains intact as well, consistently stored in the subconscious. This becomes particularly problematic when the memory is amnesial and the trauma and the need to medicate it are forgotten. After Myra described her efforts to quit smoking, I offered her the opportunity to explore the origins of her smoking within the context of her personal history. I asked her where in her body she felt this ongoing need to smoke. She immediately identified her chest area, "on the inside ... like a black emptiness." When she focused on this metaphor, she reverted to the age of eighteen. When I asked her where she was when she first felt this feeling, she suddenly clasped her hands to her mouth and said:

I'm at my best friend's house when I first felt this feeling. (Pause) Oh my God! I didn't realize that my smoking was connected to this. It was the last time my stepfather ever physically abused me. He beat me so badly that I ran away from home to my friend's house. I never went back home again; I moved out. I was so glad to be away from home and so angry at what he had done to me. Smoking calmed me down; it kind of grounded me and helped me to deal with it all. It was kind of an act of defiance too! I guess I need to talk to the eighteen year old part of myself and let her know that it's 1996, and we don't have to smoke any more to feel safe or independent. The abusive marriage that I've been in hasn't helped my smoking either. I can see why I couldn't stop. I married my stepfather. It's not about smoking; it's about safety and calm. Now that I'm on my own and creating my own life, it's OK to stop. I just can't believe it was so obvious a connection and I couldn't see it.

This is a recurring pattern with addictions and compulsive behaviors. Traumas to the emotional body lock in feelings and perceptions that leave us with an urgent need to medicate. This is true in the majority of cases of "smokers" for whom the "patch" failed. It is really quite simple. The very first stage of addiction is "psychological dependency." Physiological dependency comes later and increases over time. Traumatic experiences lock into the psyche the need, the obsession for whatever drug, experience, or behavior served to medicate the original pain. In addition, undue attention, shaming, or humiliation can "energize" even a healthy coping behavior to the point of compulsivity. Ridicule, shame, humiliation, sarcasm, and insensitivity can traumatize a person to the point where he or she will begin to obsess over the behavior – giving it more and more attention and energy, ensuring its continuance and locking it into the psyche. Indeed, **trauma can create psychological dependency – the first stage of addiction.** This theory has not yet been fully integrated into treatment modalities for addicts. If you have difficulty with a compulsive pattern, whether with food, drugs, work, sex, religion, gambling, relationships, perfectionism, or other, track it back to its point of origin. This is, perhaps, the most powerful relapse prevention technique that we have available.

The "life or death" struggle that is internalized in the psyche at a moment of trauma transmits an urgent message that says, "Unless you stop this pain, you will die.(The intensity of the experience and its content will determine the degree of compulsivity we feel in our urge to medicate.) Our rational efforts to change these "state-bound" scenes within our memories will meet with limited success. In the "right order of things," we would like to see ourselves making rational decisions from the highest level of self-understanding, with empathy for others and a healthy acceptance of our limitations, backed by a storehouse full of resources. Trauma, however, seems to throw an obstacle into our best laid plans. Yet all is not lost! Our imbalances can serve as cues or maps to direct us in the healing process. The obsessive thoughts, the compulsive coping mechanisms that we evidence in our daily lives are the likely indicators of an unresolved issue or trauma within our psyche. I have worked with many individuals who, like Myra, above, were completely immobilized in their efforts to abstain – thwarted at every turn by some inexplicable factor until they identified and resolved the precipitating trauma. They abided in this morass until they realized that the blockage was coming from an unresolved issue – a fear of abandonment, anger, neglect, physical or sexual abuse which was encoded in the emotional body from a previous trauma. These imprints in our emotional bodies carry immense energy and can easily deter the best rational efforts of our seven percent conscious minds.

It becomes clear that the conscious rationality of the "mental body" cannot resolve the patterns subconsciously locked into the "emotional body" from unresolved traumas. The mental body cannot influence the emotional body except in a limited behavioral way. It cannot change the content of energy stored in the emotional body, but it can, for instance, be instrumental in altering behavior in such a way as to predispose us for emotional change.

While studying in the seminary, my spiritual director suggested that I pursue yoga. He understood that when I could not change my emotional body (traumas) directly, I could use the postures of my physical body to improve physical and mental functioning so as to predispose me for deeper emotional and attitudinal change. In yoga, this is accomplished by certain postures and breathing exercises which improve the balance of the respiratory and glandular systems of the body. While I could not, at that stage of my life, change my emotional body by mental intention, I exercised limited influence over my behaviors and disposition for emotion. However, the trauma-induced blockages did not resolve through the yoga. Over the years I have had the opportunity to work with clients who have studied with Tibetan masters, but who could not progress beyond a certain point in their meditation. Certain blockages present in the emotional body could not be directly resolved through meditation.[9] In fact, the blockages consistently emerged as the other "bodies" moved into alignment. Meditation which effectively accesses the trauma-induced trance state and is used to resolve it can accomplish this, but this requires some initial training or facilitation. Meditation can achieve resolution if it teaches us to work effectively within holographic space – teaching us how to alter our states of consciousness so as to heal ourselves. Meditation merely as an act of the intellect or "mental body" becomes an exercise in frustration (I know this personally) and cannot, alone, accomplish the resolution of a trauma memory. As Chris Griscom indicates, we can use the mental body in a way to constrict, to control, to hide, to alter our behavior, but the mental body does not orchestrate or control the emotional body.[10] With respect to trauma or "frozen feelings," it cannot decrystallize emotions or dissolve them, because that part of the mental body operates on certain horizontal planes with a specific linearity that does not allow emotional decrystallization.[11]

The emotional body derives much of its initial power from the concept: emotion is prior in the developmental process. Thought is posterior or secondary in early childhood development. I have found it most interesting to work with very early pre-verbal trauma. Maintaining a light state of co-consciousness, the adult self with highly developed mental faculties can access and articulate the original crystallized body of emotions that occurred before the developing child was capable of formulating thought or speech. Now that such skills are developed, the stored emotions can be articulated and released.

The predominance of the emotional body over the mental body as a result of trauma induction becomes paramount when we attempt to understand why, despite our best efforts to convince ourselves intellectually of the need to change our behavior, we repeat the pattern. A mental intention to change remains only that – an intention, without the support of the emotional body. Imprints in the emotional body cannot be resolved in the mental body. Emotional imprints are on a deeper level and do not respond to the linear thinking of the intellect. Emotional imprints from trauma, in fact, are often totally incomprehensible to the intellect. The intellect may not have a clue as to why I feel the need to bathe compulsively five times a day or eat continuously, but the emotional body, when accessed, discloses that this is my way of coping with the abuse. Certain "irrational" fears, behaviors, and impulses are the cues to the imprints or metaphors of trauma encoded in the emotional body. The mental body cannot resolve what it does not know exists. We often use our mental bodies, in fact, to avoid dealing with the emotional body and its "burdens." One of my most common defenses was to avoid dealing with emotions and trauma by focusing all of my attention on the development of my intellect or mental body. Dissociation, losing oneself in the intellect or mental body, is a common defense mechanism. This intellectualization repeatedly manifests in messages like "forgive and forget," "why bother – the past is over and done with, and you can't change it," "just accept what happened and get on with your life," or "just don't think about it and it will go away." These mental messages only foster further repression and disrespect for the actual power of the emotional body and the true nature of human emotion. As a stored form of energy, the emotional body can only be changed by working within it. The sense of hopelessness suffered by many is due, in part, to our lack of respect for the emotional body and the impotence evidenced in trying to resolve trauma from the mental body (intellect). Forgiveness is, foremost, a matter of the heart, not of the intellect. No amount of "forgiveness" that simply comes as a mental act will have any impact on or heal the emotional body – and the proof is that the feelings about the event or perpetrator will be wholly unchanged. Little of the "forgiveness" that I offered as a priest had any major impact on resolving core behaviors induced from emotional trauma. The penitents soon returned seeking more forgiveness for the same behaviors locked within their emotional bodies. We know now that the emotional body must be healed <u>from within itself</u> and not merely by an appeal to the mental body. We also know that authentic access to the emotional body can resolve the old trauma-induced "triggers," phobias, compulsivities, and the emotional shadows of the past that have continued to haunt us.

Principle Three: The Emotional Body and Spiritual Body Are Profoundly Connected – Resolution of Trauma in the Emotional Body Is Often the Path to Spiritual Awakening.

During my training for ministry, it was emphasized that there are no "good" or "bad" feelings. Feelings are never "immoral." They are "a-moral" or non-moral. They simply are. What we do with our feelings determines the morality. Judgment of our feelings is based upon our associations with pain. We have come to judge painful feelings as "bad" due to the discomfort they cause. The truth is that all of our feelings have immeasurable purpose and value. To a society so bent on the avoidance of pain, this may sound like a death knell. The fact remains that the resolution of trauma would be impossible without the warning signs which point out its presence. Now we know how to identify and resolve these containers of trauma without having to relive such pain. Pain is often the first indication of something to be learned, of blockages to be resolved. Instead of responding to these cues to healing, we spend fifteen or twenty years avoiding our pain, the very warning signs that are trying to tell us that something is surfacing for attention within our consciousness. When we finally acknowledge the warning signs and choose not to medicate our discomfort, we discover that the memory surfacing has nothing to do with personal defectiveness, but, instead, involves an experience that left a distortion that is appearing in order to be healed. Few of us were taught this during our emotional development.

Emotions are the gateways to higher levels of consciousness. They provide the energy needed to propel thoughts from the inner, non-physical world into the outer, physical or "objective" world. They are relational bridges – the gateways to the nonphysical, to the spiritual body. Though I may not know everything about myself or about you, we are, nonetheless, able to enter into a relationship based on a deeper foundation – a "felt" connection. On a higher level, emotions actually transcend words and categories. They are pre-verbal in our development and often seem greatly reduced when expressed in finite language. Consider the vague uses and misapplications of the word "love," for instance. Still, emotions are an experiential and relational bridge to non-physical realities. Many of the spiritual experiences that we have felt cannot be communicated through words. Reducing them to limited expressions or vocabulary of the linear mental body does them an injustice and fails to communicate the total experiential nature of what occurred.

Throughout much of my life I was encouraged to seek the spiritual, but the impression was given to me that this path was largely contingent upon mental acuity – being intelligent enough, correctly articulating theological truths, completing a certain curriculum, learning and following the rules, talkin' the talk and walkin' the walk, etc. All the while, certain messages were communicated by family, educational, religious, and societal systems – trusted entities – about control, repression, and avoidance of emotion. Many of these messages were subtle, but they were consistent and internalized. They were precepts continued by my religious system which fostered an underlying message indicating that controlled emotional expression was allowed, but that excessive emotional displays were highly inappropriate, particularly for priests. A certain "holy detachment" from emotion was to be sought. Looking back on these messages and influences, I see clearly how they fostered emotional repression and resulted in obsession and compulsivity.

One of the essential criteria for determining whether a system is fostering spirituality or spiritual abuse is its approach to emotion. If a system is inducing fear of human emotion, the very key to spiritual development, something is gravely wrong. The incidence of religious systems which ostensibly foster spirituality while instilling messages that create emotional repression in their followers is tragic. Through a deep need for spiritual nourishment, we may entrust ourselves uncritically to those who claim to provide the keys to spiritual enlightenment. Unfortunately, "holy detachment" comes perilously close to emotional repression. I find it reassuring that Jesus found close companionship with individuals who lived emotionally "on the edge" and that he had such strong condemnation for the "whitened sepulchers" of the "hardhearted" religious of his time. "Spiritual incest" is committed when those claiming the service of spiritual ministry to others "in the name of God," utilize their power and authority to foster emotional repression. Though it may be unintentional, it is, nonetheless, abusive. Authentic spirituality recognizes the importance of honoring all emotions as keys to healing and wholeness.

Emotions allow us to experience deep within ourselves a significant sense of connection with All That Is. It is the openness to our own emotions that allows the blockages to higher consciousness to come to light. At times it seems that it would be much easier if the main channel of contact with the spiritual dimension was the mental body. Then it could simply be a matter of learning the right scriptural verse, of finding the right equation, without having to invest ourselves emotionally – taking risks and being vulnerable to pain. Authentic spiritual encounter is profoundly emotional by its nature. Over the centuries, we have excluded entire dimensions of spiritual experience from our repertoire by repressing certain emotions and/or failing to integrate certain emotional energies. Emotional repression fosters spiritual repression. We wondered, for instance, why we did not see greater manifestation of the "gifts of spirit" such as healing, while we were communicating sexually repressive messages. That very center of a spiritual being which generates the power to create and heal was being repressed in the same breath. In the Eastern religions, it is the channeling of the energy at the base of the spine – the "kundalini," that energizes the system to access the resources employed in healing and higher states of meditation. The "physics of the soul" dictates that we cannot bypass the emotional and manifest the spiritual. What one ends up with if one attempts to do so is illness and/or addiction. This is how our psyches let us know that something within is not balanced.

Upon leaving formal ministry in the Catholic church, I did not understand why my awareness of the electromagnetic fields in my hands emerged at that time. I now know that I was repressing a tremendous amount of energy in my efforts to deal, first, with the series of personal traumas that I spoke of earlier; second, to integrate the energies incumbent with celibacy; and, third, to deal with the many demands of a rapidly changing ministerial lifestyle. I now see quite clearly that the emotional blockages had to be removed in order for me to find a balance with the powerful creative energies of my life. As these blockages began to be resolved, my conscious connection to the spiritual realm intensified. My spiritual growth advanced rapidly; my hands offered proof.

As soon as we begin to open ourselves to our emotions, we can resolve the blockages present. This allows us access to our intuition. Intuition is a far-reaching knowing that resembles "feeling" in its power to transcend words. It is a heightened sense of knowing that feels greatly reduced when limited to words. Intuition cannot be fully accessed without authentic openness to our emotions. Over time we come to discover that the security we seek does not reside, primarily, in the improved functioning of the mental body, though this can certainly be used to "tide us over," but in the openness to our emotional body which provides unlimited access and knowledge about the past, present, and future. In embracing our emotions, we come into greater and greater interplay with our intuition. Eventually, we come to realize that **true security resides in trusting our intuition.**

I had always been fascinated with the wonderful things that my mother evidenced intuitively and that my religious system taught me about the "mystics and ascetics" of spiritual tradition, but I could never understand why these things were not more evident in my life and in the lives of the ministers around me. Perhaps, I thought, these intuitive abilities were just for the "gifted" or the "worthy," as my religious system had implied. I now know that they are accessible to all. In the "shutting down" of the emotional channels of our consciousness through the traumas begun during childhood, the intuitive access that was easily available to us as children diminished. For myself, as soon as I chose to begin opening the emotional valves that had been closed by trauma in the physical, mental, and emotional bodies, the energy began flowing. I feel enormous spiritual connection in my life today, and the path is becoming clearer as my intuition strengthens. This too is available to all.

I think fondly of my friend and former professor, Father Janusz Ihnatowicz, S.T.D. I was an avid student of his course entitled, "Mystics, Ascetics, and Ordinary Christians." He possessed a great wit matched by his powerful mind. I remember the peculiar feeling that I experienced when I tried to understand why the so-called "mystical gifts" were not manifest in modern times. My religious system generally explained that they were gifts given by God's mysterious choice only to a select few and that they could not be "earned." Fr. Ihnatowicz's observation was that there was an "ordinary mysticism" that was openly accessible to all. I have had the privilege to meet many active "mystics" since that time and have come to believe that we are each called to this spiritual power and mysticism. This invitation is a natural step in our spiritual evolution, an exigency inherent in our nature as spiritual beings.

By embracing our trauma memories and the emotional shadows of our traumas, we open the gateway to higher mind and higher consciousness. This means that anything that we do to nurture our emotional bodies will be profoundly spiritual in its impact and will foster well-being on all other levels. Emotions are the access to the multi-dimensional self. They open the door to access the healer within. Feelings allow us to climb the ladder to the multi-dimensional self and to unite with that aspect of self. From such a union, all things become possible.

Chapter Eleven

Man is a fallen god who remembers the heavens.
Alphonse de Lamartine (1790 - 1869)

The Spiritual Implications of Trauma

We have seen in the previous chapters that we are multidimensional beings of light and energy who are capable of sustaining varied levels of consciousness simultaneously. Such a capacity affords us the opportunity to perform many of the operations of the psyche concurrently – from long-term structuring of goals, to crisis management, creative expression, spiritual development, problem solving, pain management, emotional development, and trauma resolution, among many others. Few examples serve to advance our appreciation of this multidimensional nature as does our capacity to deal with trauma. The expert management of the overwhelming experiences of our lives is a riveting attestation to the power of this polymorphous nature. Such multi-dimensional existence means that within our minds or consciousness, "ego-states" can exist that were created to contain our overwhelming experiences. These aspects of ourselves, the orphans of trauma, have not yet been fully integrated nor balanced within the whole. This means that, depending on the number of ego states, the subconscious, which comprises upwards of ninety-three percent of our mind, will be empowered by these unintegrated forms of "I." Depending on the number, nature, and emotional content of the encoded scenes, these ego-states possess the capability to dominate our choices and virtually "run our show." This means that the conscious mind, which constitutes approximately seven percent of our mind, will be dominated primarily by the subconscious ego states that surface for expression. At the same time, however, the deeper function of the mind that we call "spiritual" seeks to draw these unintegrated aspects of self to the surface for purposes of healing. "Flashbacks" and "body memories," therefore, are not signs that we are "going crazy," but, rather, the very means by which the "Higher Self" or "self-seeking-integration" will identify for us the spiritual or integrative work that needs to be done in order to achieve wholeness. Some refer to this recurring sensation as a "still small voice." On the one hand, there is an aspect of self that has been and will always be whole (sometimes referred to as "Higher Self" or "Soul") which communicates on a profound level via intuition, feelings and experiences. The reciprocal is the wounded self which, with its finite vision, often fails to see the spiritual value of "flashbacks," "body memories," or any other painful occurrences.

The greatest spiritual, mental, emotional, and physical harm that comes from trauma occurs from the prolonged effect of carrying this arrested, static form of complex energy and memory within our nervous systems. We carry it until we identify ourselves with the trauma and lose touch with our higher consciousness. We then become the shame, the brokenness. Such is the power of our minds. What we pour our thought and energy into we become. The opposite of spirituality is not "sin." We all make mistakes and must face certain moral struggles. But the greatest opponent of spirituality is the total identification with and experience of shame that induces a sense of worthlessness and despair, separating us from our Higher Self. It is this phenomenon which fosters isolation within and estrangement from the Divine Mind which encompasses all. It is an illusion, a false perception induced by a shame experience that convinces the child/adolescent/adult self that he is not a being of light, of infinite value and worth – an expression of the One Light that encompasses and embraces all. The frozen trauma, when it presents itself to our consciousness for healing, is interpreted as: "There's something wrong with me … I must be bad, broken, dirty." This self-assessment is easy for the child whose boundaries are already fragile and whose way of learning is self-referencing (meaning that the world revolves around "me"). In the child's mind, if something bad happens, it "must be about me."

This shame induction process has been well researched by Gershen Kaufman, who wrote his doctoral dissertation at Michigan State University on the psychological impact of shame.[1] Kaufman's research suggests that shame alienates the self from the self.[2] This concept corresponds precisely with the dynamics of trauma induction described above. I believe that Kaufman's description of shame induction is really a description of the emotional dynamics of the trauma induction process. Trauma induces "shame," an internal sense of wrongness or defectiveness. This "wrongness" is often associated with moral failure, though it is pre-moral in its induction. Shame is induced on the emotional level and is more profound in its impact than any moral failure or "sinful" behavior. Shame is far more detrimental to spirituality than "sin." In fact, shame induction often begins in a dysfunctional family long before the child is capable of "sin." Psychologists place the age of moral reasoning at seven or eight years old. Children often have shame induced long before the age of moral choice. By the age of four, I had internalized a great deal of my father's shame and was a miniature version of his personality which had been shaped by numerous unresolved abuse issues. He could have been diagnosed as an "avoidant-dependent personality" when it was really unresolved trauma that resided at the heart of his struggle. Nevertheless, I imitated him; he was my developmental model. Consequently, I was "shy" like my father; which was verbally reinforced by my family. A child's internalization of another's shame is easily comprehensible when we realize that we are "designed" to learn by imitating everything that we see and hear in our early years of development. This is how we, as children, learn our primary language so quickly; we hear and repeat – initially, without fear. During my youth I innocently bore a trace of a Southern Louisiana ("Cajun") accent. Once I realized that individuals sometimes were ridiculed in school when they spoke in such a manner, I made a conscious effort to change it. We learn rapidly as children because we internalize all that we see and feel. When we innocently internalize emotionally shaming messages and perceptions from significant others, we begin to narrow our emotional, intuitive, and spiritual channels of communication. As young children, trauma induction is fostered by the following factors: 1) our fragile "boundaries" which are still in formation; 2) exposure to the unresolved abuse issues of our parents which repeatedly are "acted out" in front of us and which we internalize and imitate – for example, domestic violence, chronic depression or rage, pain avoidance through medication or denial, etc.; and 3) internalization of shame through repeated exposure to patterns of emotional repression. This last factor is even more pronounced if the negative modeling is from the same sex parent or the parent with whom the child most identifies.

A number of significant observations can be made from observing the dynamics of shame induction and resolution. Anything that leads to the release of internalized shame feelings has a profound spiritual impact. Any experience that fosters an "alienation of self from self," likewise, impacts the other two dimensions of relationality. The three dimensions of relationality-spirituality-intimacy are: 1) relationship to self, 2) relationship to others, and 3) relationship to Higher Power. These relationships are not as distinct as was once thought. They form a whole. Trauma will always impact all three spiritual dimensions. These relationships can be seen in Diagram A, p. 184. To be alienated from oneself is also to become estranged from others and from one's Higher Power. In the case of trauma, the alienation and splitting that occurs results in a loss of integration, a fragmentation. The alienation of self from the self produces the result seen in Diagram B, p. 185, designated by S1 (Self 1) and S2 (Self 2). S1 is the original state of relationship, whereas S2 is the withdrawal and estrangement that occurs as a result of the trauma. In the case of an addiction, for instance, the addict is drawn increasingly into the shame cycle and becomes more and more alienated from self, emotions, family, partner, and Higher Power. Addicts have shown me that addiction results in the repression of feelings to a level that formally constitutes "trauma" or a cumulative static emotional state, fostering denial and delusion, accompanied by increasing isolation. If this cycle continues and no intervention is made to stop the downward spiral, "emotional death" and, eventually, physical death ensues. One can see from Diagram B that this increasing isolation in the direction of S2 results in loss of relationship with self, others, and Higher Power simultaneously. This type of delusion or alienation from one's own

Diagram A: The Three Dimensions of Spirituality (Intimacy)

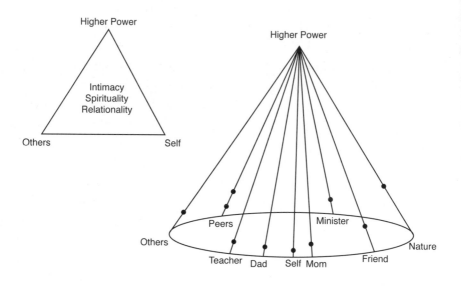

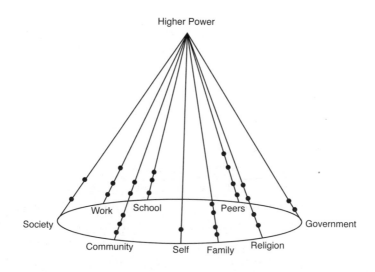

Diagram B: The Multi-dimensional Effects of Trauma

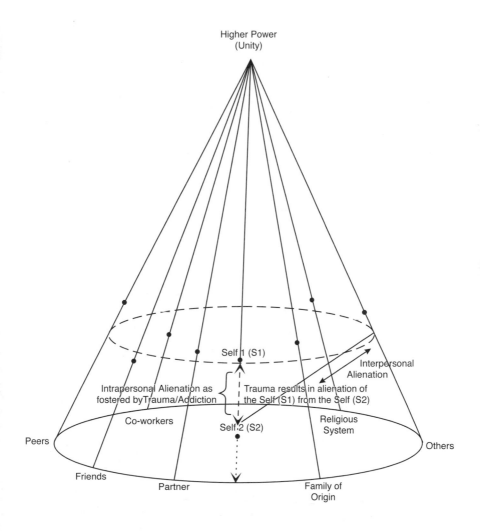

Diagram B: Increasing isolation from Self, Others, and Higher Power. While the connection with Higher Power cannot be severed, physical death can occur.

186

Diagram C: Reintegration through the Healing of Trauma

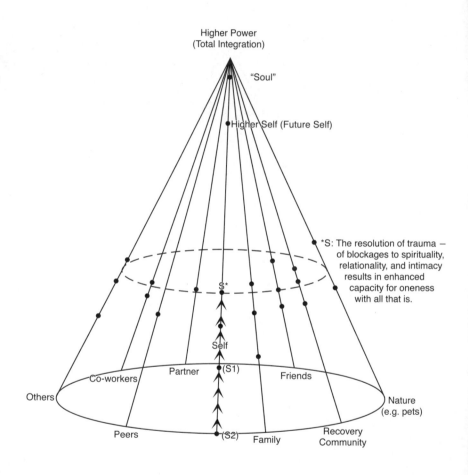

Diagram C: Trauma resolution fosters reintegration with Self in movement towards True Self. This results in increased intimacy with Self, Others, and Higher Power. Movement is from the disintegrated state experienced as S2, toward increasing integration at SI, S, and Higher.

truth will, inevitably, result in both intrapersonal (within the self) and interpersonal (between persons) loss of intimacy, even relationship. As in the case of physical or sexual abuse, to be treated as an object for another person's gratification causes a confusion or "mixed message" reaction that results in the S1-S2 type splitting. An individual may have been told throughout her life that she was "lovable and precious," but here she is being treated as a "thing" by the very persons who are supposed to be loving her. This is perhaps most poignantly seen in the case of incest, where the very persons who are claiming to provide love for the child abuse her. At S2 the victim induces the message that she is "an object for other peoples' gratification." Is it any surprise that the abused individual may then grow up to treat others as objects for her gratification?

Kaufman, in his research on shame induction, adds a most important point: "Shame is a <u>primary</u> affect."[3] This means that once induced, this feeling dominates or controls emotions and the nervous system in such a way that no other emotion can hold priority. Coming from a shame-based family, this means that efforts to compliment me will be met with skepticism and suspicion because "I know that this compliment isn't true ... I know what I'm really like inside, so what you're saying can't be true." Since healthy nurturing messages cannot penetrate this primary feeling of shame, the individual will then, by necessity, have to develop alternative ways of coping in order to survive. John Bradshaw, in his book, <u>Healing the Shame that Binds You</u>, demonstrates the many defenses of the psyche against the disintegrative nature of shame and trauma.[4] The reason that shame is a "primary" emotion is due to the dynamics of trauma induction. If shame is dominant in the psyche, it is certain that some manner of trauma has occurred.

I use a broad definition of trauma that includes: 1) the understanding that trauma is relative to the perceptual field of the observer – that is, what traumatizes a child may seem trivial to the adult, and 2) that anything that constitutes actual energy blockage, whether intentional or accidental, is legitimately "trauma." There are profound spiritual, emotional, and moral repercussions from this understanding of trauma. For example, often we see trauma survivors "beating themselves up" or being blamed because they have not been able to "forgive" or release their emotional pain. Those commanding the need to forgive frequently have no awareness of the nature of trauma induction or the power held by the subconscious mind of the trauma survivor. For millennia, survivors have been judged for not "forgiving and forgetting" when, in reality, no mental deliberation or decision could resolve a trauma induced in the emotional body. As discussed in the previous chapter, the cognitive cannot resolve the affective nature of the encoded trauma. True "forgiveness," therefore, must involve respect for the uniquely individual timetable required for the authentic healing and resolution of the trauma, not just a sincere verbalization of the concept of forgiveness.

Those who perceive and treat the spirituality of the person without regard for this multidimensional nature are likely to foster shame – the antithesis of authentic spiritual experience. This constitutes spiritual abuse!   Let us remember the millions of alcoholics over the centuries whose disease was fostered and accelerated by the moral harangue that was supposed to shame them out of their "willful drunkenness." There are many churches that continue to rely on this approach. We now know that shaming someone can, indeed, alter his behavior, but it <u>increases compulsivity</u>. By shaming us into "appropriate moral behavior" many religious systems have created and sustained the very emotional dynamics which they sought to alleviate. Similarly, many parents, with the best of intentions, continue to employ age-old shaming language in attempts to elicit attitudinal and behavioral changes in children. While the desired behavior may be achieved, the self-worth of the child is undermined.

Perhaps the most destructive of all spiritual abuses is the repression of emotion, because emotions constitute the principal spiritual bridge to higher consciousness. We may not be able to "grasp" what the Higher Power is, but we can still experience the relationship via the emotional bridge. If we waited on complete cognitive information about someone before we entered relationship with them, we would never be able to enter into relationship at all. Emotions provide the bridging needed to bond, to connect with the other. Similarly, the repression of emotions – of all emotions including anger, pain, sadness, anxiety, and sexual feelings, for instance, deprives us of our spiritual power. It is most often the emergence of anger that gives a trauma survivor the power, the gift of energy that she needs to re-enter the original scene of pain and to change it. In fact, it is the imbalance created by the inability of the victim to utilize this anger or emotional energy to protect herself during the original trauma that results in getting stuck. Anger often surfaces as we are being violated and can be used to stop or prevent traumatization. This is, however, usually not possible for the child who may have already internalized the message that, "It's not OK to be angry" or that, "Expressing my anger will only make it worse. Hence, the adult client comes into my office feeling defective because of the anger and rage pouring out in current life circumstances.) Rather than discount the anger, I recognize in it the map pointing to the specific unresolved issues and the location of the emotional energy that has been stored up over years. We can become familiar with it and use it in healing the original trauma. In addition, the amount of repressed, stored-up anger is often proportionate to the amount of unresolved trauma stored in the cells and fields of the body. When my clients cannot access anger over their abuse, we have problems with the resolution process, for this usually indicates damage to the adult/parent ego-state that is needed for resolving the traumas.)The messages conveyed by family, religious, educational and societal systems that anger is wrong fosters spiritual and emotional abuse.

Another common message, usually shared with the intention of empowering us, is the statement that "we create our own reality." While this is a profound truth from the higher spiritual plane, it is often wielded without due appreciation for the true multi-dimensional nature of the person, as evidenced in the simultaneous ego-states we maintain as a result of our traumas. This statement, intended to affirm our personal power to create, when heard, not from our higher spiritual awareness from which we strive to function, but from the wounded ego-states that frequently dominate our day, will only serve to induce greater shame about the perception that we cannot seem to change our reality. We have not recognized until recently that there was a child, adolescent, or adult that was forced to use his creative ability to "freeze" reality at some point(s) in order to survive. This freezing was largely subconscious and automatic, a product of the ninety-three percent influence of the subconscious. **The issue, therefore, is not whether we create our own realities, but how to reconcile the different and even opposing realities that we are creating simultaneously.** The statement about our unlimited power to create our own reality can easily result in further shaming when our conscious mind finds itself overpowered by the subconscious. It is to the wounded ego state that the message of empowerment needs to be communicated. This is, in fact, most effectively accomplished not by positive mental affirmations directed to the adult/parent self, but by actual intervention to recover the integration lost at the moment of trauma itself, which is predominantly a helpless child ego-state. These wounded ego states must be reintegrated under a singular intentionality if we are to cease creating diverse and opposing realities for ourselves. Through internal dialogue with our wounded selves we can actually change the emotional experience that resulted in the loss of integration and resolve the event, thereby restoring our single-mindedness and bringing us closer to the reality – a healed mind and body, for which we strive.

The spiritual implications of the resolution of trauma are tremendous. As I move from an alienated state (S2) to a more integrated position (S1), I grow in relation to self, others, and my Higher Power (See Diagram C, p. 186). The healing process will, therefore, involve experiences on all three levels. Let us examine these levels more closely.

Relationship to Self: Being present to oneself is a simple form of meditation or prayer and is integrative by nature. All of the various ways in which I foster a sense of serenity and integrate my "frozen feelings" bring me closer to my true self. Whatever I do to put me in touch with my own truth moves me closer to Truth. This means that whatever helps me to break through denial and delusion moves me closer to an authentic experience of self, others, and Higher Power. By releasing traumas, moments where I became trapped with my abuser's distorted perceptions, adopting those distortions as my own, I move from the false sense of self which inhibits intimacy and authenticity to a restored self-nurturing perspective. This posture, by its very nature, is more integrated and whole; hence, even the simplest form of meditation, such as focusing on the intake and exhalation of breath – when I take time to be fully present to myself, constitutes a powerful movement toward integration (See Diagram C, p. 186). Efforts at self-help, such as affirmations, therapy, and Twelve Step program participation, accelerate the trauma resolution process. Anything that enhances my self-integration increases my capacity for spiritual and relational growth.

Relationship to Others: The effort that I make to reach out from my trauma-induced isolation to communicate with others also brings me closer to my truth. Often it is at the initiative of others that our first steps in recovery begin. Those who love us may even "intervene on us" to bring us back from the alienation and withdrawal fostered by our unhealthy coping mechanisms. When I am unable to bring myself back, a Twelve Step meeting or communication from a friend will often restore me to a healthier sense of self and dispel the sense of estrangement. Research in clinical sociology now indicates that the success of the Twelve Step programs in addressing addictions is due to the social support system that is created to break through the sense of aloneness and foster reintegration. Spiritual reintegration also occurs through this social transformation. This is not a new concept. In the spiritual literature of many cultures, the "spiritual intimacy principle" affirms that wherever two or more "gather in the name" of the Higher Power, that Power is present. As seen in Diagram C, increased intimacy through others moves me toward greater unity with Higher Power. In Christian literature, the biblical account is given of a man whom Jesus heals through the intercession and faith of two friends who lower him into Jesus' midst by making an opening in the roof of the house (Gospel of Mark 2:1-12). Jesus recognizes the faith of the friends and heals the paralytic. The social intervention of others can bring healing to the self.

Our socialization began with our parents or primary caregivers. Our first experience of intimacy, spirituality, and reality was mediated by them. The realization that our parents are our first "gods," our first "Higher Powers," has profound implications. When, for instance, my father sought to teach me to swim by throwing me into a body of water when I was two and a half years old, my perception was that he was "trying to kill me." This trauma instilled a barrier of distrust between us, but also led me to be suspicious of a god (a "father," I was told) who would let his son die on a cross – the latter just felt remarkably similar to my own abandonment experience. Here again, I rationally and theologically knew better than to believe this, but I could not help but be distrustful of father figures who let their sons die. This distrust was the overriding emotional (subconscious) impact of the trauma. A primary emotional trauma on the level of relationship to others deeply impacts the vertical dimension of relationship to Higher Power and also the relationship to self. Subsequent to my experience with my father, I was terrified of water and certain that something was, therefore, wrong with me. I was also amnesial following the experience and did not understand the origins of my fear, believing, rather, that I was defective. This feeling of personal insufficiency was reinforced when I found myself distrusting my father with no conscious explanation for my feelings.

I have found the following exercise to be very helpful: List five adjectives which describe the mother and father of your childhood. Then list five adjectives to describe "God" as you conceived of him (usually told he is a father or of male gender) during your childhood. If you can come up with no image or description, check to see if there was an absence of the primary caregiver (e.g. death, separation, divorce, etc.). It is not unheard of to find the "abandoned" child in an atheistic or anti-religious (even cult) stance at some point, particularly in adolescence, as an expression of anger based on abandonment. Compare the three lists for possible correlation. For myself, the working definition that I had in my emotional body about what a Higher Power was corresponded to my most common experience of my father – namely, a (usually) gentle physical presence that cared for one's material needs but did not "do" feelings. Here one can see how the spiritual trauma induced by the primary caregivers from the horizontal dimension impacts the vertical, the rapport with Higher Power simultaneously (See Diagram B, p. 185).

For the majority of individuals, the most intense experience of love that they have ever experienced was mediated through other people. Our parents mediated our first experience of love. My self-esteem was first "mirrored" to me through the eyes of my mother. I internalized her expressions, feelings, messages, accent, and attitudes. This formed the foundation for my self-esteem. We were not born co-dependent, we were born dependent. If we did not get the nurturing and love that we needed at certain developmental stages, we became stuck in that stage – the naturally outward-looking posture of the child. This created the pattern called "codependency." **Codependency is the child of trauma** – the product of certain unmet needs and "stuck points" in development. In my life I discovered that the unmet needs from childhood left me looking outward for the solutions, whether that was for surrogate nurturers or for my Higher Power. These realities were surely to be found outside myself, I thought, because my own sense of unworthiness or low self-esteem excluded the self as the place where love would be found. I did not consider myself to be a resource. But just as these early traumas imprinted me with false messages about self, life, love, relationships, and where Higher Power was to be found, so too the healing of these "stuck points" removed many of the obstacles to intimacy and authentic spiritual experience (See Diagram C, p. 186).

With respect to resolving the obstacles to intimacy, it is important to note that there are many solutions now available to us through the creative resources that we are learning to access through the subconscious mind. In light of the fact that the majority of trauma is contained within the subconscious mind, it is not always necessary, even if it is possible, to reconcile face to face with those who traumatized us. (Because of the power of the subconscious mind, it is possible to reconcile or resolve issues even with those who have died or are emotionally or physically inaccessible.) Some of our abusers, to this day, are inappropriate for a face to face confrontation. Alcoholic parents may be less available than they were during our childhood if their disease has progressed, for instance. Irrespective of the level of recovery of another, we can heal. Our subconscious minds readily bear our perpetrators intact and provide the locus needed for the inner confrontation and for resolution. This point also relates to the healing function of dreams which we will examine in Chapter Thirteen.

Relationship to Higher Power: The model that I present of the tripartite relationship between self, others and Higher Power actually originated in the patristic era, around the third century AD. At this time, the "fathers" of the early Christian church were struggling to articulate their understanding of these interrelationships to "God." Their objective involved trying to put their profound spiritual experience into words in order to communicate it faithfully to others. There was much theological speculation and philosophical discussion centered around the language to be used to articulate the truths that they wished to share. It is of our very nature to seek understanding of these "higher" realities, but true understanding resides not so deeply in cognitive apperception as in the total experiencing of the reality itself. True understanding means to see or stand within the "frame of reference" of the other; this means that understanding includes not just the mental, but the emotional as well. While theological speculation can open our minds to consider higher realities, the ultimate objective is experiential. It is in this respect that the vertical dimension of spirituality needs to be addressed.

Anything that fosters relationality fosters spirituality. Further, any experience that enhances my capacity for intimacy will impact my relationships to self, others, and Higher Power. Whatever builds relationship to self and others necessarily builds relationship to Higher Power. I think fondly of the "Anonymous Christian" concept of the theologian Karl Rahner. This concept cedes that whoever evidences authentic love of self or others also manifests the "Spirit of God." According to this principle, when an individual evidences love of self or others, the "Spirit of Christ" is present; hence, we have an "Anonymous Christian" who, irrespective of the religious, atheistic, or philosophical label she may consciously wear, still can be seen securely within the model of spiritual experience as defined above. This tripartite model, it should be noted, is not the "property" of any one religious system. It is far more comprehensive.

When applied to the understanding of trauma, the implications are profound. Rather than become preoccupied with defining exactly what Higher Power is in order to experience spiritual growth, I come to realize that every step I take that brings me closer to myself or other people is a spiritual experience – that even if I have no idea from my upbringing about what a "Higher Power" might be, the experience of Higher Power is fully accessible to me. Spirituality and intimacy are founded on the ability of the human individual to internalize and externalize the reality of love. Trauma induces spiritual and relational blockages that inhibit our experience of our birthright, our heritage as beings of Light, as children of the Divine. Anything that I do, therefore, that fosters the release of the trauma experiences stored within me, whether it is giving myself permission to remember, allowing myself to cry, deciding to go to therapy or treatment, owning my depression, anger and the other warning signs of trauma, asking for help, saying a prayer, journaling, meditating – or any other of an infinite variety of expressions, is a healing or integrative movement toward the Divine. The three-dimensional model that I have presented to you demonstrates that we can have authentic spiritual experience without becoming preoccupied by our thoughts and cognition – our definitions of Higher Power. Religious systems and even Twelve Step programs frequently have been so defensive or protective of the vertical dimension of the model that they have failed to realize that you cannot have the first (self) or the second (others) without also experiencing the third (Higher Power). This may not be conscious, as Rahner's concept of the "Anonymous Christian" pointed out, but why be so preoccupied with labeling when we need only look from our own inner vision to see the Light that is present? With our histories of trauma, it is understandable that many of us have experienced difficulty with the notion of Higher Power. Some of us were even abused by ministers eloquently wielding the scriptures and the name of God to support their own compulsive behaviors. Those who are religiously addicted can also do much harm to those who are spiritually and emotionally needy.

The model of spirituality-intimacy-relationality that I suggest states emphatically that we are one with Spirit when we are single-minded, when we are united with ourselves and others. This tripartite model affirms that all is of the Divine Mind, but that from within this growth process toward oneness with all creation, estrangement can occur. This, however, is different from the spiritually abusive and shaming messages that we received as children and adults that suggested that total rupture of the spiritual relationship is possible. Only estrangement is possible. As seen in Diagram B (p. 185), the life-line only gets longer, more distant from the center where all things are one. It is not, however, severed. There is no death in the realm of Spirit, and the spiritual is all-encompassing. Trauma is an invitation to transform "negative" experiences into opportunities for growth and spiritual awakening.

Frequently, addicts seek treatment for "simple detoxification" from alcohol. The lucky ones come to realize that the core of the recovery experience is in the recovery of the **true self**. With the clearing and restoration of the self comes the healing of relationships to others and Higher Power. Confronting in ourselves a disease such as alcoholism often serves as the catalyst for healing. I commonly hear addicts express their anger and disappointment about the years "wasted" with their addictions, but there is no time wasted when the experience of pain finally leads to the integration that is our primary lesson on this plane of existence. Integration and unity is the objective of all of our lessons – our losses, traumas, and addictions. While we are immersed in these "negative" experiences, however, it is oftentimes difficult to maintain that vision of hope.

My "pyramid meditation" helps me to remain hopeful. During this meditation I sit in a lotus position and imagine myself as the cone or pyramid diagrammed in this work (See Diagram A, p. 184). I begin by identifying my present state of feelings about myself and imagine the first line (anchored in the right knee), representing myself, and feel myself moving upward from this position toward greater integration (above the crown of the head). I then identify any unresolved or strong feelings that I have toward others – those whom I love, those with whom I need to reconcile, those who need or ask for my prayers or support, all whom I have ever offended or assisted; these I move upward (picturing a line from the left knee) toward integration (meeting the other line above the crown of the head). The third line reflects my connection with my Higher Power, perceived as the core energy sustaining me and running along my spine (the third line). I often pause at this point to focus on this felt link with my Higher Power. Finally, all three lines connect and become one within my mind, at my "third eye" (brow). All converge at the top of the pyramid where All Is One, where all prayers are "answered." My care for myself, my love for others (my "other-selves"), and my relationship with my Higher Power all converge to find a single point, an infinite point, a "gateway to intelligent infinity." Language is lacking to describe the profound sense of unity and oneness of knowing that all is really so perfectly simple, so unified. That there is really no love of self that is not love of others and Higher Power; there is no love of others that is not also love of self and Higher Power; and there is no love of Higher Power that is not also love of self and others. There is reciprocity and unity. All is One; all is the Divine Mind. Just as I have within my own mind ego-states or fragments of myself that become estranged or stuck and need to be reintegrated, so too, on a larger scale, we are ego-states of the Divine Mind that have become disenfranchised. This estrangement is primarily discovered through traumas and our endured disintegrative experiences. In traditional spiritual teaching, this was called the "via negativa," the negative path to the Divine, to Truth. This has been, by far, the more common path for most of us. From what we have just seen of the tripartite dynamics of our spiritual nature, all movements, in any direction, hold spiritual meaning and value.

    I awoke Thanksgiving morning with this tripartite relationship as clear as crystal in my mind. The model that I set forth is actually a greatly reduced understanding of the dynamics of the "Divine Mind" and our return home. The study of the implications of trauma reminds us of our spiritual, creative nature and destiny, as well as our multidimensionality. It helps us to manifest our personal truth in concert with others. As such, it is also the path to healing and wholeness.

Chapter Twelve

Recovering Spiritual Awareness After Trauma: Twelve Principles

The energy that we expend in the effort to heal ourselves from trauma inevitably leads us in the direction of "spirituality." This is true for a variety of reasons. Since trauma tends to reduce our perceptions of ourselves to something that is "less than" our true nature and potential, the resolution of trauma reveals our authentic self. It forces us to expand our understanding of ourselves to include higher dimensions, potentials, and experiences that we term "spiritual." Spirituality provides us with a new understanding of Truth not yet embraced by present levels of scientific knowledge. We are not limited to our measurable, observable physical bodies; we can not be distilled down to our intellects alone; nor are we simply our emotions. We are something more than all of these – a consciousness that extends far beyond these concepts. As the Gestaltists believe, the whole is greater than the sum of its parts.

My history of trauma is a journey emerging as a spiritual path that has necessitated and provided an opening to higher realities. It is a path of spiritual awakening that explains why many of these traumas happened to me. When I review my trauma experiences and those of others, I realize the many gifts which I have received. Traumas have taught me, gifting me with some very important spiritual truths that give order and meaning to what was once a chaotic and untrustworthy

world. The resolution of my own traumas and the participation in the
healing of others' has restored my faith and trust in reality as a spiritual
experience that leads to wholeness. While in the midst of this morass,
it was difficult for me to see this. Looking today at my recovery, I see a
process of spiritual growth that has emerged. In order to facilitate that
process for others, I have outlined the principles that served as stepping-
stones in my healing process.

I identify twelve spiritual axioms which together form a picture of
a process. I originally recorded them while witnessing well-intentioned
therapists attempt a "Christian therapy spirituality program" in a
psychiatric hospital in a city where I worked as a psychotherapist. While
I supported their intention, I could not condone providing a spirituality
program and imposing on all the patients the "Christian" forms of
expression. This constituted spiritual abuse to those whose spiritual
paths were different from "Christian" doctrine. In addition, a number
of clients with whom I had a therapeutic relationship had been abused
by ministers and "religious addicts" who used their beliefs and threats
of damnation to manipulate and further abuse the members of their
spiritual family. Though I came from a strong Christian background, my
paternal great grandfather was Jewish. I have an appreciation for beliefs
different from my own and contend that "authentic Christ-likeness"
honors the variety of spiritual paths. Jesus affirmed this in his references
to the loving acts of the Samaritans (as in the Parable of the "Good
Samaritan" in Luke 10:33ff) who typically were viewed as heretics and
"worse than the pagans" by the religious of his day. Spirituality is not
the "property" of any system, and any attempt to contain it by such a
reduction obviously will fail because it violates the principle of love by its
exclusion of the different beliefs that combine to constitute spirituality.
"Truth" is not the property of any one system. The principles that I
outline in the next twelve sections are simple tenets by which we may
approach and understand spiritual experience without betraying our
natures and the core truths that existed generations before the "systems"
that we are familiar with were constituted.

Historically, these core truths existed long before "religious"
history commenced. The "religious" systems with which we are familiar
have existed for approximately five thousand years. Spirituality and

the core principles which we will be examining existed in "pre-history" – in the hundreds of thousands of years that preceded the emergence of organized religious systems. The claims of our religious systems seem presumptuous and proportionately finite compared to the vast pre-history of the spiritual traditions, the heritage that gave rise to them. And there may be steps in this spiritual evolution, links with which we have, yet, to reckon. Presently, scholars and seekers embrace the possibility that the spiritual search may have a pre-history in other worlds, in civilizations older or "more advanced" than our own.

Spiritual evolution is a process that has neither ebbed nor halted for an instant. We may forget the ongoing nature of the process amidst our personal, societal, and global traumas. We can also lose sight of this unfolding in our efforts to feel more secure by convincing ourselves that we possess all the truths we need in our convenient "systems" of belief. Since the development of "systems theory" in the 1950's, we have come to realize that every system, by its very nature, contains both healthy and unhealthy elements. In our efforts to feel more in control of our lives, we manage to convince ourselves that we possess all the truths we need in our conveniently packaged systems. We lose sight of how vast the salvific plan really is. We tend to focus on the steps that we can grasp at any given stage and become secure and content with that information. Once entrenched in the "comfort zone," the scientific principle of inertia deters expansion beyond our settled condition. Trauma survivors know that it is this "settled" feeling that precipitates the clamoring of the next unresolved issue to be addressed. Our natural exigency is toward wholeness, and illusions of security will not stop this inward movement. Our spiritual nature will not settle for complacency or reductionism. It will not allow us to stay "stuck" for long without objecting in some manner. This unquenchable drive for the highest development possible—for autonomy, will provide the fertilizer for growth and expansion when we become stagnant. Trauma is born when the divine energy that creates us is arrested and held by complacency, neglect, or abuse. The resolution of these frozen moments reveals to us our underlying nature – as pure creative energy. Trauma resolution reveals to us fundamental spiritual truths about ourselves. These truths, born in the release of our emotional pain, disclose our true nature, beauty, and power.

Each of twelve principles is listed, followed by a reflection of the relationship between each postulate and trauma characteristic.

1. **To Be is to be Spiritual.** Trauma is a distortion that profoundly impacts, but cannot destroy our core spiritual identity.
2. **I am the Locus (place) of all my spiritual experience.** Trauma often leaves us outward-looking in our search for wholeness, though the truth remains within.
3. **Admission of my own powerlessness and unmanageability directs me toward right relationship to the ordered universe.** Traumas are moments when we lost our power which can now be restored.
4. **Each of us possesses the vision needed to heal ourselves.** Traumas are occasions to access our "healer within."
5. **My feelings are a primary medium of my spirituality.** Our feelings are the cues to unlocking our traumas and opening to higher states of consciousness.
6. **Affective blockages are spiritual blockages.** Traumas impact us simultaneously on emotional and spiritual levels.
7. **All forms of abuse – of alienation of the self from the self are, at the same time, spiritual abuse.** Abuse also creates spiritual traumatization.
8. **Spirituality involves the healing of our intentionality – our decision-making ability.** Trauma involves the entrapment of a "false intentionality" within our consciousness which subsequently influences our decisions.
9. **Spirituality is both a growth process and a permanent relationship state.** Our spirituality grows and continuously supports us in the healing of our traumas.
10. **Spirituality is simultaneously intrapersonal (within me) and interpersonal (social) in nature.** Trauma resolution is profoundly spiritual, simultaneously healing relationships to self and others.
11. **Spirituality is naturally unitive.** Spiritual reintegration occurs through the resolution of trauma.
12. **Spirituality is a unique vehicle of truth, a major experience in the comprehension of reality.** Spirituality can give meaning to the most disturbing of our traumas.

In the following sections, I will share with you my experience and understanding of these principles as they have emerged through my spiritual growth process. I draw on experiences both personal and professional. Together, these principles reveal an intimate personal process, a purpose, and a plan. I invite you to discover the pieces to your unique puzzle as we journey through these principles.

1. **To Be is to be Spiritual.** (Trauma is a distortion that profoundly impacts, but cannot destroy our core spiritual identity).

Oftentimes growing up, the message was communicated that our worth was contingent upon our performance. The truth is that our integrity and value are not merely constituted from our actions and behaviors, though these certainly flow from who and what we are. "Being" precedes "doing." All of our actions flow from and are expressions of our identity.

Our earliest behaviors were basically the reflection and imitation of our physical, mental, and emotional heritage. As we learned moral responsibility as children, our behaviors reflected this heritage which was imprinted in our consciousness and in the cells of our bodies. And we were always more than our behaviors. Hopefully, our parents communicated this to us prior to disciplining us. If they did not make the distinction for us between "personhood" and "behavior," we may have interpreted the disciplinary act as personal rejection. In addition, as we grew and developed, many other primary systems that influenced us placed emphasis on "the right behaviors." Some of us received clear messages that, unless the "right actions" were produced, the love we needed would not be forthcoming. Others were taunted with the notion that unless certain behaviors were performed and others restrained we "would not go to heaven." Ironically, many of the approaches of our religious systems (and their influence on our families through our parents' religious beliefs) diminished our actual energy levels by weakening our sense of self through the use of shaming tactics and language. While attempting to "save" us, they often "shamed" us; and, in diminishing our spiritual integrity, they fostered compulsivity for "doing the right things." We now know that such shaming can, indeed, produce behavioral changes, but the cost is increased compulsivity and diminished sense of worth. In fostering a preoccupation with behaviors, the first spiritual principle is violated – that we are spiritual beings, first, because we are. When, for instance, increasingly shaming language like "mortal" sin, meaning "deadly," was used by religious systems, it took no great effort for us to confuse issues of personhood with a behavior – because of this "bad" behavior, my "being" will cease; I will die. The language itself reflected confusion between person or being and behavior. This excessive focus on behaviors, before our spiritual integrity was affirmed, produced an imbalance in our spiritual development that commonly resulted in 1) a preoccupation with "doing the right things" and 2) an inability to feel our inherent spiritual nature and worth. We became "spiritual doings" before we recognized that we were "spiritual beings." This may have produced the need to be perfect and right in all behaviors, for there was no sense of internal integrity to keep us alive if we made a mistake, were less than perfect, or sinned "mortally." Today this imbalance is fostered as behaviors continue to be assessed and adjudged without considering the spiritual nature of the being who performs them. Several religious systems give the impression that spiritual being equals spiritual doing. It is most important to remember that being precedes doing. We see this demonstrated in the beauty, innocence, and goodness of the newborn infant whose integrity is evident. Jean Jacques Rousseau (1712-1778) posited that a child develops like a plant, a flower, in all things intellectual, physical, and emotional. He added that a child is innately good in spirit. A child's behaviors mirror his experiential lessons from home and environment. For a child, "moral responsibility" is not present until age seven or eight.

Religious systems, particularly in their earlier stages of development, focused on morality as the key to wholeness and salvation. In Christianity the excessive focus on behaviors was fostered by translational problems. To "be perfect as your heavenly Father is perfect," as translated in New Testament Greek, meant that the <u>one</u> Greek word for "perfect" would be employed in both parts of the statement. This set up a parity or equality of behavioral expectations for the divine and human natures. Talk about a set-up for failure! In the older Hebrew language, there were two words used for "perfect."

One was used for "God," the other for humans and other living things. The Hebrew terms meant perfection according to your appropriate nature. Divine perfection without error or mistake was certainly not to be equated with human perfection, where mistakes were an acceptable part of human nature.

An excessive emphasis on acts violates the very nature of spirituality. The illusion that we are "wasting time" with experiences such as meditation reflects the stress on measurable productivity. Meditation, which allows us to become centered and puts us in touch with our "beingness," actually fosters "right action." The basis of meditation is found in this principle. There are those who dedicate their lives to prayer and meditation for others. They assist us directly on the level of "being." The true value of their efforts is in the nurturing and affirmation of our personal and collective identity. From such spiritual nurturing, our actions and decisions flow more easily.

Our spiritual nature cannot be measured by traditional standards of "productivity." Experiences such as paralysis or illness in the physical body, while seen as threatening to the quality of our life at first glance, can enhance the productivity of our lives on other planes of equal importance. For example, when Franklin D. Roosevelt first aspired to politics, hoping to follow faithfully in the footsteps of "Teddy" Roosevelt, he was struck with polio and nearly despaired of his personal aspirations. Instead, when he incorporated his experience of illness, he became the champion of the handicapped and disadvantaged – forming the platform for a unique contribution to our country and our government. Many of our most important governmental services were borne from his experience. Even paralysis itself can become the vehicle for spiritual growth and manifestation. We recall the more recent case of Christopher Reeve, whom I met before his "accident" – a man chosen for his "superman-like" appeal on the screen – now confined to a wheel chair by paralysis. His courage and example provide us with profound lessons to ponder. Milton Erickson, a pioneer in the development of hypnotherapy, was confined to a wheelchair from an early age due to polio. Is it so strange that some of the most inspirational people we meet are those who have been the most traumatized?   My attraction to work with addicted populations was generated from this paradoxical phenomenon: where pain and trauma are found, nearby is Spirit.

Many people believe that among their most powerful "spiritual" encounters are those which occur in their subconscious dream states. They suggest that, in altered states, well beyond the reach of performance assessments, conscious agendas, and rational thoughts, we are more real – beyond the interference of our limited logical minds. Since our conscious awareness constitutes only seven percent of our mind, while the subconscious comprises ninety-three percent, this must, in fact, be the case.

A friend, David Abadi, recently summarized this notion of "being." He stated that, "We are here simply to learn to <u>walk the face of the earth</u> … and to do so without attachment; any pain that emerges in our lives is our resistance to life." After scrutinizing most of my physical and emotional pains, I have found this philosophy to be true – most of my pain was the by-product of unresolved traumas. Trauma creates subconscious attachments. Our ego becomes bound to these states of pain which, subsequently, color our choices and perceptions.

I have come to believe that trauma induces a distortion or blockage that is so profound in nature that it is often perceived as a distortion in "being." I have yet to encounter a rape survivor who has not induced a false sense of being – a "dirtiness" or defectiveness, though she had nothing to do with the behavior perpetrated against her. The transfixing which occurs at a moment of trauma induces a conflicted and distorted sense of being, for the encoded scene contains, not only the trauma victim's personal reality, but that of the perpetrator as well. In a moment of trauma, we become stuck with a sense of powerlessness and deficiency from our intense interaction with those in the scene with us. We often feel this misrepresentation in our nervous system from the moment of trauma onward. In order to survive this spiritual violation, however, the subconscious mind stores it until we are ready to release it. Trauma does not destroy our spirituality, but it causes a false message to be induced about who we are – about our true spiritual nature. We can carry this false sense of being (dirty, bad, wrong, defective, or powerless) with us our entire lifetime. Trauma resolution involves the restoration of our true sense of spiritual being. I have found the resolution process to be one of the most liberating and the most spiritual of all experiences.

Spirituality is not merely a momentary experience, a place, an activity, or a feeling. As spiritual beings, we are not limited to our activities, addictions, feelings, or traumas; we are something more. Spirituality is a state of relationship that exists simply because we are. Having examined the spiritual priority of being, let us look next at the "where" of spiritual experience.

2. **I am the <u>Locus</u> (place) of all my spiritual experience.** (Trauma often leaves us outward-looking in our search for wholeness, though the truth remains within.)

While this principle may appear simple at first glance, its internalization and acceptance can take a lifetime. To trauma survivors whose concretized feelings convey a sense of wrongness about something inside them, the "self" is often the last place that they would expect to experience spiritual reality. Since trauma and abuse result in an alienation of the self from the self, it seems much more plausible that love is to be found "out there" somewhere in external reality, rather than inside the self where feelings of low self-worth, defectiveness, depression, and shame reside. For years the notion of "Divine Indwelling" – that "God" is to be found living within, seemed totally incomprehensible and irreconcilable with my experience of self. I knew how I felt about myself, and this surely excluded any possibility of such spiritual access. Over time, several relationships offering unconditional acceptance helped me to recognize the truth of my integrity and worth, but, ultimately, the solution was found within me. Others can mirror these truths to us, but unless they awaken our own sense of worth, unless they displace the shame that has accumulated inside, this sense of defectiveness will continue to block our spiritual awareness. If love is not internalized or cannot be internalized due to preexisting trauma, our relationships will look more like addiction, for we simply are using something (someone) outside of ourselves in order to temporarily feel better. These codependent solutions are not healing in the strong sense and will do little to resolve core issues. We will use these medicating experiences, however, to sustain us through our pain or to avoid it entirely.

Recent studies indicate, for instance, that one of the single strongest contributing factors to alcoholism in women is a history of sexual trauma. In cases where severe abuse has occurred, as in the case of incest, it is easy to comprehend reliance on such defenses. How can a child (or adult) survive betrayal by the very persons who held the primary responsibility of representing love? Once this level of trauma is induced, defenses are established that allow the child to survive, but, as the child matures, if the walls are not removed, they will become more strongly fortified, manifesting as behavioral, emotional, relational, or medical problems. Such walls serve to keep out further pain and abuse, but they also restrict experiences of love. The abused child frequently develops addictive or outward-looking solutions to substitute for what is lacking inside. In some cases, the child turns the pain and the blame inward on self, fostering depression and a host of ineffective coping mechanisms.

The healing of trauma requires intervention to resolve the alienation that has occurred. The most effective and empowering solution for this alienation is to have our own adult-parent or nurturing self intervene on the wounded child within us. In such a manner, we discover our power to restore the integrity that was robbed at the moment that the shame was induced. Others can facilitate this process, but it must be the self that heals the self. Only in this manner will the truth be brought home to the psyche that "I am the place where love happens."

As children we were born dependent – naturally outward-looking for our nurturing and sustenance. As we grew according to plan, we were expected to internalize enough love and nurturing so as to move from "insecurity" to "security." Physical, mental, emotional, social, sexual, and spiritual "boundaries" were to be formed that would allow us to function securely in life. Boundaries are the phenomena that provide our sense of identity. If Kuwait loses its boundaries, for example, it ceases to exist, as do we. Very few of us experienced enough nurturing in the areas identified above. Hence, where the specific boundary was not formed, an "insecurity" arose. The healing of these wounded boundaries results in the restoration of power, self-confidence, and awareness. The most effective of these processes is not where someone outside "fixes" us, but where we discover within ourselves that we are meant to heal ourselves and, in so doing, bring the power back to where it was conceived and expected to remain: the self. Authentic spiritual healing occurs when the self finds empowerment.

For years I gave all my spiritual power to the people and systems outside of me that claimed it. As a trauma victim, this seemed natural. Where else would it be found if not outside of me? There were also people and systems more than ready to claim my power and use it "in my best interest" and "for my well-being" since they knew better than I what I needed. I did not realize that this "set me up" for additional abuse and allowed the continuation of the original trauma. I knew that my family system was dysfunctional and sensed the need to individuate from the emotional enmeshment with my mother, but I was completely oblivious to the notion that those in my religious system could use their power and authority to abuse me. I experienced more overt abuse within my religious system than I suffered within my family system. I had few "boundaries" toward what I had expected to be a "spiritual" system. I did not know the difference between spirituality and religious systems. I did not know that all systems possessed functional and dysfunctional dynamics. This naivete left me vulnerable to abuse. My parents, who themselves did not know about the nature of dysfunctional systems, encouraged my association with priests and bishops that they thought, naturally, were "safe" and reliable role models. Their blind trust and the complete surrender of their power to the religious system had been interpreted and esteemed as obedience and fidelity for many generations. No cautions were necessary; God was present.

Denial about instances of sexual advances and abuse from priests in authoritative positions allowed my classmates and me to survive, to continue on toward our goal of ordination and service. Later on, once I had established some distance from these experiences and from my dependency upon religious and educational systems, I was able to identify specific instances of abuse. During the early years of my seminary training and, even as a priest, I continued to strive to do the "right things," fulfilling my call to obedience and service, while experiencing a growing sense of emotional death. Over a period of time, I felt as though I was losing more and more of myself by not dealing with some elusive inner pain. I became more workaholic, less and less in touch with my feelings. Soon after I was ordained, my mother died, a close priest-friend died, and my best friend left ministry. All of the most important systems that had shaped my life dissolved quickly. Looking back, I can see a profound force that was at work at that time in my life to help me break through my own denial and delusion about myself and my emotional pain in order to bring healing. At the time it felt more like death. It took four additional years for my unacknowledged and unresolved grief to become fully conscious and for me to muster the necessary strength to begin drawing my power back to myself. I did this by taking leave of a system that had become my "reason for existence."

Immediately upon resigning from parish ministry and committing to my own healing process, I began to feel the same keen sense of spiritual direction that I had felt regularly guiding me throughout my life. As I continued to focus on myself and sort out my spiritual sense from the traumas that had occurred, I became aware of a purpose underlying all of these losses. I had used my priesthood addictively to provide a sense of worth by "doing the right things" and by focusing on service to others. But what I had never fully possessed throughout this formative period was a definite sense of self. To love others as self is possible when one is in touch with one's own sense of worth. Jesus was able to do this because he took the necessary time to know who he was, to love himself, and to know himself as beloved before immersing himself in his service to others. To love others before one has come to love oneself or to use others to gain this sense of self is called "codependency." Of course I was codependent in my relationships; that was how I had survived. But it was no longer sufficient. Withstanding the losses of loved ones, it became easier to bring the focus back to the place where the solutions needed to happen: myself. These events drew my attention back to me and my own power. Now I had to differentiate between the abuse and the nurturing – to relinquish what had impeded my growth and embrace what had helped. I began to seek, rather than fear these occasions for healing and empowerment. Studying the patterns of dysfunctional systems and addictionology enabled me to resolve the abuse and recover my spirituality. I felt ill when I realized how much power the traumas in my family, educational, and religious systems had usurped from me. I became angry when I realized that those claiming to mediate the "love of God" had used their authority to dis-empower me. I felt humbled when I realized that I might have done the same to others. While this had not been done intentionally, it was, nonetheless, abusive and traumatizing. It became more difficult, prior to my leaving ministry, to preach "morality" when I now recognized the faces of addiction and trauma in the congregation; moralizing to such individuals intensified shame and accelerated the addictive cycle. The original search for "Truth" suddenly became bigger than my traditional religious, educational, and familial parameters could sustain. The understanding of these dysfunctional dynamics allowed me to begin to distinguish between spiritual illness and authentic spirituality. I was able to claim what had been helpful and relinquish what had not. It was as though my life had been designed to teach me that the answer was not "out there" in a job, another person, in "religiously appropriate" behaviors, in pleasing others, forgetting self, or in ignoring or repressing my own feelings. The solution was and remains right here: <u>I am the place</u> where the answers are to be found. I am the locus, the place of all my spiritual experience. It is no longer acceptable to give that power away to others. We are here to discover, explore, and experience this spiritual indwelling, and to know that this occurs within us.

3. **Admission of my own powerlessness and unmanageability directs me toward right relationship to the ordered universe.** (Traumas are moments when we lost our power which can now be restored.)

This principle will resonate with many of you who are familiar with the Twelve Steps of Alcoholics Anonymous and the various applications of this spiritual process to other areas of addictive behaviors. If you have had difficulty with the notions of "Higher Power" or "God" as they appear in the Twelve Step philosophy, do not be dismayed. As we shall see, the efficacy of healing is not contingent upon our cognitive grasp of the notion of "God" or "Higher Power." Nevertheless, healing is available to us. Additionally, this third principle does not require adherence to Twelve Step philosophy. It is more basic, and it relates to trauma.

One of the most painful issues for me was the loss of personal power that occurred in my life, robbed from me as a result of trauma. Each of us, I have come to believe, has experienced some such diminution as a consequence of trauma. Even the simplest of traumas involves the encoding of incredibly complex and subtle forms of energy as I outlined earlier in this work. This fixing of energy in our nervous systems precipitates a loss of power. If the cells of our bodies take on and hold this "negative" charge as a means of self-protection, they are no longer available to carry the "positive" energy that would otherwise be accessible to us. Increased trauma results in decreased power. The continued induction of shame that occurs as the addictive cycle progresses, for instance, results in even greater repression of emotion. As more and more of the cells of our bodies are used to store this static energy, the dynamic flow of energy throughout our bodies slows. If this process is allowed to continue without intervention, death occurs. The identification of these blockages is essential if emotional and spiritual growth are to flourish. Admitting the existence of these blockages, even if we initially believe that we are at fault, is an essential step toward healing and restoration. Trauma commonly leaves us with the feeling that something is "wrong" about us. This is understandable since the trauma is stored in our bodies. Maintaining illusions of control and manageability over the traumas stored in our bodies results in the need for these traumas to "speak louder" in order for them to be healed. I originally became a trauma therapist because of this phenomenon. Using traditional therapies, I found my clients returning to therapy with the same, and, frequently, more intense symptoms when actual resolution was not accomplished. This experience quickly taught me which therapies were effective and which fostered retraumatization. Without initial acknowledgment of our pain, however, any intervention is vastly reduced in effectiveness.

Our admission of powerlessness does not dictate that we identify or understand the origin of our powerlessness and unmanageability. A significant percentage of the addicts that I work with have no conscious recollection of the origin of their need to medicate their emotions. They commonly identify the emotional "triggers," but are often oblivious to the precipitating trauma itself. Powerlessness typically indicates a blockage of some type. Admitting one's powerlessness is the access to the block that may manifest as depression, addiction, compulsivity, destructive relationships, personality disorders, etc. As human beings, perfect children of the universe, we are not meant to be powerless. Our spiritual nature is, inherently, an empowerment process. Left unattended, energy obstructions will manifest in order to reach our consciousness so as to be released. Our natural exigency is toward power in a balanced, spiritual order. All that is within us will work to bring our "stuck points" to our attention. We addressed these fixed feelings in Chapter Ten, "The Hierarchy of Healing." As we identify our experiences of powerlessness, we learn that these are springboards to power itself – that the resolution of trauma provides greater energy flow. We quickly discover this, for when we reintegrate with ourselves and others, we feel this empowerment on all levels – the physical, mental, emotional, spiritual, and social.

This third principle states that honesty or "admission" "directs me toward" my proper place in the universal order. It does not state that the admission alone accomplishes the task. Admission alone is insufficient to restore the balance, but the healing or resolution of the blockages can be initiated once they are identified. Admission is the first step toward the restoration of balance and the power that accompanies it.

For those of us who have come to identify ourselves with powerlessness and unmanageability after living with these feelings for many years, final admission of their existence and their insufficiency feels like a threat to our lives. We become attached to our pain. There is great fear associated with such a shift in awareness. An additional anxiety arises: what if, when we concede our powerlessness and unmanageability and surrender to this admission, there is no underlying source of power to sustain us?

Spirituality enables us to address our fears from a position of power. It provides the vision that is necessary to move beyond our natural fears and to step above them. Spirituality provides us with that very "organizing principle" that discloses to us the "ordered universe" that we have doubted again and again amidst our traumas

(See Principle Twelve also, below). We will consider this now in the fourth principle.

4. **Each of us possesses the vision needed to heal ourselves.**
   (Traumas are occasions to access our "healer within.")

Built into human consciousness is the capacity to make "leaps" – to bridge the seeming gaps in our knowledge or experience and to make connections. The Hebrew word that lies at the origin of this vision or "faith" concept is 'aman. This word means "to be firm or solid" and, thus, "to be true." That which is firm and true gives security. Part of the spiritual revolution taking place is the movement from basing our assessment of reality on the "Newtonian notion of solidity" instead of the certainty that comes from trusting our intuition and our multidimensional awareness as facilitated by quantum physics. Through evolution we have come to associate security with the limited vision of our five-sensory awareness and have missed the security that comes from intuitive knowing. "True" inner vision or faith includes the capacity to grasp realities beyond our five-sensory limitations or awareness. It is a delusion to believe that reality is only that which our five senses present to us. But even our five-sensory awareness hinges on the capacity to make leaps. For instance, in the fraction of a second that it takes for our optic nerves and brain to process incoming data, our senses have already "moved on" to the next instant of perception. What we, therefore, treat as current or present is, in fact, already obsolete. On the basis of what has been most currently perceived, we project forward "in faith" and anticipation that the next experience or perception will be reliable. We have come to rely upon these habits of perception to present to us what is true, real. We learned this reliance upon five-sensory awareness as infants. Developmentally, we first internalized the "vision" of our parents and those around us. Their way of "making leaps" became our way of "making leaps." Their fundamental way of perceiving reality became our own. But inherent in this capacity to make sense of reality is something more. Quantum physics is teaching us that we are not the passive observers of independent, objective realities, but that, by our vision, we create our reality. This capacity extends far beyond the limits of our five senses and gives us access to a multidimensionality that transcends the limitations imposed by traditional Newtonian thinking. This allows us new dimensions of possibility for personal, societal, and universal expansion. It offers us unlimited possibilities for growth on all levels. Life is the opportunity to open ourselves to greater perception, to multi-dimensional awareness, and we are each, due to our human nature, capable of this change.

It has proved a great personal challenge and adventure to go beyond the narrow expectations that I inherited from my traditional systems — my family, religion, educational institutions, and peers. As a child I was labeled "shy – like his father." As an adult, I was shocked when I realized that I had become or had always been more extroverted than introverted. Once I had outgrown the educational expectations of my family, for instance, and had not only completed college but continued on with my post-graduate studies in Rome and Jerusalem, my family seemed "at a loss" when it came to relating to my experience. I had gone beyond their program for me. Having inherited the family's vision of excessive caution and fear, I was challenged, for this limited vision could no longer sustain me. I was in new territory. When I began my thirteen years of archaeological work in Israel, a nexus of controversy and political upheaval, family members were amazed and worried for my safety. I learned to trust and follow my own vision by listening to my heart and confronting my fears – as well as those fears which I had inherited. I came to understand that there was a force stronger than fear, and that this force could sustain me. I actually enjoyed unlearning my fears, conquering my inherited "shyness" or "shame," and discovered increased confidence and power in each experience. Over and over I created a new vision of myself, not the one induced from childhood and trauma. I shaped a new vision and faith in myself confronting the fears and discovering their "unreality," their illusory character. The emotional parameters which bound me could be released!

Somewhere in this process I learned that the "faith" or vision that I was living was originally constructed from the beliefs of others – Mom and Dad, family, church, teachers, and society. I realized that certain of those beliefs were constrictive and inhibited my growth. Many of the significant influences had shared their own "truths" with the best of intentions, but they did not accurately reflect my personal truth. Underlying this discernment process, however, was a strong spiritual connection that continued to sustain me and provided the vision to transcend the limitations of a reality that, oftentimes, was too narrow – a vision that I had "inherited." My father's spirituality had been a consistent, daily, gentle, but strictly traditional one. My mother's had been highly intuitive and flexible – deeply connected to feeling and emotion. I am the child of both – a bridge of sorts between a very traditional history spanning many generations and a profoundly intuitive culture even more venerable and ageless.

Many gifts were provided by traditional forms of spiritual expression. This traditional spirituality awakened in me the fascination with mystery and the use of symbolism to facilitate spiritual encounter. This same history gave us the great mystics who served to elevate the mass consciousness to unprecedented levels: Francis of Assisi, John of the Cross, Teresa of Avila, Catherine of Sienna. They expanded my vision and explained my particular experience. My mother, however, was the one who brought it home, and quite literally. Her gift to me, among many, was her special gift of faith – her vision. How ironic that, on her death-bed the one self-criticism she shared about her life was that she feared that she had not expressed enough "faith." Mother, who could feel the events that happened to us separated by vast distances, who wrote poetry and loved spending hours on False River fishing – she brought home to me a vision and belief that was both simple and profound. In every sense, it was the purview of the poet, the insight of the mystic. Her perspective stimulated my quest to explain and understand these phenomena for myself. It challenged my vision to expand to include the multidimensional nature of humans. I did not know that it would be this revelation that would provide the foundation for the work that I do to facilitate the healing of trauma. To my developing belief system, the fact that she could actually feel the traumas occurring to others seemed a most incredible phenomenon. Little did I suspect that within a few years I would experience this discernment myself, daily.

This learning experience began as part of a constant, gentle, growth process. I started, as each of us did, as an infant learning to trust my sensory perceptions. This simple, mechanical approach to grasping reality, based on the influence of Newtonian physics, holds that "what is observable" is real. Such mechanical thinking, however, was limiting and failed completely when faced with Mom's intuitive demonstrations. Hence, it was fairly easy to discover the restrictions of Newtonian physics. There were realities that entered my life that were not actually "observable," but were, nonetheless, real. Cases like Deidra (see Chapter Four) taught me about the limitations of Newtonian physics – of relying exclusively on measurable and observable phenomena to diagnose and treat illnesses and depression. The belief systems that had shaped my personal hermeneutics (science of interpretation) and my professional training, including the educational systems and the medical profession, continued operating from a foundation of Newtonian physics. This resulted in a negative labeling of "psychosomatic" illness when all the mechanical explanations failed. Subjection to these purely mechanistic or somatic approaches which failed to resolve trauma-induced somatic pain left many individuals additionally traumatized with a deepening sense of hopelessness and despair. In the worst case scenarios, as in the example of Diedra, bodies were permanently damaged.

Personally, a great shift occurred when I discovered the consistent reporting of my clients' traumas in the form of holographic metaphors which were often described in great detail and accompanied by intense somatic sensations. These sensations frequently were not verifiable by the medical profession – that is, the "lump in my throat" did not appear on the X-ray; the "weight on the outside of my chest" could not be measured by any instrument yet developed by the medical profession; and no cause could be found for the recurrent migraines which, my client would report, "are always located over my left eye." The consistency of the locations where these traumas were identified, the detailed description of their forms as they appeared to my clients, the connection of these details to certain specific behaviors, phobias, and compulsions, all suggested a neurologically linked process that had not been addressed by medical science. Unresolved traumas were causing illness and presenting themselves for diagnosis and resolution, but our technology was limited to medicating or addressing the symptomatology on a physiological, mechanical, Newtonian level.

I have described some of the more dramatic cases in the previous chapters. These cases altered my understanding of disease and pathology, generating a new vision of the human person, marked by a dynamic consciousness that unceasingly works to protect us and contain our pain in order that we may survive. A frustrating hiatus or gap remains between the level of credibility and power attributed to the medical profession and its grasp of trauma. A vast number of those in the medical profession, overwhelmed with the rapid growth and changes in medicine and in their specialized fields, remain surprisingly unaware of the dynamics of trauma induction and its impact on the bio-psycho-social-spiritual unity that is the human person. It is time to bridge this gap. Sufficient research is now available to allow articulation between trauma resolution experts and medical personnel. A vast body of literature exists relating to the dynamics of trauma induction and the role of electromagnetic fields in the treatment of illness. Discounting these highly effective therapeutic modalities simply because they do not meet the criteria of Newtonian physics serves to retard the effective healing processes. It would appear that the technology to provide the verification of this highly sophisticated neurological process will be the product of quantum physics. Already, scientists have developed the technology to measure the energy fields of the body. The electrocardiagram (EGG) measures electrical currents from the heart, while the electroencephalogram (EEG) measures electrical currents from the brain. Electromagnetic fields around the body can now be measured with a sensitive device called the "Superconducting Quantum Interference Device" (SQUID).[1] When measuring the electromagnetic fields around the body, the instrument does not even touch the body.[2] Dr. Samuel Williamson of New York University indicates that the SQUID provides more information about the state of brain functioning than a normal EEG.[3] The means to measure and monitor the subtle dynamics of trauma induction and resolution are available to us.

Obviously, the split between science and spirituality is considerably smaller when considering that the findings of quantum physics are expanding our knowledge and capability to explain what was previously inaccessible. This is serving to remove suspicion and allow for the bridging of spirituality and physics. Gary Zukav's work, <u>The</u>

Dancing Wu Li Masters – a sort of layman's guide to quantum physics, has helped many thinkers to integrate these disciplines.[4] In this work, Zukav comments on physicist David Bohm's holographic vision of the universe:

> Bohm asserts that the most fundamental level is an unbroken wholeness which is, in his words, "that-which-is." All things, including space, time, and matter are forms of "that-which-is." There is an order which is enfolded into the very process of the universe, but that enfolded order may not be readily apparent.[5]

As Zukav and Bohm indicate, this requires a perceptual shift in our consciousness to accommodate a new vision of reality. Zukav continues:

> Bohm's physics require, in his words, a new "instrument of thought." A new instrument of thought such as is needed to understand Bohm's physics, however, would radically alter the consciousness of the observer, reorienting it toward a perception of the "unbroken wholeness" of which everything is a form.[6]

Zukav indicates, however, after discussing the importance of this new "instrument of thought," that such an instrument already exists. Indeed, in the convergence between eastern and western religions, particularly in the discussions of "mysticism" or "mystical experience," there is a fundamental compatibility with Bohm's physics and philosophy. It is my belief that, in the notion of the hologram, we already have this new instrument of thought. In his text, The Holographic Universe, Michael Talbot observed the following about the origins of this unified holographic view of the universe:

In short, long before the invention of the hologram, numerous thinkers had already glimpsed the nonlocal organization of the universe and had arrived at unique ways to express this insight. It is worth noting that these attempts, crude as they may seem to those of us who are more technologically sophisticated, may have been far more important than we realize. For instance, it appears that the seventeenth-century German mathematician and philosopher Leibniz was familiar with the Hua-yen school of Buddhist thought. Some have argued that this was why he proposed that the universe is constituted out of fundamental entities he called "monads," each of which contains a reflection of the whole universe. What is significant is that Leibniz also gave the world integral calculus, and it was integral calculus that enabled Dennis Gabor to invent the hologram.[7]

Here we see the distinctions between science and spirituality dissolving in service to a unified vision. In the Hindu <u>Avatamsaka Sutra</u>, its author compared the universe to a visionary network of pearls said to hang over the palace of the god Indra and "so arranged that if you look at one (pearl), you see all the others reflected in it."[8] The author of the Sutra then explained that, "In the same way, each object in the world is not merely itself, but involves every other object and, in fact, <u>is</u> everything else."[9] Fa-Tsang, the seventh-century founder of the Hua-yen school, employed a similar analogy when trying to communicate the ultimate interconnectedness and interpenetration of all things.[10] Fa-Tsang, who held that the cosmos was implicit in each of its parts, likened the universe to a multidimensional network of jewels, with each one reflecting all the others ad infinitum.[11]

The suggestion here includes the simple holographic principle that the vision of the part is also the vision of the whole. This way of thinking is not entirely new to us. We have long been able to utilize our multidimensional awareness on an intrapersonal level – within the self. I rarely encounter trauma survivors who cannot utilize, within seconds, their inner holographic perception to locate the holographic fragments of their unresolved traumas within their own bodies. The immediate access and precision of this expanded perceptual capacity validates that we are, indeed, at home with this holographic vision. In The Holographic Universe, Talbot reminds us that great scientists like David Bohm, the protege of Einstein and one of the world's most respected quantum physicists, and Karl Pribram, the neurophysiologist at Stanford University and author of the classic neuropsychological textbook, Languages of the Brain, independently and simultaneously arrived at the conclusion that the holographic model best explained the phenomena of quantum physics and the previously unexplained neurophysiological puzzles of the brain.[12]   In addition, Bohm and Pribram realized that the holographic model explained a number of other mysteries, including the apparent inability of any theory to account for all the phenomena occurring in nature.[13]   This model also made sense of a wide range of phenomena considered well outside the province of scientific understanding, including: telepathy, precognition, mystical feelings of oneness and interconnectedness with the universe, and psychokinesis (the ability to move physical objects with the mind).[14] The holographic model helped to explain nearly all paranormal and mystical experiences.[15]   Based on the holographic model, leading researchers in psychology, psychiatry, and physics have begun to make sense of previously inexplicable phenomena within the following areas: 1) near death experiences as well as death itself appear to be nothing more than the shifting of a person's consciousness from one level of hologram to another; 2) only a holographic model of the brain can explain archetypal experiences, encounters with the collective unconscious, and other phenomena encountered in altered states of consciousness; 3) the holographic model explains lucid dreams in which the dreamer realizes that she is asleep, and will ultimately allow us to develop a "physics of consciousness" to explore other-dimensional levels of existence; and 4) the phenomena of sychronicities – "coincidences" that are so unusual and meaningful that they do not seem to be the product of chance alone, can be explained by the holographic model that affirms the interconnectedness of our thought processes with the physical world.[16] Additional support for the holographic model surfaced in 1982 when researchers at the Institute of Theoretical and Applied Optics, in Paris, demonstrated that, "The web of subatomic particles that compose our physical universe – the very fabric of reality itself, possesses what appears to be an undeniable holographic property."[17]

The perspective that the universe itself is something of a giant hologram and that it is projected from a level of reality that is beyond both space and time emerges from the study of the holographic paradigm. In other words, the perceptions of "apparent" separateness and solidity that the limitations of our five senses produce are simply projected images. On the level of multi-sensory awareness, these illusions begin to dissolve, and interactions on a much deeper level become possible. We can begin to accept that it is "normal" to possess the capacity to "look within" ourselves or scan for electromagnetic distortions in our "bodies" if these bodies and the universe itself are really holograms. Eventually, we may begin to reframe our beliefs to include the fact that we can also discern the emotional and energetic realities of others. A new depth and understanding of intimacy then emerges. We are no longer limited to the "confines" of our physical bodies or our old Newtonian thinking. "I," therefore, am not as far away from "you" as I was led to believe. The "intrapersonal" and "interpersonal" dimensions of reality are no longer distinct. I can begin to realize that there is an interconnectedness of all reality if the "illusions of separation" fostered by the old paradigm begin to dissolve. As much as some of us would prefer to remain in our isolation and false sense of security, we are unavoidably immersed in a living, fluid, unified, interconnected universe.

The well known Yale surgeon, Dr. Bernie S. Siegel, author of <u>Love, Medicine, and Miracles</u>, provided a clue to the nature of our resistance to paradigm shifts, to changes in the fundamental way we view reality, when he stated that people are addicted to their beliefs.[18] We become dependent upon our beliefs to create a sense of security, stability, safety, and comfort. We become increasingly invested in them and the principle of "homeostasis" sets in. Homeostasis is defined as, "a state of physiological equilibrium produced by a balance of functions and of chemical composition within an organism."[19] The term derives from the Greek words <u>homeo</u> (like) and <u>stasis</u> (stand firm), meaning to "stay as it is." It is my belief that the "resistance" to change that manifests as an "addiction to our beliefs" is easily explained when we realize that the intensity of such attachments is fostered by the homeostatic energy created when memories, thoughts, beliefs, and perceptions are transfixed at moments of trauma. Resistance to change may simply be the extension of the same "freezing mechanism" by which our beliefs and perceptions were so urgently encoded **in order to keep us alive** during a traumatic experience. How often have we felt that a challenge to a particular belief left us feeling that we would perish if this belief were compromised? This "threatened" feeling that arises for us when certain beliefs are challenged may disclose the origin of many of our unresolved traumas. It is normal for "resistance" to manifest when retraumatization of the wounded ego state feels imminent. To our wounded ego states that are already fragile, it is easy to understand that control of the inner world becomes the key to survival. We cannot control our perpetrators, particularly when we are children, but we can exercise control over our inner holographic world and its perceptions. We can transfix and contain the trauma within our personal holographic space; we can seize and maintain control of our "vision." Once we protectively encode these threatening experiences, we continue to hold onto them until we possess sufficient resources to connect with the "healer within" – using our holographic perception to locate, identify, access, and resolve the scene that was encoded in self-defense.

But how many traumatic scenes can we store holographically in such detail? Scientists estimate that we carry the capacity to hold 280,000,000,000,000,000,000,000 bits of information during an average lifetime.[20] Holograms have an incredible capability for information storage.[21] Using holographic recording, researchers have calculated that a one-inch-square of film can store the same amount of information contained in fifty Bibles.[22] The electromagnetic fields of the body are infinitely more complex than such film. At the moment of traumatization, all of the perceptions of consciousness – the environment, clothing, emotions, and sensory data are all stored intact. Beliefs we hold about ourselves are also stored and encoded at such moments. For example, "body image distortion" can occur as the result of being frozen in a scene with a belief that "I am fat," and this view can be carried intact into the present, although I may now be quite "skinny." When I look upon my body, I may actually see myself as fat, though this is no longer true. In a similar fashion, ideas about core issues such as worthiness in relationship, gender roles, physical appearance, sexuality, and safety are all encoded in my nervous system when a trauma occurs. All three dimensions of relationality: self, others, and Higher Power are affected when trauma is induced. When we are abused, a false conception of self, others, and our spiritual worth is induced. We feel guilty, dirty, unworthy as a result of storing the transaction within ourselves. We begin to see how, from the standpoint of a holographic mind, intrapersonal and interpersonal realities are profoundly connected. Our speech, our gestures, our touch carry far more impact in the holographic model than in the old model that did not inform us of the capacity to "internalize" others – their beliefs, their shame, their intentions, their energy, their spirituality. Our holographic nature enables us to internalize any perception, attesting to a remarkable power. From the standpoint of healing, the holographic model also indicates that we have the power intrapersonally to heal the interpersonally induced traumas to our consciousness. Though our abusers may have died long ago, the holographic mind preserves them intact and accessible for the moment when we are ready to release or transform the memory. This profound capacity to heal ourselves is simply an extension of the holographic mind's capacity to create its reality. As quantum physics affirms, we are creators, and, as such, possess our own "inner healers." These "healers within" possess the perspicacity to scan our nervous systems, to locate and resolve trauma scenes that they have held until we were prepared to heal or release them. No one but you from within your own mind possesses the capacity to return to that specific moment in space and time, to that specific set of feelings to find the perfect solution for the scene, for no one but you knows that wounded part of self completely. With such perfect understanding of our "inner patients," is it any wonder that we are, in fact, our own best healers. The complex solutions our traumas require are easily identified by the infinitely complex mind that so wondrously encoded them. Our traumas are invitations to step into our holographic vision and use this new instrument of thought to its full capacity, and, in so doing, to realize our true spiritual nature.

5. **My feelings are a primary medium of my spirituality.** (Our feelings are the cues to unlocking our traumas and opening to higher states of consciousness.)

The single, most important piece of information for successful resolution of trauma is the identification of key emotions. As demonstrated in the cases reviewed earlier, from the affective residue of a trauma it is possible to access the memory fragment, to return to the scene, and to resolve the problematic feelings. Through resolution of the feelings we free ourselves from the trauma memory's hold over us – liberating us from the pain that bound our consciousness to another place and time. The resolution of this affect results in an empowerment that impacts us on all levels.

The role of emotion in the human psyche has been historically and scientifically undervalued. Many of our most influential systems – family, school, peers, religion, and others, conveyed messages that fostered emotional repression. Some of the systems even implied that such repression was essential for maturity and spiritual enlightenment. In my personal spiritual development, there was an intense emphasis on intellectual development, but even my "greatest" insights did little to enhance my communion with the spiritual. It is emotion that enables us to grasp the non-physical. Emotions are a powerful relational bridge. They transcend the limitations of time, space, and finite knowledge. I may not know everything about you, for instance, but I can maintain a relationship with you through my feelings for you and the connection that this bonding creates. This is even further enhanced if the feelings are mutual – if the relational bridge is mutual. Our deepest friendships seem to transcend space and time and to "pick up right where we left off" as though there has been no separation. Emotions assist us in providing a relational bridge far stronger than the intellect can supply.

As infants, our earliest messages were not mental; they were emotional – they were felt experiences, founded upon attitudes we read from our primary caregivers. In Chapter Six, citing Julian Hawthorne, we saw that without emotion, the mind remains inoperative – a blank; emotion is developmentally prior.[23] Our earliest perceptual experience was not so much a thought as a feeling. When asked about their most "spiritual" experience, most people will describe a profound emotional encounter, not an intellectual transaction. My most profound spiritual experiences have been moments when I have felt the presence of unconditional love. These experiences have often defied my ability to describe them verbally. By their nature, they transcend the limitations of language. Recalling these encounters, however, I can immediately connect with those persons and places. Emotions are incredible bearers of experience and contact that go far beyond the limitations of language and thought.

All emotions are opportunities for spiritual experience. Anger is, for instance, the emotion that has proved most useful in the resolution of trauma, serving as a signpost, a mnemonic to memory. It is the energy that accumulated during trauma induction that we were unable to apply appropriately and were incapable of accessing at that time. The anger remains with us as a guide and warning sign that the original trauma is yet to be resolved. It is the energy that, when used effectively in the original context, will allow total resolution of the memory, giving us the strength to heal. The amount of anger that we hold is proportionate to the amount of unresolved trauma, past or present, that we bear. Inappropriate venting of "buried" anger does not genuinely release the anger because it will only "resolve" when released at its locus of origin. Our subconscious minds will not allow us to prematurely release the anger that we will need to heal ourselves. When the anger is applied in the appropriate place and time, the resolution is expedient.

Shame, similarly, is a reliable indicator that unresolved events remain in the psyche. This feeling usually leaves us with the impression that there is no relational bridge with ourselves, others, or a Higher Power. We feel defective, broken, bad, isolated. In actuality, this feeling serves the very important purpose of pointing out the exact location of the traumas in our emotional bodies. We are not born with shame. It is always induced, initially, from the outside. By locating this feeling of shame, we can discover the source of the damage that has occurred to our psyche. Unfortunately, we have been taught to judge our emotions and to fear them. And in being taught to fear our emotions, we have been taught to fear our spirituality. The fear of emotion is the most powerful contributing influence to the traumatization of humankind. Such fear "sets us up" so that, instead of identifying the "feeling distortions" that are the keys to our healing process, we remain emotionally and spiritually paralyzed. We then try to appeal to our "spiritual" resources from the mental level and wonder why healing is not forthcoming. All the while we fail to see our emotions for what they really are – the key to understanding and resolving the problem, blockage, or illness. The only way for us to continue to heal, without this permission to feel, is for our bodymind to force our attention to this "stuck" point. Instead of allowing ourselves to feel and release anger and resentment held in our chest area, for example, we may develop breast or lung cancer. There is compelling research emerging that substantiates this theory.

Many of us have been seeking spirituality for a long time without the willingness to do the emotional groundwork. In my own case, I used my religious lifestyle to avoid certain emotional realities. A ministerial lifestyle that wields such authority and power over the minds of others, whether used in service to others or self, can be employed to avoid painful experiences within the self. We can busy ourselves with performing the "right actions," speaking the "right language," and "studying" the spiritual truth while dying emotionally. Many of us have experienced shame in our development and yet refuse to look at our feelings. We resort to misusing the spiritual tools available, like our religious systems, to avoid the very contact that we are seeking. This is fairly easy when "ritual" is involved. Ritual, by its nature, provides a security and reliable expectation of a positive, predictable outcome. Once habituated, however, it can be used to maintain homeostasis and to avoid growth or change. Ritualization is also a stage in the addictive process. I saw how easy it was to utilize the beauty of ritual or to hide behind its external trappings while avoiding the responsibility for personal growth. I saw many individuals using sacramental rituals (like "confession" – the "Sacrament of Reconciliation") to avoid emotional realities, particularly addictions. In the "Charismatic Movement" of my own religion I saw countless individuals who were sincerely striving to integrate their emotional content within their religious experience, but who were still looking for a quick vertical solution without doing the necessary internal, emotional work. The emotional body must be fully honored. There is no by-pass to spirituality without embracing the emotional. This may be terrifying for those of us who were taught to repress our emotions as proof of character. While this was not a conscious message in my family, it was, nonetheless, clear in its subtlety, particularly with respect to gender roles: Mom deals with the feelings;

Dad works and makes decisions. But what kind of healthy decision is anticipated from a process that excludes the essential spiritual and relational bridge of emotion?

For trauma survivors, the principle that spiritual access is to be found in working through our feelings may seem quite frightening. It is essential to remember that we have now reached the point where it is not necessary to "retraumatize" a person in order to resolve the original memory. I have never attended a client who authentically embraced his feelings (using the trauma resolution process described in this work) without receiving an accompanying sense of empowerment. In a way, we could conclude that the amount of emotional pain that we feel as a result of unresolved trauma is proportionate to the spiritual empowerment that awaits us when the trauma is resolved. This would be true in the case of a "predictable, closed energy system." In reality, since the human energy system is necessarily open, the empowerment will actually be <u>greater</u>, for, once the trauma-induced limitations on consciousness are removed, we return to our natural spiritual state where "grace" and abundant, unconditional love are found.

Openness to our emotions allows us access to the treasury of spirituality. These emotions allow us to bond with that which transcends our intellect and to experience that higher connection in consciousness, though it may elude our intellectual comprehension. Experiential understanding is possible even when intellectual comprehension is lacking. Our feelings are a precious vehicle for this communication, a primary medium for our spirituality.

6. **Affective blockages are spiritual blockages.** (Traumas impact us simultaneously on emotional and spiritual levels.)

The origin of our affect and our spirituality is our parents. Our parents or primary caregivers are the first "powers greater than ourselves" on whom we are dependent for life. They are the first to model and define love. Our earliest messages are felt messages of perception. This early emotional conditioning creates our predisposition toward reality, relationships, and self. My own development has affirmed the potency of these early emotional influences.

Over ten years ago I came to realize that, as a means of dealing with my fears and my pain, I had emotionally "shut down." As I discussed earlier in this text, I had effectively internalized my father's unhealthy coping mechanisms by the age of four and learned to avoid and repress any overwhelming fear and pain. Such repression and introversion enabled me to divert my "negative" feelings in order to survive, but it also prevented me from me from experiencing authentic love and intimacy. Having acquired this survival mechanism primarily through imitation, I was unaware of spiritual implications of this subconscious influence until I decided to explore the origins of my defenses. My discovery amazed me; its implications for spiritual development are enlightening.

Working with a therapist, while searching for effective trauma resolution techniques to assist my clients, I discovered a "body memory" that originated at age two and a half. My father threw me into a swimming pool to teach me to swim – the same way that his father had taught him. As a young child my perception was: "He's trying to kill me." This trauma created a distrust that impacted me throughout our relationship. For a considerable portion of my life I neither remembered the event nor realized its spiritual implications. I had been taught that "God is a father who sent his son Jesus to die for our sins." Theologically, this was all explained very nicely. On intellectual levels everything was quite comprehensible and orderly. On the emotional plane, however, whenever I heard that "God is our father" who let his son die for us, I had a negative emotional reaction that triggered this inexplicable feeling of distrust or caution. As you may glean from my earlier descriptions of "trauma triggers," this was a powerful, early trigger. A childhood message proclaimed "fathers are not to be trusted and may even threaten our lives." Since my mother and father mediated my earliest spiritual messages through affect, it now made sense that I was unconsciously transferring this emotional blockage to my relationship to my Higher Power. My emotional trauma had become a spiritual trauma. Healing the trauma with my father, consequently relieved the confusion and feelings of distrust about Higher Power. This experience also taught me that we apply those early messages directly and that they intimately impact our belief system, especially our spirituality. It is important to note that the blockage impacted me on an emotional level, but this also inhibited open access to my spiritual potential.

Emotions constitute a primary relational bridge to spirituality; likewise, emotional blockages create spiritual blockages. This is not to be interpreted, however, as a total rupture in the relationship to Spirit. Nothing can totally sever the bridge that links us to spirituality. We examined this truth in Chapter Eleven, where we saw that trauma, shame, addictions, and other emotionally repressive experiences can estrange us from conscious contact with our spirituality, but, even in these emotionally "shut down" conditions, spiritual access is never severed. As many of us heard quoted: "What can separate us from the love of God?" (See Romans 8:39; see also Diagram B, p. 185). Frequently we were given the impression, often at the direction of our religious systems, that total separation from spirituality, from our inherent connection to all things was possible. This, itself, was a "fear-based" notion. Traumas induce false perceptions and leave us uncertain regarding what to believe about ourselves, others, and our Higher Power. Traumas are moments when the nervous system acts to protect us from an overwhelming perception – often a feeling that we are going to die. Such fear, once encoded in our systems, can distort our rational thinking and result in desperate and compulsive behaviors. At times, our familial, educational, societal, and religious systems justified the use of fear and shame-inducing parenting techniques. We now know that threats of condemnation serve to induce emotional trauma and reduce open emotional access to the very spirituality that these systems seek to foster. In other words, many of the systems charged with our care have used emotionally and spiritually abusive techniques to foster spiritual growth. Absurd! They are mutually exclusive concepts.

One demonstrative case involved Daniel, who was in the hospital dying of AIDS. Daniel had long ago made peace with himself and his "Higher Power" regarding his situation and knew that he was dying. He asked that his family members be contacted and come to see him in the hospital; he had "some things" that he wanted to say to them. When Daniel's brother came to visit him in the hospital, he refused to make eye contact with Daniel and began quoting biblical passages, erroneously cited, indicating that his brother was already condemned for being homosexual. At no point did his brother allow Daniel the time to share what he had wanted to tell him – namely that he loved him and that he was sorry for any wrongs that he had ever done to him. The brother completed his well-planned and executed sermon and immediately left the room. When the priest arrived to talk with Daniel, he cried and shared his anxiety and concern about his brother: "I'm worried about my brother," he tearfully stated. "I believe he's religiously addicted and, though he doesn't drink any more, he's more out of touch with his feelings now than when he did, and now he justifies this in the name of God." Where is the spiritual growth evidenced in this example?

Emotional blockages are spiritual blockages. This is apparent in Daniel's story. It is hypocritical and an addictive use of religion to use these resources intended to foster spiritual growth to avoid dealing with emotions. We can use religion to avoid spirituality, to avoid our own vulnerability, to avoid love. It has long been stated by innumerable spiritual traditions that "God is love"; love is also identified as an emotion. There is a profound connection implied, without moving into discussion of the misuses of the word "love." Anything which represses our emotions impacts us spiritually; that which inhibits our capacity for love impacts us spiritually. This has become most evident through the study of addictions.

Addictionology has vastly expanded since the identification of alcoholism as a disease in the 1950's. We now recognize that the common denominator underlying all addictions is the repression of emotion. We call addiction a "spiritual illness." As the disease progresses, this individual spends more time in a "mood-altered" state; shame is increasingly induced, isolating the individual and intensifying the need to medicate. This increasing cycle of emotional repression reduces conscious contact with the spiritual. Anything that removes us from conscious contact with ourselves or others constitutes "spiritual illness." The repression of emotion does this.

In her book entitled, When Society Becomes An Addict, Anne Wilson Schaef states that we are an addicted society; we have become radically pain avoidant.[24] We are too focused on alleviating our pain to recognize that painful emotions are the gateways to accessing our spiritual truth. In our earnest efforts to avoid pain, we close our ears to the voices that speak to us from within, voices that direct us to those places within our physical, mental, emotional, and spiritual bodies that are in need of healing. We have been taught to distrust our emotions – especially the so-called "negative" ones. In reality, pain is the single most important key for the identification and subsequent resolution of traumas. It is the bodymind's way of telling us where, when, and how to resolve the trauma that was induced. Pain is the pointer that directs us to the exact location for the trauma to be resolved. It is the unfinished trauma manifesting in physical form. It is a two, four, nine, eleven, thirteen, seventeen, twenty-two ... year old within us frozen in some terrifying moment that feels like impending death – crying out for help to the only one who can hear. But, instead of attending to these voices crying to us through our pain, we medicate.

With my clients I repeatedly emphasize the need to remain present to the pain long enough to determine if the physical discomfort is trauma-induced or memory related. Once a trauma survivor learns that great healing can result from remaining present to her pain, both the conscious and subconscious minds begin to support the resolution process. Many clients observe that, "while in the waiting room," or "just when I got up this morning," some somatic pain arose cueing them to an opportunity for healing. For most individuals, the "cramps, back and neck pain, sinus problems, headaches, migraines, tightness, heaviness or knots" in their body are fragments of encoded memories, trance states surfacing for resolution. In over eighty percent of the cases, the subconscious mind is facilitating the healing process by presenting a "body memory" to the conscious mind as the initial cue to identify a trauma to be addressed. Upon resolution, many survivors comment that their pain was surfacing daily and, in some cases, for years. Without guidance or understanding of trauma, they found themselves "clueless" as to the means of addressing or resolving their pain.

We have not learned to listen attentively to the voices of our bodymind – to give our holographic mind sufficient trust and attention. However, we have gained expertise at expending our resources for medicating our symptoms. Many of us have spent extraordinary amounts of time and money on medical care that did little to resolve our suffering, without a clue to the pain's origin in the pathology of trauma.

We have become adept at medicating our pain with relationships, substitute addictions, prescription medications, religion, "forgive and forget" messages, even by trying to recover our worth through the lives of our children. We have failed to recognize the warning signs of trauma in our system, even as they broadcast more and more loudly – to the point that our bodies finally erupted, demanding our attention through cancer, a stroke, exhaustion, a "nervous breakdown," migraines, panic attacks, and countless other illnesses. Even in these acute states we did not recognize the underlying face of trauma. This is not a moral judgment, but an observation that we have been restricted in our solutions and approaches as a result of our lack of understanding about the dynamics of trauma induction and storage. We have not always seen this profound connection between the physical, the emotional, and the spiritual bodies. In our inattention or medication of our emotions and our somatic warnings, we have become blind to the opportunities offered us for spiritual and emotional healing. Additionally, we may have become angry and frustrated with a Higher Power that did not heal our condition, seeing our unique pain as a sign of rejection rather than the perfect invitation to heal our blockages – our traumas. We do not expect Higher Power to come wearing the face of pain. This, as you may recall from previous mention, was called the "via negativa" in ancient times and was always esteemed as a valid spiritual path.

Because it is true that affective blockages are spiritual blockages, perhaps it is also true that affective messages (i.e. painful feelings) are spiritual messages. If we could but learn to listen to ourselves differently, with reverence for all our emotions, we would discover the truth that authentic security is to be found in accessing and trusting our feelings and our intuition, not in finding better ways of avoiding our pain. Intuition is a direct and immediate knowledge, often described as a felt knowledge; it is more about feeling than logic. By opening to our emotions, we open to our intuition, our most powerful access to the spiritual. Anything that fosters distrust of our emotions restricts our intuitive abilities. We have often wondered why the high level of intuition that was so evident in childhood seemed to disappear. I believe that this is directly correlated to messages taught about repressing feelings. How is it phrased? ... "Unless you change and become like little children, you will not enter the Kingdom of God?"(Mt. 18:3) In Buddhist practice the use of koans (paradoxical statements) purports to force the mind to abandon logic and rely on second-sightedness. The key to the spiritual lies within our emotion and our intuition. Anything that inhibits this, inhibits our spiritual connection, our experiences of intimacy.

7. **All forms of abuse – of alienation of the self from the self are, at the same time, spiritual abuse.** (Abuse is also spiritual trauma.)

As we examine this principle, we must first ask: what precisely do we mean by abuse? Any experience that causes an alienation of the self from the self constitutes abuse. Most commonly we think of physical, verbal, emotional, spiritual, and sexual abuse … and we associate these with the most violent or intrusive acts. One of the earliest revisions to my traditional thinking involved my concept of what constitutes trauma. That which traumatizes or abuses us is not always intentional. Sometimes it is due to oversight, insensitivity, forgetfulness, distraction, ignorance, or benign neglect. The electromagnetic fields of our bodies that mediate consciousness and memory are incredibly subtle and sensitive. I did not appreciate this until I felt the intense pain that could be generated from a memory that, at first glance, may have been considered of minor importance.

A most instructive case in this regard was Jennifer, who came to me reporting a fairly healthy and happy childhood. Nonetheless, there was something causing her to question her own worth – feeling low self-esteem. When I asked her what this felt like, she stated that, "It feels like shame."

"When you feel this shame, where do you feel it in your physical body?" I asked.

She replied, "It's over my shoulders; it's dark and heavy – about the shape of a large coathanger surrounding my shoulders and weighing them down." She became tearful as she described this heavy feeling of shame.

After defining the metaphor – the fragment of the original scene that was used to encode and store the memory, I asked her, "How young are you when you first feel a dark, heavy feeling of shame over your shoulders in the shape of a coathanger?"

She stated, "I'm seven years old."

"And where might you be when you're seven years old and you're feeling this?" I continued.

"I'm at home," she replied.

"And what happens then when you're at home and you're seven years old?" I questioned.

"I go up to Daddy and ask him for a hug."

"And what happens then, when you ask him for a hug?" I added.

"He won't hug me," she responded tearfully.

"And what happens then, when he won't give you a hug?" I inquired.

"I feel like he doesn't love me," she sobbed in reply.

The trauma which Jennifer identified in this experience startled me. She later explained that her father was alcoholic and non-demonstrative. He never gave her hugs or held her. When this profound need was repeatedly denied, she unconsciously induced a feeling of shame, a dark heavy feeling closely resembling the shape of a hug, an embrace in her shoulders – what she had described earlier as the shape of a "coathanger." This confirmed a principle that I had learned earlier: if certain developmental needs are not met at the appropriate time, shame or trauma is induced. We continue to grow, but those areas that are deprived or stunted become more evident as time elapses. It is not unlike a young sapling needing certain amounts of rainfall and nourishment to grow. If sunlight is blocked from one side of the tree, the other side that is receiving full nourishment will outpace, outgrow the side that is deprived, but overall growth will continue. We develop in much the same way. Certain aspects of ourselves freeze through lack of nurturing and trauma. The imbalance that is created often leaves us with the feeling that something is wrong, out of balance, and in need of attention. The increasing tension from such imbalances is our system's natural way of pointing out the blockage or trauma for resolution. Neglect and abandonment induce dark and heavy, debilitating feelings of shame in the nervous system. Jennifer's case taught me the intricacies and sensitivities of our nervous system – that our whole body is really memory, and an incredibly sensitive recorder of memory it is! In resolving her trauma, Jennifer reentered the memory as her nurturing adult/parent self and assumed the responsibility for the care and healing of the seven year old, beginning with a hug. She was able to resolve the unmet needs from her childhood and release the shame feeling that she had carried on her shoulders for many years.

When we hear the word "abuse," we usually think of overt physical, verbal, or sexual abuse. These are only the extremes of the continuum. Each of us experiences deficiencies in our development. It is impossible for parents to meet all of a child's developmental needs. This is a more pervasive problem today with single parent families or with both parents working. More and more early nurturing is being entrusted to other primary caregivers like those in day-care centers. But let us consider the fact that, even when parents consistently are present for their children, they cannot respond in such a precise manner as to prevent any trauma or deficiencies from occurring; nor are parents expected to do so. A parent is the trustee, not the owner of the child. Ultimately, the only persons with the emotional capacity for ownership to undertake the reframing and resolution of the unfinished business of childhood, adolescence, and adulthood is ourselves. In the reframing and reconstruction of the subtle energies of memory, we become fully empowered. Our parents were not intended to complete this process for us. We are perfectly (and I use this word with respect and for its precise meaning) designed to assume this responsibility, for, there is no one who can understand the exact needs of my wounded seven year old self, unless it is I who share the same nervous system with that wounded ego-state. Our own development "sets us up" to have to assume the responsibility and to become empowered by so doing . It should also be noted that there is a true perfection in the nervous system's operation. How astounded I was when I first learned that <u>no</u> energy appears to be lost during the electrical transmissions of the nervous system; they are "perfect"– complete.

Our culture has supported an incredible awakening during the last five decades in our understanding of the dynamics of "abuse." We discovered the disease of alcoholism in the 1950's and at the same time developed "family systems theory" – an understanding of the dynamics and interactions of functional and dysfunctional families. We later identified other addictions, diseases, and behaviors that foster the emotional repression that creates dysfunction. Recently we have changed our beliefs substantially about the frequency of sexual abuse, particularly incest. I do not believe that this is a movement toward hysteria or an effort to justify our addictions or our "victimhood." Rather, I believe that this "awakening" is necessary for us to recognize that we have, indeed, been living "unconsciously" due to our traumas and, therefore, need to heal our past. If there is no recognition that our individual or collective growth has been deficient in any way, there is certainly no access or motivation to reframe these memories or heal the deficiencies. In reality, the attention that is drawn to abuse and which is constantly before us in the media serves a much deeper spiritual purpose; this relates to an increasing dissatisfaction with anything less than our full potential.

We are discovering that we have been "designed" to complete our own nurturing and development – that we can reenter our own memories and place in those cells and fields of our bodies the positive nurturing that needed to be there during our early developmental stages. We are learning to utilize our "quantum" mastery over space and time. We are growing tired of giving our power and attention to therapies, systems, philosophies, and authorities that foster victimhood. This is the invitation that underlies all abuse – to discover our power to heal the damage done and become creators who are able to live fully in the present. The recognition of our traumas is never to be seen as an end in itself, but as the occasion for the emergence of our "shadow selves" into the sunlight in order to dissolve these illusions fostered by trauma and all forms of abuse. We all experience traumas and abuses which serve to awaken in us our need and ability to self-heal and to foster the healing of one another. With the insight and means for healing, we can look at the more subtle issues and forms of abuse without feeling frightened. I have seen the look on parents' faces when I share the case of Jennifer (above) – where the child induced shame from not receiving a hug, or the case of Lorraine – the seven year old whose father would not answer her question. They appear terrified that they might have unknowingly "traumatized" their children or harmed them. All parents have traumatized their children at one time or another, at least inadvertently. This is understandable, in part, due to the encompassing sensitivity of the nervous system. Pretending that parenting does not involve such trauma induction fosters emotional repression and impedes the trauma resolution process. The goal of parenting is simply to do one's best and to trust in the self-healing abilities that we are now learning. Eventually, as we master trauma resolution, we will teach our children the practice, enriching their legacy, improving their birthright. With opportunities and effective methods for healing the self, we can then look at forms of abuse and trauma without the frightened, avoidant, and dissociative reactions that we have used to "just survive" in the past. We can learn more effective healing practices.

With new options for healing our emotional wounds, we can look honestly at the effects of abuse and trauma. As we have seen, one of the most powerful effects of trauma is that it imprints us with illusions and false perceptions that seem to contradict the truth: that we have the power to heal ourselves. This is part of the spiritual deception that repeatedly accompanies a traumatic experience. All traumas encode as experiences and declarations of powerlessness within our psyche. Trauma and abuse foster spiritual confusion by introducing frozen or false beliefs which introduce into our psyche a conviction of powerlessness; such trauma-induced deception contradicts messages declaring our nature as powerful, creative spiritual beings. They introduce a splitting in the belief system that, unless resolved, will result in a loss of power and centeredness. If it is true, as we have observed: "I am the locus of all my spiritual experience," anything that alienates me from myself will also affect my spiritual integrity. The shame-inducing experiences of our lives profoundly impact our spirituality.

As Gershen Kaufman has effectively indicated, shame alienates the self from the self.[25] When we are shamed, we pause to look at ourselves and question our integrity. It is as though we look into the mirror and do not know whether to believe the message that we are OK or the shame message that tells us that we are defective. Shame is fragmenting; it generates civil war within us. This has happened to each of us, whether as children or as adults – a moment when we were shamed and received a message that contradicted what we previously had been told about ourselves. This splitting of our ego results in confusion, for it introduces opposing messages: "Am I handsome as I was told, or is there something wrong with me like these people are saying?" As we saw earlier, shame is a primary affect.[26] Once induced by a trauma, it becomes internalized and estranges us from our inner truth, establishing a lack of self-trust. This distancing effect is the alienation of the self from the self. Anything which results in the induction of shame fosters self-alienation. Obviously, physical, emotional, mental, verbal, sexual, and spiritual abuse produce this kind of alienation. When shame is induced by abuse from another, we lose touch with an integral part of ourselves.

Earlier in this work we defined the interdependency between the three dimensions of spirituality: relationship to self, to others, and to Higher Power. It makes sense that abuse from other individuals creates similar repercussions in the remaining two dimensions (See Diagram B, p. 185). Once abused by another person, we also feel alienated from ourselves and from Higher Power. One of the first questions that I hear from trauma survivors is: "How could God let this happen to me?" I also see that the internalized shame, originally induced externally, is commonly felt and interpreted as an intrapersonal defectiveness, although its origin was interpersonal. The point of origin of self-esteem is, initially, inter-personal. Our parents first mirrored to us our value; through their eyes we began to see our own worth. We began to record these messages, and, hopefully, they were uniform and consistent in their affirmation and validation of our unconditional value. As these affirming experiences became more common, we began to internalize them. We identified with these reinforced messages filling our consciousness, filling the cells of our bodies with memories of gentle touch and nurturing, consistent and reliable satiation of our basic needs, and sounds of caring and gentleness. On the other hand, we also may have received conflicting messages: gentle touch and abusive touch, satiation and neglect, nurturing and abandonment, words of affirmation and criticism. As we internalized the emotional or verbal abuse, we came to experience this externally originated conflict within ourselves. As children, against what were we to measure the validity of these assertions, particularly when they originated within our primary care systems? When they came from outside the family, it was to be hoped that our parents provided the grounding needed to correct the intrusive and false messages about the self. Clearly, when self-esteem is undermined, this affects all other dimensions of our being. When shame is internalized, we feel "down" on ourselves, less worthy of relationship with others or of contact with our Higher Power. Addictions, as "spiritual illness," inevitably affect the comfort of the self in seeking or maintaining contact with a Higher Power. This is logical as we understand the dynamics of shame induction and the profound sense of worthlessness, dirtiness, isolation, emptiness, and embarrassment that it deposits. When we become alienated from ourselves through trauma or abuse, we live with opposing beliefs about our worth, value, and purpose. Our creativity becomes subverted because our perceptions are skewed. Subsequently, we proceed to create reality according to these opposing beliefs and altered frames of reference; this creativity is both conscious and subconscious.

In the book, <u>Getting the Love You Want</u>, the author, Harville Hendrix, talks about the "unconscious marriage."[27] When there are considerable unmet dependency needs from our childhood, we continue to seek resolution for the old scripts, repeatedly acting them out in our contemporary relationships. We unconsciously seek our original profile of love, recreating "love" experiences as witnessed, imitated, and internalized from our primary caregivers – as healthy or unhealthy as those may have been. We recreate the same patterns that we unconsciously recorded from our childhood. We may try to heal or "complete" the pattern, seeking partners like our parents, or, perhaps, opposite our parents – individuals who we hope will heal the original breach in nurturing. Such "codependent" solutions do not work. Marry someone like your father or mother, when Mom or Dad could not meet your needs growing up, and you will find yourself recreating the same emotionally unfulfilling relationship. I have noted during trauma resolution work that many survivors, when it comes to the moment of finding the appropriate, safe person to enter the trauma memory to retrieve the "wounded child," instead of recognizing themselves as the ideal healer, first turn to their current spouse and, sometimes, even to their own children to heal them (which may be construed as emotional incest – i.e., using your children to meet your emotional needs instead of meeting theirs). The thought that they could accomplish this nurturing themselves simply does not occur to them. One wonders what the marriage is like when the unmet dependency needs arise from childhood. I have felt resentment when I have found myself playing the role of parent or therapist in interpersonal relationships. Partners wanting equality in relationships resist playing a parental role to their significant other. It is the primary thinking and neediness of the child within that continues to orient the consciousness to external forces for answers and solutions. As trauma sufferers and survivors, is it any surprise that it does not occur to us to think of ourselves as the solution? Given the influence of the subconscious mind, it does not surprise me when the early outward-bound gaze of the child dominates the thought processes and healing efforts of our lives. The emotional power of our memories is tremendous. When the cells and electromagnetic fields of our bodies were utilized to stop a threatening situation, to prevent death, they became preoccupied with this task and were no longer available for other creative endeavors. This is the effect of trauma and abuse. Our spiritual power, our creative potential is greatly diminished when we are, thus, alienated from ourselves.

8. **Spirituality involves the healing of our "intentionality" – our decision-making ability.** (Trauma involves the entrapment of a "false intentionality" within our consciousness which subsequently influences our decisions.)

An understanding of spirituality necessarily includes the tripartite relationship between self, others, and Higher Power as well as the choices we make which shape this rapport. Trauma, in its direct impact on the nexus of consciousness – the self, the foundation of all relationship, significantly alters outcomes and our decision-making process. Crucial for the healing process, therefore, is a grasp of the importance of decision-making.

Beneath every creative act and every decision is the notion of intention. Each choice that is made is one of intent, and it may be conscious or subconscious. Intention is the focused manifestation of consciousness that underlies every choice, action, or thought. Trauma produces a fragmentation of consciousness that results in both conscious and subconscious intentionality. Though we may desire healthy relationships for ourselves, we continue to be attracted to persons sharing a likeness to our abusers because of the unresolved bond with the abuser or the abuser's profile that is still intact in our subconscious. This relational bond is the frozen scene of trauma. This scene is an ongoing part of a survivor's reality, of her nervous system. The amount of emotional energy stored within the holographic scene empowers this intentionality. I shared with you earlier in this work the case of Claire, who, upon hearing that her husband was going to divorce her, proceeded to go to the kitchen and eat raw flour. This childhood coping mechanism was part of a very powerful history of abuse that was still stored intact – untouched until the memory was tapped by the feeling of abandonment from the impending divorce. The adult Claire thought that she was "going crazy," but the overwhelming feelings emerging from the divorce announcement overrode her conscious, adult intentionality and activated a very potent, though childlike, repressed objective. This is the power of trauma. The fragmentation within the psyche that occurs from trauma creates diverse and often opposing intentions. One part of us may desire healing and release of an unhealthy behavior pattern while another part holds onto the experience from some hidden place within us. This was the case with Claire's attraction to "raw flour." Powerlessness is further manifested when we are not at all conscious of the intentionality encoded at the moment of trauma, demonstrated by Claire's amnesia. We cannot choose our intentions consciously if we are unaware of these ego-states frozen with their unique and precise intentions. One indicator of trauma is the fact that we find ourselves saying one thing and doing another. Frequently we can deduce the existence of these opposing intentions by simply observing these patterns in our lives.

I recall an experience of a visit with a friend. After hours of conversation with him, following clues from his comments, I asked if he had ever been abused. Briefly avoiding the question, he stated that it was "funny" that I should ask. He explained the reason for his surprise: after more than two years of therapy, his psychiatrist had decided to utilize hypnosis to assist him in exploring a childhood sexual abuse experience. I was not very surprised. I had spent two hours listening to him tell me about his previous relationships in which his partners had each abused him. When he showed me pictures of them I could not tell the partners apart. They were all older than he and looked virtually identical to each other. When I asked him to describe his original abuser, he suddenly gasped and made the connection for himself. He also admitted that, given the affective deprivation that he had experienced at home as a seven year old, the abuse from the older fifteen year old male neighbor was perceived as love and attention. With this subconscious bonding in place, his choices all manifested this early definition of love, programming him for pursuit of these look-alike, unsatisfying, abusive relationships.

Reviewing my life, I am amazed that I repeated behavior patterns so many times before I became conscious of buried intentions and their precipitating traumas. I have increased the trust level of my ability to expose my subconscious intentions; this occurred with discipline over time. I have worked with individuals who were married as many as eight times before identifying their traumas and their potent but sabotaging intentionality. Recognizing patterns in a timely manner and discovering their origins in our trauma histories can greatly assist us in reclaiming our lost intentionality and precious years of living.

This process of reclaiming lost intentionality is not promised to be easy. I have found wounded ego-states within me content to isolate from family and friends, as well as to avoid painful feelings. I have found that I cannot bully or force these ego-states to cooperate. They can be integrated effectively only when they are loved back into a participative consciousness. This means that the reintegration of subconscious intentionality is only possible when a certain purpose is defined. Another opposing, aggressive, or abusive intention will only result in reinforcement of the original trauma. I have seen survivors evidence an adult-parent self eager to access and resolve memories of abuse, only to find the wounded child-self trapped in the frightening scene, overwhelmed and distrustful of all attempts at intervention. In such cases, the nurturing adult-self must proceed with extreme patience, gentleness, and understanding. Trust must be restored with sensitivity to the individual's timetable for healing. This is not simply an exercise in creative imagination. The wounded child ego-states within our multidimensional consciousness are real – just as quantum physics tells us. The fact remains, however, that the most competent person to approach the wounded child is the one who carries the capacity for perfect understanding of that child, and that person is the survivor-self who knows exactly what this child has experienced. There is no other who possesses the capacity to feel this younger ego-state's experience and to understand it completely; there is no other who can understand or feel this pain and its consequences as well as the survivor who shares it so totally.

The goal of evolutionary process individually and collectively is the same: wholeness, oneness, unity, integration. The journey is, of course, more difficult when certain fragmented parts of our psyche utilize their decision-making power to remain set in their original defenses while other parts seek wholeness and integration. Increasing exercise of conscious, singular intentionality is the goal for trauma resolution. As we identify and subsequently resolve our "stuck points" in intentionality, we experience increasing consensus in our aims. This increase in power results in more consistent creativity and intimacy. We become more effective as conscious creators of our realities. Until now we have not had the tools to reclaim the subconscious intentionality lost through trauma. As Gary Zukav states in his book, The Seat of the Soul, "Unconscious evolution through the density of physical matter, through the experiences that are created unconsciously by unconscious intentions, has been the way of our species to now." [28] We are entering the age where the discovery of our lost intentionality is upon us. We have come to discover, through our insights into more subtle forms of illness such as addictions and family systems dysfunction, the dynamics which underlie our loss of power as creators. The hidden dynamics of trauma have long held the secret of our ability to create opposing designs which then manifest as loss of power. Over these last decades our society has come to identify itself as a victim. The increasing frustration with this "victim mentality" has only served to make us more aware of the disparity between this perception and our true nature. Just as a tree manifests increasing tension between the branches that are stuck and unable to grow and the parts that thrive, so we have come to the point where we are increasingly eager to recover and focus our intentionality as the creators that we are meant to be.

In freeing myself from the constrictions that had stunted my development, I found that I could exercise creative power over the past (as it was stored in my nervous system). I recognized the power to shape my reality by my decisions. As I began to reintegrate the wounded parts of myself, I found my intentions to be more singular, thus decision-making seemed less complicated. The conflicting voices that had previously hindered or clouded my decision-making were no longer clamoring for my attention and energy. I found increasing harmony within myself and, consequently, in my relationships with others and my Higher Power. An intuitive clarity emerged from this process that endowed me with a sense of spiritual guidance within my decision-making milieu. From an increasing position of spiritual power, it became easier and easier to focus my resolve and to foster integration on all levels. Distortions in the emotional body now hold less energy and are viewed as occasions for further empowerment, rather than dreaded moments of pain or impotence.

Our nature is spiritual. It seeks integration and unity. Emotions that speak of disintegration and powerlessness are cues to wholeness. This process simply requires a decision to pause to listen to our cues, to recognize Spirit speaking to us through our manifest conscious and subconscious intentions, through our seemingly irrational behaviors. I can make the decision to honor all of my emotions; I can track my emotions and bring the hidden intentions to consciousness. In so doing, I exercise responsible choice and greatly accelerate healing and movement toward wholeness. On all levels, spirituality can be fostered by my decisions, and by my growing intentionality.

I have discovered that, even in our weakest moments, our spiritual nature holds onto a design which, despite severe trauma on emotional, mental, and physical levels, will yet provide a profound strength and focus that invites healing. During my early spiritual formation I read Victor Frankl's book, Man's Search for Meaning.[29] I was deeply impacted as he chronicled his imprisonment in Nazi concentration camps at Auschwitz and Dachau. He described the loss of his wife and children, his occupation, his possessions, his health, and his emotional strength. His description expanded my concept of trauma beyond anything that I had imagined. From torment Frankl grew to believe that purpose and meaning can be found in the experience of trauma. In describing his therapeutic approach (called "Logotherapy," from the Greek word <u>logos</u>, which denotes "meaning") which evolved from his experience in the concentration camps, he stated the following: "In logotherapy's attempt to make something conscious again it does not restrict its activity to <u>instinctual</u> facts within the individual's unconscious, but also cares for <u>spiritual</u> realities such as the potential meaning of his existence to be fulfilled, as well as his will to meaning."[30] This "will to meaning," which formed the foundation of Frankl's work, is the foundation of our spirituality. As seen from his own example, there is a personal resolve that exists within our spiritual nature that cannot be eliminated by traumatization. There is fundamental choice that remains and can provide the grounding necessary to survive devastating assaults to our psyches.

   This vision or "will to meaning" capacity allows us to remain in contact with that greater knowing which reminds us that we are connected on levels that transcend the pain and limitations imposed by time and space. From the standpoint of the Higher Self, there is no "real" death. There are only lessons of meaning and stepping stones to greater creativity and consciousness. We can survive tremendous trauma to the emotional, mental, and physical aspects of ourselves with the higher understanding that all forms of trauma are manifestations of energy that can be transformed from negative to positive, from "death" to "resurrection." It is our inherent spiritual nature that helps us to identify and access these opportunities to discover, manifest, and explore the creator potential within us. During moments of intense trauma, when the emotional body is crying out for assistance, we have resources that allow us to tap into that creative power to lay the groundwork for the healing process. We now realize the magnificent capacity we possess to pause time and space so that we can access the appropriate resources for healing. Instead of viewing my memory loss from traumas as defectiveness, I recognize that I have orchestrated my life, giving myself the time and emotional space needed to develop sufficiently in order to complete the healing process. Amnesia from trauma serves the timetable and purposes of self-healing.

Among the greatest privileges that I experience through my work with trauma survivors is sharing that moment of awareness when they realize that the awful traumas that occurred in the past have all remained only a fraction of a second away from consciousness, and that they can now readily free the wounded self from the past and from its outdated messages and intentions. A great understanding dawns when the deeper spiritual purpose of these frozen scenes comes to light. Though we used our subconscious intentionality to numb the moments of impending death during our childhood or adulthood, we can now utilize our conscious intentionality to recover the use of those powerful cells of memory for creative work today. In so doing, we discover the perfection of our "design." We were intended to discover our own creative power and to reparent ourselves, to recreate our past as it should be. There is no one who knows the intricate details of our histories better than ourselves. Some of us might respond, "Oh, yes there is — God!" But the reality of it is that Higher Power chooses to heal us first from within ourselves, not externally. To attempt healing from "outside" would only foster illusions of separateness and "spiritual codependency." And the person most appropriate to facilitate this healing is not a divinity that resides "outside" of us, but that self where all three dimensions meet. Within the self is the promise of an experience, a unity so complete that self, others, and Higher Power could manifest as singular consciousness. (Look at the top of Diagram A, p. 184). At the apex of consciousness, self, others, and Higher Power are one. St. John of the Cross, one of my favorite mystics, dismissed the distinction between "primary" and "secondary causality" – in other words, it didn't matter whether God created all things first, for instance, and then allowed our parents to share in this creative act secondarily. When we move beyond the limitations of space and time, there is only one creative act, one creative energy in which we all participate. Though Higher Power may, indeed, possess one hundred percent knowledge about us, we also bear this capacity in our "design," for, between our conscious seven percent and our subconscious ninety-three percent awareness, we possess complete knowledge of ourselves. Perhaps, like John of the Cross, we need to dismiss the "causality" that creates the conflict in our minds about the identity, location, and source of all healing. It is one and the same.

When I ponder that who I am today is the result of the memory of one cell – one complete DNA/RNA helix, I marvel at the promise of creative power when trillions of cells, all carrying this capacity, are brought under the influence of my conscious intentionality. If the cellular mind so rules the physical body, then what is our creative, healing potential? There is a resolve, an intention, a design, and a power manifest on all levels of our being.

When we are overwhelmed by our trauma experiences, and are unable at a given moment to grasp this overpowering intentionality, we remain with the "will to meaning" capacity of our spirituality intact. So often I remind the newcomers in the treatment center that, though they may feel the hopelessness or discouragement that led them to treatment, the fact remains that something has shifted on a profound internal level to bring them, despite their diseases, resistance, and fears, to a place and time of healing. Something has brought them to this occasion for transformation. There is a fundamental resolve that remains amidst the power loss. We can choose, for instance, to place our bodies, which hold these overpowering emotions, thoughts, and sensations, in situations that promote healing and relief. We can choose to connect with a sponsor, therapist, friend or spiritual resource that can help us to find the underlying purpose and meaning in today's painful experiences. As seen from the description of spirituality (See Diagram A), there is not just the one vertical avenue available through Spirit, there are three: access to healing through connection with self, through others, and via "Higher Power." Though we may have felt spiritually separated from our creative power for years, we can still make choices from within the limitations imposed by trauma. Oftentimes we would like to simply use our "willpower" and resolve our traumas and blockages ourselves, without "outside" intervention, but the exigency of our broader spiritual nature may not allow us to resolve these traumas alone. A more empowering resolution often occurs through the decisions that foster spirituality and healing in all three dimensions. Repeatedly individuals enter treatment with a belief system stating that spirituality involves the vertical dimension only, and with great frustration and disillusionment that Spirit did not intervene at their request and preempt the need for "external help." We can spend years seeking the solution to our traumas in the vertical dimension. It makes more sense, however, that resolution of trauma should include all three of the dimensions that were present when it was induced: self, others involved, and Spirit. Attempts to access and use spirituality to avoid what will prove our most effective and thorough methods of healing will not, of course, succeed; our Higher Self will see to that.

Spirituality ensures that we transcend our fluctuating emotions, our finite thoughts, and our physical pain. As we move through our traumas, our intentionality becomes more focused, our decisions more supportive of our truth, our creativity more powerful, our relationships more nurturing, and our lives more centered.

9. **Spirituality is both a growth process and a state of relationship.** (Our spirituality grows and continuously supports us in the healing of our traumas.)

Working with a chemically dependent group of clients, I asked each member to define spirituality as he understood it. A young man who had overdosed twice on cocaine "accidentally" and had to be resuscitated said, "It's a gift – I'm already saved and know that I'm going to heaven; it doesn't really matter what I do." Another of the patients quickly objected. He had been raised a "traditional Catholic" and felt tremendous guilt and shame about his inability to control his drinking. In his Catholic education, "drunkenness was a sin." He stated, "That's a bunch of bull … you have to do certain things to get to heaven – you have to follow the rules." I then posed the question to the group: "What do you think? Is spirituality a gift, a given, a permanent state of relationship? Or do you think that it's more like a growth process?" After considerable debate and discussion, they reached a consensus: "It's both – it's always there, but you can lose touch with it. You can take it for granted because it is always there, but it's also a growth process that includes changes and learning from mistakes."

Principle Nine follows closely from the first principle that stated: "To be is to be spiritual." Spirituality – the natural, dynamic interaction of relationships to self, others, and Higher Power, is a permanent state of relationship. It is always present. It can, however, be intensified or diminished by our choices. In Diagram B we saw that, although estrangement may occur as we experience trauma, addictions, and other experiences which seem to draw us away from the integration for which we are intended, the spiritual connection cannot be totally broken. This means that the stages of our lives that lead to personal and interpersonal integration or disintegration constitute a growth process with opportunities to experience the effects of our conscious and subconscious choices. This journey through intentionality begins before the age of moral choice and proceeds as a movement toward ever-greater consciousness. It is multi-dimensional and paradoxical.

We are always one with a Source that is unchanging, but we also grow and evolve. This is paradox. The relationality that we call spirituality is constantly here. On higher levels of consciousness we are never separated from contact with this Source. This becomes apparent when, from our woundedness, we suddenly discover the infinite resources immediately available to us for the resolution of age-old blockages. Repeatedly we have surrendered our own inherent power and self-knowledge to the notion of an omniscient god that was "out there" when the answer was within all along. "Spirit" is closer to us than our conscious selves are able to admit. St. Augustine said: "God is closer to us than we are to ourselves." The gap, however, is understandable from the standpoint of trauma. When those powerful emotional energies overwhelm us, they often leave us with a profound sense of powerlessness and spiritual isolation. The internal splitting that occurs precipitates what spiritual tradition has referred to as the "dark night of the soul" experience, where we "feel" cut off from higher consciousness. While this can be helpful for giving us emotional warning signs of the when, where, and what of an unresolved trauma, it is not our "intended" state of being from the perspective of Spirit. Since spirituality is a permanent, abiding state of relationship, experiences like the "dark night of the soul" can serve as a "spiritual wake-up call" to remind us that life is intended to be more than darkness. "Man is that he might have joy." We know intuitively that we are meant for something more than the static moments pervaded by darkness and feelings of despair or hopelessness. Given our spiritual nature, a restlessness sets into the darkness when we have dwelt overlong in its pseudo-security. The cool darkness of the cave into which my two and a half year old wounded inner child withdrew eventually manifested as a shackle which hindered my adult capacity for intimacy. The emergent feelings of discontent and restlessness signaled the need for liberation of both the wounded child and the impeded adult.

Through our spirituality, we have access to that vision which senses the purpose of this growth process. The Higher Self already sees the outcomes from beyond the limitations of space and time and helps us to become "unstuck" when we encounter the hurdles of trauma. These hurdles increasingly condition us for the next stage of the journey. The goal of the journey is consciousness. The reward is the experience of spirituality-intimacy-relationality.

As multi-dimensional beings, we have, in one sense, already transcended space and time. From this higher vision, the goals, tasks, and process are already accomplished. This is the source of the permanent state of relationship that cannot be altered. We have already reached the apex of spirituality (See Diagram C) from the perspective of our immortal "soul" or Higher Self. On the other hand, there is the manifestation of consciousness which I experience in this lifetime now. This experience of consciousness presents itself as still in progress, still evolving. From a temporal perspective, failure to honor the growth process merely delays its movement and evolution in time. As demonstrated in the case of the young addict who overdosed, trying to use: "I'm saved!" to avoid facing the spiritual and emotional hurdle of addiction – "side-stepping" will only serve to intensify and foster the progression of the addiction. The failure to honor the challenge to ascend through our traumas and our addictions will produce increasing feelings of tension, inconsistency, and imbalance. The upward thrust of our spiritual nature ensures that higher consciousness will, ultimately, be achieved.

The belief that spirituality is a "growth" process inviting an expansion of consciousness, assists us in placing both emotional and physical "death experiences" in their proper perspective. "Death," from the standpoint of the multi-dimensional being, is simply a shift in holographic awareness; it is a stepping-stone, an invitation to participate in a much greater process. Death does not involve the cessation of consciousness. When, however, we become immersed in the illusions of our addictions and traumas, losing touch with the permanency of our spiritual consciousness, it is possible to forget that these experiences are invitations to expansion. In our fixation and immersion in the "emotional" body, we fall under the illusions of these perceptions of "impending death." Trauma activates inherent defenses that foster hypervigilance and defensiveness for survival. With a sufficient amount of trauma stored in the nervous system, it is possible for us to become invested in remaining "stuck" in our addictions and other illusions of safety, thereby avoiding further change or growth. Such patterns must then be brought to our attention through manifestations in the physical body as illness, disease, or body memories. This awakening will be accomplished through the exigency of our spiritual nature. All within reality serves the spiritual growth process. All is, ultimately, movement upward in consciousness.

There is no "punishment" as a part of this growth process. There are fewer "demons" than we thought. But our spiritual natures will allow the full experience of our own imbalances as part of the healing process. Even the external interference created by trauma and abuse from others becomes an opportunity to access our own power – to create our reality and not be "victimized" by false beliefs. It is very reassuring to see more and more clearly the underlying flow of our lives as we resolve the obstacles that impair our vision. At certain points in the process we cannot see this completely, but, as we learn to clear each of the hurdles provided by trauma, we gain greater and greater access to our intuition, allowing us to feel the flow. The hurdles come to form patterns which point us toward our underlying spiritual purpose. As we come to recognize and heal the painful patterns that emerge, we learn to trust and to be patient that our moments of trauma hold lessons and meaning. As we practice and learn to rely upon our inner guidance, "trauma" occurs less and less frequently, since our inner strength allows us to cope more effectively. We, eventually, come to trust that underlying flow and to realize its inherent strength. The "Higher Self" – that true form of ourselves that has already learned these lessons and transcended space and time, reassures us as we journey.

As access to our intuition intensifies and we move increasingly from five-sensory perception to multi-sensory perception, the underlying flow becomes palpable. Such transformations prove more difficult from the limited five-sensory awareness on which we relied in the past. Just as the trauma survivor finds a pseudo-security in the controlled, frozen scene of trauma, so too the five-sensory personality finds a false security in limiting reality to the capabilities of five senses. This sensory-bound illusion of "solidity" is <u>not</u> security. I have heard repeatedly in my own thoughts, dreams, and meditations: "True security lies in trusting your intuition." This means moving into an increasing reliance upon our multi-sensory awareness. This may contradict the old Newtonian assumption that security was equated with that which is "solid" and accessible to the "five" senses. "Real" for me now is found outside the limitations of these five senses. The traumas of others are largely imperceptible to the five senses, though they can certainly be deduced from observation. When we move, however, into the creator-potential of the mind to freeze time and space, to store it intact within the nervous system, to quickly access and change these electromagnetically stored forms of memory, we move into multi-sensory awareness. The spiritual growth process is readily perceptible to the multi-sensory personality. Traumas are easily identifiable to the multi-sensory self. In my trauma work, I find increasing effectiveness and power directly related to the development of my multi-sensory awareness. This feels like my true nature. I do not believe that I am intended to live for eternity within the limitations imposed by this physical body. We are intended for an experience of intimacy and wholeness that allows us, as beings of light, to, ultimately, know the meaning of true "understanding" – to move into the very space or holographic consciousness of another individual (with permission) without loss of self or injury to the other. I feel this in the interaction of my own energy consciousness with that of others – sharing the pain of their overwhelming experience and feeling the serenity that follows its release. The magnificence of experiencing intimacy through multi-sensory awareness defies description. That compassion could mean feeling the actual trauma of others in my hands as the hidden, trapped pain is finally released from their bodies, has been the most profound of all my experiences and lessons. Likewise, for the trauma survivor, to know that another person can feel and validate her buried pain and sense its release is, at least, equally profound. Discovering the power and authenticity of our "wounded selves within" provides a gift of self-understanding that defies words and provides the agency for healing the repetitive patterns of dysfunction, compulsivity, and the blockages to intimacy. Sharing such transactions with others, one cannot but be transformed.

While these experiences greatly broadened my notion of the human potential for intimacy, they necessitated changes in lifestyle. In order for my own multi-sensory awareness to continue its evolution, and, in order to not "take on" those heavier energies released during trauma resolution, I found myself searching for more effective ways of maintaining my personal energy levels in order to remain balanced. I learned, for instance, that, if in the process of helping others to release their pain, I internalized it within my own system, the pain levels would force me to discontinue facilitation. On two separate occasions I felt the client's pain move up my arms as the release process began. I discovered that I was developing a throat infection and experiencing, as a result, a noticeable decrease in energy. Through these lessons I learned to attend to my body's cues for exhaustion, suppression of immune system function, and onset of illness. In my self-care efforts, I implemented practices to enhance and maintain the energy fields of my body, like "kundalini yoga," as developed and taught by Yogiraj Vethathiri Maharishi.[31] Immediately upon implementation of the physical exercises, I enjoyed higher energy levels and increased multi-sensory awareness. As an additional effect of this practice, I felt a heightened awareness of the continuous exchange of energy between myself and my surroundings. I began to feel an intensified sensitivity as I interacted with my clients, with nature, and with all of creation. I sensed an enhanced interconnectedness and an increased awakening to the unification of all reality. Such enhanced multi-sensory awareness helped me to see that this profound relationality can be accessed and felt on a conscious level. This intensified perception has both improved my work with trauma survivors and has also helped to keep me grounded – particularly amidst work with more intense cases of trauma. While causing me to feel the sensitivity to the various frequencies of energy more keenly, most notably in cases involving the extremes of violence, emotional, physical, and sexual abuse, ritual abuse, and near-death experiences, it has also provided many new avenues for strengthening and support. Heightened perception of the conscious exchange of energy with everything around me has served to motivate me to contribute all that I can to the enhancement of this collective energy field and to assist others in transforming the trauma states that keep us immersed in "lower" energies in this lifetime. There is a great need for us to access our multi-sensory awareness if we are to transform our lives, our world into an experience of wholeness, healing, and well-being. If we continue to function from the limitations of five-sensory awareness alone, we continue to foster the illusions of separation that do not see the spiritual responsibility that is also part of our creative power and challenge.

As an ongoing state of relationship, multi-sensory awareness is accessible to all. My clients are amazed when they realize that they have always had the ability to scan their bodies identifying the holographic forms that the traumas or electromagnetic distortions take. It was they who first taught me about this capability. It is a very short step from realizing that I can scan my own body within seconds, defining the parameters of my headache, to discovering that I can also perceive the distortions in the energy fields of others. In discovering our own natural multi-sensory nature, we can use this awareness to assist others in their own spiritual growth. In "seeing" our bodies as the energy fields that they are, we suddenly see the "illusions of separation" dissolve, for we are no longer "solid," as Newtonian physics led us to believe. We are and have been involved in continuous energy exchange on very profound levels. We can learn to honor these exchanges of energy when we operate from **multi-sensory awareness.** Remaining in denial by focusing only on **five-sensory awareness** leaves us isolated and unaware of our connectedness to spiritual realities. Multi-sensory awareness offers continual reassurance that we are not alone; it assures us that the Divine Energy is continuously present to sustain us at all times. This awareness is readily accessible to all.

An episode affirming this accessibility occurred while I was working at a treatment center in New Mexico. I was in session with a woman suffering a terrible migraine. She had great difficulty concentrating or visualizing, so I assisted her with the use of the electromagnetic fields in my hands. This is commonly referred to today as a form of "Therapeutic Touch" or "Healing Touch".[32] Within minutes, her migraine was gone, and she was able to return her focus to treatment. The next day, as I entered the nurses' station, a Native American patient was using the same technique on a fellow patient. I observed for some time, noting the quality of his skills, and later asked him where he received his training. He responded by stating that, "I just saw you do it." He subsequently shared with me that he was a descendant of a long line of "medicine men" of the Navajo Tribe and had witnessed much of this type of work when growing up. It is my impression that multi-sensory awareness is not new, but, rather, was commonly utilized in times when there was less dependency upon machines and "external" technology and a much greater reliance upon intuition and Spirit as the mediator of experience. While there was much that was not known then from a "scientific" standpoint, the experience of oneness and interdependence with the earth was a daily, ongoing part of the belief system. The earth was a mystery; the human person was mystery. Mystery surrounded and enveloped primitive man. He believed that "Spirit" connected the whole of reality and provided access to spirituality, relationality, and intimacy. There was honor for the Spirit inherent in all. All was connected in the mind of ancient man, without a clue that this thinking was, in essence, "holographic perception" – seeing the whole (Spirit) in its manifold parts. Only now are we emerging from our technological grandiosity to the simple truth of the interconnectedness and interdependence of all forms of consciousness, from sub-atomic particles to the expanding universe and beyond. This interconnectedness is a simple truth to the multi-sensory personality. This is our invitation; this is our birthright. Spirituality-reality-intimacy is both a growth process and a state of relationship. We need only move beyond the old limitations imposed by five-sensory awareness to recognize this.

10. **Spirituality is simultaneously intrapersonal (within me) and interpersonal (social) in nature.** (Trauma resolution is profoundly spiritual, simultaneously healing relationships to self and others.)

At one stage in my personal spiritual development, I experienced a period of romanticism marked by a hunger to understand the paths tread by the great mystics and ascetics of history. These, I mused, would be the guides to lead my journey to spiritual growth and enlightenment. In studying religious history, the notion of monasticism – of cloistered communities separated from society for the purpose of exclusive devotion to the "service of God," fascinated me. This phenomenon was evidenced in nearly every culture in some form. The Essenes of Qumran along the Dead Sea, Buddhist monasticism, and Christian monastic communities in the East and West are some of the most familiar forms of this spiritual lifestyle. The idea of retiring to a quiet, secluded location, far away from "worldly" influences, to spend my energies in total commitment to "service to God" seemed almost ideal. In reality, I think that the attraction was influenced by the illusory promise that such an atmosphere would eliminate the need to face those feelings that seemed "less than spiritually uplifting" such as greed, envy, jealousy, lust, and rage. Surely, I thought, by entering such a "sacred" atmosphere one could eliminate the intrapersonal stressors, distractions, and temptations and simply focus on service to God and others, forgetting self. Such thinking was naive at best. I recall my visit to the Trappist monastery of Gethsemane outside Louisville, Kentucky, where Thomas Merton had resided and written many of his works. After a few days of silence, I was sensitized to every thought, feeling, emotion, and sound around me. Rather than escape from my internal reality, or reduce its intensity, the solitude heightened awareness, eliminated the distractions that I had used to avoid my inner world, and brought long-buried issues to light. The silence seemed to heighten every movement, every chant, every toll of the bells. Finally, when I managed to see my friend with whom I was traveling, we could hardly wait to converse about our experiences and to break the intense introspection created with external obstacles removed. I learned on that occasion that a deeply interpersonal spiritual lifestyle, such as monasticism, was simultaneously and immediately a profoundly intrapersonal experience and could not be used to evade intrapersonal struggle; if anything, it accelerated the self-confrontation. Revisiting my years of spiritual infatuation, it is clear that I assumed an extrinsic orientation – seeking to escape self. With an awareness that this outwardly "idyllic" community would force me to face my own internal "demons," I knew that I was not ready to enter such an atmosphere for any prolonged period of time. The intensity was too great. This was one of the first experiences that taught me the intimate relationship between the interpersonal and the intrapersonal realms.

Spirituality is a state of balance between my experience of myself and other-selves. As seen from our definition of spirituality (See Diagram A), there is no interpersonal growth that does not foster intrapersonal growth. The fact that our earliest experiences of intimacy and love were mediated through our parents attests to the importance of this social dimension for our formation. Our parents were our first gods. They were the starting points for our self-esteem. What they mirrored to us about ourselves and reality became the foundation for our intrapersonal and interpersonal realities. Neither were we born with self-esteem, nor a sense of deficiency. Our earliest social and affective impressions left a profound impact on our understanding of relationality. If we were given the appropriate nurturing and social support, we became more secure with ourselves and our relationships, possessing a stronger foundation for intimacy and communication. Each intrapersonal experience, likewise, has a profound impact on the interpersonal dimension.

This last point has become most precious to me. If taken to its full implications, it suggests that intrapersonal spiritual experiences can produce profound effects on the social level. Christianity has long posited that Jesus' intrapersonal transformation simultaneously changed the nature of interpersonal reality. If our holographic principle is correct, insofar as every fragment contains the whole, then, the transformation of one human person should, indeed, have some impact on the entire species. Perhaps it is true, therefore, that, "to save one man is to save the world." Furthermore, if a consensus of change is established by an entire group, the impact on the species would be greatly amplified. Within nature this holographic interconnection has been suggested. The "Hundredth Monkey Principle" attests to this. According to this notion, described by Lyall Watson in his text, <u>Lifetide: The Biology of Consciousness</u>, a group of monkeys learned a new behavior, whereupon other monkeys on other islands, with no possible means of "normal" communication, spontaneously learned or demonstrated the same behavior.[33]   I can testify, personally and professionally, that change within the self is profoundly linked to social change. In quantum physics, Bell's Theorem suggests that subatomic particles transcend time and space – that is, what happens to one particle immediately affects other particles; "time" is not needed for the transmission. It indicates that there is an instantaneous interconnectedness that underlies the whole of reality. This underlying interconnectedness enables multi-sensory perception and the "synchronicity" present in our relatedness.

From the standpoint of memory, it is clear that traumas which are induced interpersonally are stored immediately and holographically in the self – that is, intrapersonally. It often takes less than a minute in working with my clients to access the unresolved interpersonal traumas that are prominent within the cells and electromagnetic fields of the body. These fields within the body are the storage places of our interpersonal experiences. All that occurs outside of us is holographically stored intact within this sophisticated system of memory. These social perceptions are encoded and stored within our "personal" reality and leave imprints which we bear with us even in our most isolated states. We are the constructs of the profound social and inter-relational imprints that were mirrored to us and became the foundations of our self-esteem.

There is another manner in which our intrapersonal reality impacts our relationality. The intrapersonal boundaries that exist within us determine how we process our relational experiences. My internal belief system that affirms my right and ability to express my feelings, for instance, will contribute greatly to determining if a new experience becomes an opportunity for emotional growth or an incidence of trauma. My internal boundaries or belief system, already founded on my history of interaction with others, is continuously and intimately tied into my perception of reality. Changes in my "inner world" have direct and immediate implications in my "outer world." How often have we awakened from a frightening dream to find our "outer world" colored by this frightening internal experience. From the study of trauma, it becomes apparent that we must remain awake to both inner and outer worlds. By being attentive to these dimensions we discover clues for furthering our personal evolution. Walking down a street we may suddenly become aware of a smell, a sound, or a person that triggers within us an unresolved issue or experience that escaped our attention. Sitting in meditation, we may suddenly have a thought or a feeling surface that was previously unknown, consciously, and which points to an unresolved trauma that is ready to surface for our healing. Now that we are strong enough to deal with the issue, our subconscious mind will allow it to emerge for resolution. Looking at our behaviors in the outer world, we can see the structure of our inner world. Incongruities between these two worlds provide opportunity for further spiritual growth.

We cannot, ultimately, succeed in using our relationships to avoid intrapersonal realities. The intrapersonal and interpersonal are too closely connected. All relationships serve to mirror to us aspects of ourselves. That which we attract reflects something of our inner states. Our earliest relational imprints leave us with certain predispositions based on what we did or did not receive. I still laugh at the discovery that my older sister and I unknowingly and simultaneously dated members of the same family while we were living in a city of over 275,000 people. Our childhood experiences leave us with certain subconscious messages about love and relationship that continue to form the operative basis of our decision-making until they are made conscious and/or changed. Healing our intrapersonal reality will always lead to healing of the interpersonal dimension as well. Observing our interpersonal patterns, we can actually learn to develop a roadmap of the intrapersonal work that remains to be done. Using holographic awareness, we learn to scan our nervous systems to locate and identify operative programs that form the basis of our powerful subconscious attractions, to backtrack to their points of origin within our histories, and to resolve the dynamics which will lead us to recreate these same patterns until they are resolved. Healing our intra-psychic blocks to relationality and intimacy leads to profound changes in these interactions.

Another example of the spiritual interrelationship between self and others concerns healing. Initially, I explored my "energy sensitivity" by "working on myself." I began experimenting with my own ability to "feel" my headaches and to resolve them. Once I became more comfortable with these sensations and their effectiveness, it was a short step to allowing myself to use these personal resources to assist the healing of others. Work on myself greatly accelerated the development of the technique and led to its application in service to others. Many of us have come to realize that we possess the ability to listen to or scan our bodies and to identify early imprints from trauma, but we have stopped short of consciously using this same perceptual ability to serve our fellow human beings. Extension of our intra-healing ability to serve others is now a perceptual adjustment and challenge that we face as we move from five-sensory awareness to multi-sensory awareness. From the standpoint of multi-sensory awareness, the distinction between what is "intra" and what is "inter" begins to dissolve. We perceive ourselves as parts of a whole and realize the responsibility and power that comes from such a singular vision of reality. Today we are learning all that this "corrected vision" of reality offers us. For myself, it has completely reshaped my thinking about what the human person is and how we may best facilitate each other on this journey. It means that I can utilize my holographic awareness to step into your consciousness (with your permission), as manifest in the energy fields of and around your body, and help to release static energy states that are detaining you on your journey. It has also helped me to redefine my concept of intimacy. Intimacy moves into new levels when we realize that we are able to extend consciousness beyond the limitations of our physical bodies. The "tantric" experience of the East, where the energetic lessons are brought down into the physical body now becomes possible. The highest form of tantra, called "Samaya," has nothing to do with any ritual or any form of worship involving sex, as some practitioners have led us to believe.[34] It involves discovering the balance between the "male" and "female" energies within us and integrating this core energy which originates at the base of the spine. The integration of the "maleness" and "femaleness" within us removes obstacles to intimacy, as does multi-sensory awareness. With the removal of obstacles to intimacy and the "illusions" of separation that led us to feel and view ourselves as disconnected and isolated from each other, the spiritual journey becomes an exciting new adventure. As my sensitivity to the energy forms of memory have increased, I have felt a "transparency" taking place that leaves me more and more sensitive to even the thought forms of the survivors whose work I facilitate. Powerful energetic reactions have occurred within my own relationships, from something as simple as being in physical proximity to another. The evolution into multi-sensory or holographic awareness has concrete, practical implications based on the dissolution of false or isolated concepts of self and other. We are dawning, beginning to move into new experiential definitions of intimacy, relationality, and spirituality.

11. **Spirituality is naturally unitive.** (Spiritual reintegration occurs through the resolution of trauma.)

I believe that what is truly "spiritual" fosters unity and wholeness. The foundation of this unity I view as the Divine Mind which manifests as the holographic universe. This is the foundation for the mystical vision of all known religions. The dynamics present in spiritual experience (See Diagram A, p. 184) show the interconnectedness and interpenetration of self, others, and Higher Power. All occurs within the Divine Mind. Authentic spiritual awareness moves us into greater integration with this unifying consciousness and the felt perception of oneness with all. Observing ourselves through journaling, meditation, stress reduction, visualization, relaxation, breathing exercises, artistic expression, music, jogging, intentional prayer or self-reflection is instrumental in seeing the "fruits" of our spiritual labors and discerning that path which leads us to greater spiritual "authenticity." In this light, all of our actions which foster self-unity are also considered forms of prayer.

There are many belief systems that have claimed to hold the key to "authentic spirituality." However, as my very intuitive niece Brittany once stated at the age of seven, after an instructive conversation with one of her "angels," "God didn't make many churches; man did." All systems are comprised of both healthy and unhealthy elements. One hermeneutic or interpretative key to determining the authenticity of a supposed spiritual experience is the actual integrative effects of the experience. If, for instance, someone claims that his experience of the Bible is spiritually nurturing, but he is actually using this inspirational work to move further into isolation and denial about addiction, family problems, emotional pain, etc. (See Diagram B), this use is disintegrative and addictive. "Religious addiction" is the manifestation of this disintegrative pattern under the guise of "spirituality."

Treating religious addiction has taught me that the same words, whether from the Bible, or our own personal spiritual reflections, can be directed by diverse intentions. It is often this intent which determines the integrative or disintegrative effects of such communications – and this includes the objectives of both the bearer and the receiver. Often we gain something positive from a potentially negative experience as a function of our purpose. Healthy spirituality fosters awareness in communication so that our experiences lead to integration despite unhealthy designs that may be present in the systems with which we interact. If, however, we find ourselves having to continuously exert greater and greater determination in order to remain balanced and centered while in the system, community, job, or relationship, it may be necessary for us to examine the viability of continued spiritual growth in this atmosphere. In such situations, I have found that listening to Spirit within myself provides the guidance needed to make the necessary "system shifts." This sometimes requires adjustments in relationships, living situations, religious communities, jobs, and plans. The key, however, is to rely upon that Spirit which speaks through our intuition and leads us to "true" security.

Very often, in our woundedness, we have left ourselves open to the first promise of security that offered itself. We have sought to shape our lives around the salvation promised by these various systems, even when feeling an increased loss of power and disillusionment. As a culture, we have empowered unhealthy systems out of our personal need so that many of these megasystems no longer pretend to foster the spiritual integration that they once offered. We are moving toward the re-creation of spiritually nurturing communities and relinquishing our unhealthy attachments to megasystems that have become addictions in themselves. These systems have become addicted to themselves and are considered by systems analysts to be too large for safe, successful intervention. With the power of holographic thinking, however, we come to understand that intervention can come from one person who bears the support of Spirit. Spiritual stagnation will always be challenged due to the inherently integrative nature of the Divine Mind.

Stagnation cannot coexist with spiritual atonement. Spirit supports these confrontations. There will always be a Martin Luther to confront the sale of spirituality or a Martin Luther King, Jr., to confront the enslavement of Spirit. Spirituality possesses its own inherent system of checks and balances. Spirit will not allow itself to be contained by trauma on individual or collective levels. It will always move us toward centeredness and integration.

When I speak of "spirituality," my use of the concept may seem broad. This is so because spirituality is all-embracing. Anything that fosters truth fosters spirituality. This does not mean that I need to disclose to a significant other all of my deepest secrets, for this would not necessarily foster personal or interpersonal integration. Such a display would, more likely, be a manifestation of unresolved feelings of guilt. There are more effective ways of achieving resolution. When I speak of "truth," I speak of anything that moves me toward authentic integration (See the apex in Diagram C). This means, for instance, that admitting I have an "addiction" can allow me to return to a more authentic awareness of my "true" self if, in fact, I am an addict. The discovery of the disease of alcoholism facilitated the spiritual awakening of millions who were living with labels of "moral failure" when this was untrue and was actually fostering shame and further spiritual deterioration and separation. The fact that religious systems were among the main proponents of the "moral failure" model reminds us of their capacity to foster spiritual disintegration "in the name of God." The discovery of "addictions" provided an important "truth" that returned those who became conscious of their diseases back to the mainstream of spiritual evolution. The Twelve Steps of Alcoholics Anonymous has greatly facilitated this healing and return to personal growth. The awareness that whatever is "true," ultimately fosters spiritual integration emerges from this example. The Fifth Step of Alcoholics Anonymous is: "Admitted to God, to ourselves, and to another human being the exact nature of our wrongs." Inherent in this principle are, quite clearly, the three dimensions of spirituality and a statement about the role of verity in the healing process. The Fifth Step provides us with the implicit definition of spirituality, based on "open, honest admission" of truth, upon which the Twelve Step philosophy is based. This principle honors the fact that maximum spiritual growth occurs when such truths are made conscious on all three levels. Such progress often begins, however, with confrontation from others regarding this reality about self, or the self-realization that I have a problem. The First Step of A.A. states that, "We admitted we were powerless over alcohol – that our lives had become unmanageable."[35]   Any admission, any opening of the mind to authenticity begins the integrative process and starts the movement inward toward centeredness and greater connectedness with Spirit. If Spirit is truth, then all movements toward verity are movements toward Spirit. The empowerment that occurs in the honoring and fostering of truth must be recognized.

From the standpoint of trauma, this means that facing any unknown, previously unremembered, triggered, or known trauma holds the potential to reveal Spirit to me. If trauma is a part of my history, the promise is that the disclosure and resolution of this event will provide authentic knowledge, understanding, and recovery from a moment in space and time when I was trapped within the reality of another. In a sense, we can see that trauma does trap us with the "spirit" of another present in that moment within our consciousness and that their reality is merged with ours. This "spiritual" confusion commonly manifests in the "dirty, defective, guilty" feelings of the trauma survivor that are actually created by the internalization of the perpetrator's shame and disease at the moment of the trauma's induction. Spiritual integration does not occur by attempting to transfer our pain or shame to another, but by owning it and releasing it within our own consciousness – the only place from which it can be released completely. I am the locus of my spirituality; I am the only place where my traumas can and will be released.

It is important for us to "own" the truths about ourselves. In facing our traumas, we come to realize that the empowerment that follows is worth the pain of ownership. On a more profound level, we come to the experiential awareness that we are **not** our traumas. We are **not** our addictions. Trauma resolution reveals to us that we possess compulsive ego-states as a result of these overwhelming events, but that we must not over-identify with these realities – we are not merely our wounded ego-states. My friend Robert Odom, in his book entitled,

Your Companion to Twelve Step Recovery, cites the following "ego-selves" and their distinguishing characteristics:

Higher Self: All knowing, all loving, all accepting, all supportive, divine, eternal, healing, wise.

Competent Adult Ego-Self: Honest, concerned, capable, sacrificing, intelligent, wise, conscious, self-loving.

Young Adult Ego-Self: Committed, striving, critical, competent, curious, supportive, demanding, loving.

Adolescent Ego-Self: Curious, frightened, bold, impatient, risking, critical, ego-selfish, demanding.

Inner Child Ego-Self: Loving, cuddlesome, accepting, curious, sharing, ego-selfish, impatient, forgiving.

Addicted Ego-Self: Fearful, judgmental, ego-selfish, tyrannical, demanding, unfulfilled, suspicious, self-hating.[36]

Our spiritual destiny is not to live as fragmented ego-selves, but to become singular in our consciousness – unified in our experience of self, others, and Higher Power. In facing the truths about ourselves, about our addictions, traumas, and mistakes, we realize that these are experiences which dissolve under the powerful light of our spiritual nature. They are opportunities for us to transcend the "illusions of separation" and to discover our true nature as divine, eternal, loving, wise, multi-dimensional beings of light. Addictions, traumas, "frozen feelings," "stuck points," all become opportunities for more profound conscious unification with the Higher Self. We are unaccustomed to thinking that our Higher Self might reveal itself to us from behind the mask of our traumas. This path, however, has long been know and recognized as valid; it is the aforementioned "via negativa" of ancient spiritual tradition. All experiences which lead me to the revelation of truth about myself foster spiritual growth. Whatever leads me to what is true about myself is spirituality and promotes wholeness, integration, connection, and health.

12. **Spirituality is a unique vehicle of truth, a major experience in the comprehension of reality.** (Spirituality can give meaning to the deepest of our traumas.)

Throughout history, spirituality has been a vehicle of truth. Since the most primitive times, spirituality has served to communicate humankind's most intuitive knowledge. Spiritual connection has served to bring order out of chaos, to draw meaning from confusion and mystery. The vast body of our scientific knowledge, far from eliminating the spiritual nature from our lives, has served to point out its unique contribution. Science has often forgotten its profound link and even indebtedness to spirituality. Michael Talbot reminded us of this in The Holographic Universe when he described the origins of the hologram itself and the influence of the Hua-yen school of Buddhist thought (See p. 219). Leibniz, familiar with this school of Buddhism, gave us integral calculus which enabled the invention of the hologram.

I have seen the attempts to divorce science from spirituality in a variety of related circumstances. When I was actively engaged in archaeological excavation in the Middle East from 1979-1992, I saw the question arise over separating "Near Eastern Archeology" from "Biblical Archaeology" in the effort of Near Eastern archaeologists to distance themselves from the old biases and religious preconceptions that were related to the "unscientific" approaches of the early "religiously motivated" excavators. It was the perception of the contemporary archaeologists that these early excavators were biased in their fervent intentions to validate biblical data, disqualifying their work as purely scientific. To a great extent, the contemporary scientists were correct. However, they discounted their indebtedness to these early interests in the pursuit of truth. While it is fact that the early excavators were already invested in validating their own belief systems, the initial intent and underlying process were grounded in the spiritual pursuit of truth. In addition, the scientific parameters of their time were distinct from today's. Looking back on the history of archaeology, it was as though the archaeological community was embarrassed by its own stages of historical development. I wonder what Near Eastern archaeology would have become had this early interest not been present and financial motivation not been inspired by those early biases? We do not grow by forgetting or disowning our traumas, but, rather, by integrating and learning from them. The spiritual search for truth has contributed significantly to the evolution of science.

Spirituality is a vehicle for intuitive truth, a level of knowledge that cannot be replaced by science. The reason for this is that spirituality provides a unique experience of truth that, far from rivaling or giving way to science, complements it. It is absurd to think that even independent pursuits of truth will, ultimately, produce anything other than compatible results. Is it surprising that fourteen hundred years after Fa-Tsang we are coming to confirm the interconnection and interpenetration of all things through scientific research? At times it appears as though we are simply trying to prove the reliability of our own intuitive knowledge. Spirituality will always outpace the dialectic process of science, if only because it precedes intellect in the hierarchy of consciousness.

Spirituality, which discloses to us the essential interconnection and interpenetration of all things, forms the basis for our underlying search to comprehend the mystery of life – it's joys and tragedies. In Man's Search for Meaning, Victor Frankl was correct when he spoke of a profound craving for meaning deep within the human psyche. It is our spiritual nature to seek and find this underlying truth. I fondly recall a line from a favorite science fiction movie, Starman, when Jeff Bridges, portraying the "alien" states:

> *You humans are interesting … you are unique among the species*
> *we have studied … you are all so different from each other … and*
> *you seem to be at your best when things are at their worst."*

It is this inherent ability to find meaning amidst trauma that reveals to us our true survival nature.

On the conscious level, our awareness of this underlying meaning and linking has undergone various stages of evolution. We are moving toward conscious awakening after eons of evolution with predominant subconscious programming and imprints. As more and more of the cells of our bodies move under our conscious influence, and away from the older, dominant subconscious programming, the questions that guide us become more focused. Our intuition is granted a voice. We are discovering our power as the creators of our reality. We are experiencing the validation and the support of science in this creative journey, particularly the foundation supplied by the concepts of quantum physics. The integration of our minds and bodies – of our spiritual, mental, emotional, and physical expressions of self are all aspects of this growing consensus of consciousness. As these coalesce in greater harmony, our mastery over the physical body and physical reality increases. We will examine this last point in more detail in Chapter Fourteen, "The Healing of Disease."

Spiritual awareness greatly facilitates our comprehension of reality. Without a sense of underlying meaning, purpose, and the interconnectedness of all things, we would drift from scene to scene, hypersensitive to any imminent threat without assurance of continuity or purpose. Spiritual mindedness assists us by grounding us in such a way that we can benefit fully from the growth and evolution possible in each moment of our lives. Spirituality, as the intuitive access to our Higher Selves, is a unique vehicle of truth, a major key to the comprehension of reality.

Chapter Thirteen

> *Once I dreamt that I was a butterfly, fluttering here and there; in all ways a butterfly. I enjoyed my freedom as a butterfly, not knowing that I was Chou. Suddenly I awoke and was surprised to be myself again. Now how can I tell whether I was a man who dreamt that he was a butterfly, or whether I am a butterfly who dreams that she is a man?*
>
> *Chuang Tzu*

The Healing of Dreams

To speak comprehensively of "healing dimensions" or "holographic space," a discussion of dreams must be included. Dreams are an obvious proof of the functioning of the brain and the universe as hologram. They are also remarkable opportunities for healing and integration. While our physical body remains at rest in sleep, we proceed through a variety of "altered states" of consciousness that present themselves to us as a vivid multidimensional reality.

These states of consciousness are measurable as brain waves which scientific measurement standardly categorizes as ranging from 0 to 21 Hertz. According to my training, the altered state that we commonly associate with dreams involves electromagnetic brain waves designated as "Theta" (ranging from 4 to 7 Hertz [Hz.]) on the brain wave scale. Theta waves are present during "rapid eye movement" (REM) sleep when most of our dreams take place. Creative and artistic resources, intuitive information, and deeply rooted imagery are the hallmark of the Theta state. The Theta range (4 to 7 Hz.) falls within the parameters of the subconscious mind (identified with 4 to 14 Hz.). In our sleep states we can range from the dreamless Delta states (0.1 to 4 Hz.) associated with the "superconscious mind," to the lighter rest of the meditative

Alpha state (7 to 14 Hz.), experienced during focused, alert meditation. Earlier in this work we defined trauma as a "self-hypnotic" state created to contain an overwhelming experience. As an altered state, trauma largely encodes in the brain wave range (4 to 14 Hz.) of the subconscious mind. Trauma resolution, as facilitated self-hypnosis, involves access of these same subconscious frequencies. Because our dreams access the Theta state and tap into our subconscious, holographic processes, they hold the potential, like hypnosis, to access the subconscious mind and to assist in the healing of trauma.

Dreams are remarkably potent altered states; they possess a fluidity and emotionality that we, frequently, can only approximate in "historical time." While we reside within the holographic dream world, that is our reality. The following are the principal dream types that I have experienced either personally or in my work with trauma survivors:

1. Dreams that are comprised or reflective of current, familiar life experiences;
2. Dreams that derive from "proximate" or readily accessible subconscious (stored) memory;
3. Dreams that are drawn from "remote" subconscious memory; (Note: these first three types derive from historical experience.)
4. Dreams that are "creative" or "intuitive" in origin and derive from no known historical reality;
5. Universal or "archetypal" dreams that derive from the collective mind;
6. Dreams of insight or "clear communication" that provide instantaneous and profound solutions to previously insoluble problems or dilemmas;
7. Trans-temporal or trans-spatial dreams that provide information or experience beyond the limitations of time and space (that is, "precognitive" or "forewarning" type dreams);
8. Ecstatic or enlightening dreams that are profound, integrative lessons or spiritual experiences beyond the limitations of "historical" time;

9. Didactic dreams experienced as instruction from higher levels of one's own consciousness or from the consciousness of another;

10. "Healing" dreams in which one is "worked on" by oneself or by others for the purpose of resolving blockages or fostering growth;

11. Dreams of visitation that are profoundly spiritual and emotional in nature and may be of either a "positive" or "negative" orientation;

12. "Numinous" or spiritual dreams that involve encounter with the Transcendent, as the individual perceives it.

One of the most fascinating works produced on the subject of dreams and their application to the healing process is Dr. Patricia Garfield's work, entitled: The Healing Power of Dreams.[1] In her work, she provides numerous case studies and techniques for using dreams to identify health problems, promote recovery, and accelerate healing. She describes the "seven stages of recovery from physical trauma" and their accompanying manifestation in dreams. She identifies and demonstrates the dream stages as the following: 1) forewarning dreams, 2) diagnostic dreams, 3) crisis dreams, 4) post-crisis dreams, 5) healing dreams, 6) convalescence dreams, and 7) wellness dreams.[2] Her insight and demonstration of ways subconscious resources are activated within our sleep states to promote healing is of great importance. I do not believe that there is a moment, whether conscious or unconscious, where our spirit is not seeking to move us toward wholeness and balance. In her work, Garfield provides a wide variety of tools for accessing, interpreting, and applying the resources provided by dreams to foster healing. I have found a number of her approaches helpful for providing greater access and utilization of dreams for promoting my personal growth and healing.

Within the context of this work, it is important to recognize the unlimited creative potential provided by dreams. As seen from the variety of possible dream types, nearly every imaginable scenario needed to provide access or cues to distortions in our body, mind, and spirit can be found in the holographic dimension of dream space. The dream itself provides a bridge between the conscious mind and the subconscious mind, much as the facilitator provides in the healing process outlined in this work. I learned this in a most startling and remarkable way.

In my personal training and experiential work with psychologist David Grove, I accessed the memory of the traumatic episode of my father attempting to teach me to swim by throwing me into the water. While accessing the original memory fragment, a second image, a "large piece of red granite," suddenly appeared in "my own holographic space." The red granite appeared in the form of a torso with head and arms removed threatening to weigh me down and drown me – a metaphor for my father, who failed to reach out to me at certain moments in life and in water, and who considered himself inadequate intellectually. The surprise occurred when I realized that the "red granite" motif originated from an earlier dream I had experienced immediately after suffering three traumatic losses in 1983: my mother, my priest-friend, and my best friend. In this prior dream, I am in a dried "wadi" (riverbed) in Sinai (now Egypt). Suddenly, a torrent of muddy water begins to pour in and I am unable to escape; the only way out is through the sides, but these are steep red granite cliffs which make it virtually impossible to escape. The muddy water threatens to inundate me. I frantically and blindly scramble up the sides with the water and mud pouring down. I am blinded and unable to see how close to the top of the cliff I am; I am on the verge of despair. Suddenly, in shock, I realize that a companion (of indeterminate identity) and I have reached the top. There is a fleeting moment of ecstasy and delight. Shifting suddenly, a tall red granite rock formation which has stood in position for eons, collapses killing the beloved "companion." The recent feelings of ecstasy, still flowing through my system, are instantaneously converted to horror and disbelief. I subsequently felt the sharp release of all fear, and feelings of acceptance and understanding filled me. In my mind I heard: "In life, there will always be uncontrollable factors … you can only strive to do your best … fear is helpful if it assists you; all other fear is useless … trust the underlying flow of your life to sustain you."

During my resolution of the "swimming lesson" trauma with my father, a subconscious connection was made with the three traumatic losses of 1983. Under the holographic metaphor of the "red granite," all four losses were integrated into the trauma resolution experience. The early childhood trauma laid the foundation for a terror of abandonment which was triggered by the traumas of 1983. My dream provided the holographic metaphor for the integration of all four traumas during the healing process. Resolution occurred when I returned to holographic space to retrieve a very young child "hiding in a dark, overwhelming red granite cave, distrustful of adults and fearful of being weighed down and drowned by life." In a moving scene, which I hold vivid in my recollections to this day, I converted my anger from the abandonment experiences into a sense of protection and safety for the child who recognized in me the resolution of all abandonment. When I framed this scene and moved it through my body, all somatic pain vanished, and there has been no return of the "heavy, red granite" feeling and the accompanying terror of abandonment. Only afterward did I realize that I was resolving, not just the original trauma, but the closely juxtaposed losses that were consolidated and recapitulated under the metaphor from the cliff dream. Included in the resolution was, not only the "core" or foundational trauma, but all the traumas that the dream had managed to bring together from different places of my perceived experience in space and time. With multiple, enmeshed scenes of emotional abandonment, it was not possible to resolve such a profound level of trauma by addressing each individually. These traumas had become associated or linked in the subconscious and needed to be addressed collectively. While this was not possible in "historical" time, it could easily be accomplished through the versatility of "dream space," of holographic space, for here my mind could easily consolidate and produce a metaphor which actually carried the accumulated weight of those many years of subtle trauma. The realm of such holographic metaphors, is, therefore, an immensely powerful locus of healing.

Working within the dream space of my clientele of trauma survivors, as the facilitator, I have learned that my task is a simple one – to help them employ the remarkable metaphorical resources which they already possess to heal themselves. The incredible diversity of healing resources that can be provided by dreams is not to be underestimated. We are learning to consciously enter "dream space" or "holographic space" and use the tools of our own creative imagery to transform the frozen moments of trauma – integrating them to foster nurturing and growth, rather than allowing them to continue manifesting in our bodies as disease and pain. Utilizing the processes detailed in this work, it is possible to "step into the dream" and to transform the unresolved dream from one of pain, fear, and trauma to one of safety, self-nurturing, and health. Dreams are magnificent vehicles for providing access needed to identify blockages and to resolve them completely, as the subconscious permits. As trauma survivors we are often eager to describe our intense dreams and frequently seem to feel an urgency about processing them. On a deeper level, we sense the importance of a particular dream as a possible solution for some unresolved trauma or issue. Personally, I have found that the resolution to a disturbing dream will be achieved in one of two ways: 1) either the healing work will proceed within the context of the dream itself, or 2) the dream will provide the key to the feeling that provides access to the original event that caused the dream. In the latter case, resolution of the precipitating trauma scene will, obviously, eliminate the need for the dream or nightmare to recur. When making this determination, I approach the client by asking: "When you think of this dream, how do you feel?" After locating the feeling and defining it in its holographic form, I subsequently ask: "And how young might you be when you first feel a feeling like that?" The response to this question will be either: 1) "my current age – in the dream that I had the other night," or 2) "when I was ____ years old." In other words, tracking the key feeling and its metaphorical form (as previously outlined) will, ultimately, either bring us back to work within the holographic space of the dream itself, or to the holographic scene of the original trauma that precipitated the dream. In either case, the process proceeds with the goal of transforming the unresolved scene of pain or trauma into a scene of serenity, self-nurturing, and health. Once the frozen scene is consciously corrected, that affect need no longer surface subconsciously through our dreams to get our attention. It is resolved.

The majority of our dreams or some aspect of them originate in historical time – from the present, from the proximate past, or from the remote past. Some dreams, therefore, appear identical to the original trauma. In this sense, they are the original trauma – as recorded and stored holographically in the subconscious mind of the perceiver-survivor; the sleep state provides access to the encoded memory. It is often important for the trauma survivor to ascertain whether a dream was a matter of historical recall or a construct of the creative subconscious mind. This question is most readily answered when the client grants himself permission to work within the holographic space of the dream and to make a determination based on the somatic evidence. An actual trauma leaves an imprint in the nerve center(s) where the pain was felt most profoundly at the moment of traumatization. My own sensitivity to the energy released during the resolution process offers a certain level of discernment that provides data confirming the presence or absence of a trauma-induced trance state. When this pain is accessed in the nerve centers, the survivor is left with few doubts as to the authenticity of the experience. As stated previously, since a trauma is an altered state, entry into the metaphor of a stored memory will reproduce the symptoms present in the nervous system at the moment of freezing (T-1). Traumas originating in "historical time" will present with the intense and varied physical sensations that accompanied the original experience. Once the sensory data and somatic memories are accessed by the trauma survivor, the intricate details provided and the intense somatic sensations felt usually eliminate remaining doubts about the authenticity of the experience. If a dream or nightmare is itself the source of the trauma, the symptoms presenting will be less severe since a trauma induced in a dream state does not typically possess the same physiological intensity because much of the body is still "at rest." Rapid eye movement (REM), the normal indicator of a trance or dream state will occur, however. Originating from the dream state or historical time, the solution for the trauma will be the same, regardless: the scene must be resolved for the individual to feel whole and complete, with no remaining affect to provide future triggers for retraumatization. Quantum physics validates that, regardless of the origin of your perceptions, your perception creates your reality and must be resolved within your perceptual framework.

Dreams often synthesize our experiences and provide a more simplified means to resolve our traumas. Since dreams bridge the conscious and subconscious minds, they have the advantage of access to the unlimited resources of our spirituality and the entire one hundred percent of our memory which can serve the task of balance, healing, and integration. Dreams can also prepare us for the resolution work of healing by providing metaphorical experiences which we can use consciously in the trauma resolution process. In addressing certain critical issues in our lives, it is not unusual to find a dream or series of dreams that provide the "hermeneutic" or interpretive key for resolving these situations. Dreams often arise as the genesis of a healing process. Unresolved feelings or issues may surface for the first time when our "external" defenses are down, as in the sleep state. To most trauma survivors, dreams are considered less threatening than the "flashbacks" that intrude into waking consciousness, interrupting our lives or activities. Dreams are vehicles that provide a gentler access to unresolved feelings and memories.

A recently discovered phenomenon in the trauma field is the impact of unresolved childhood nightmares. These agitating experiences can be recurrent over years, even throughout a person's lifetime unless they are addressed. While facilitating visual access to my clients' traumas using the electromagnetic field technique, I have seen the sudden recall of an entire series of childhood nightmares that fostered intense feelings of fear and insecurity that lasted well into adulthood. Just as there are many different types of dreams, there are many different sources for nightmares. The essential task is to effectively access and appropriately address the specific nightmare engaging the emotional self.

Recurring nightmares frequently originate in the fears of children who, irrespective of what stimulated the initial fear that precipitated the dream, are terrified because there is no one there to comfort them appropriately. Nightmares are reinforced by feelings of being discounted, abandoned, or isolated. The nightmare is frequently encoded as trauma at the moment the child realizes that there is no one available, willing, or able to spend the necessary time to reinforce safety and alleviate the fear. The precipitant for the encoding of the trauma is not so much the nightmare itself as the failure to protect the child from the terrors emerging in dream space. The child's safety needs are called into question by the manner in which the primary caregiver responds to the situation. A child's safety and security needs may already be threatened or compromised by recent events in the home. The nightmare is then encoded as trauma, not only because of the "nightmarish" content of the dream itself, but due to the fact that no one was there to "believe" or process this "real" experience with the child. To tell a child that "it was just a dream … go back to sleep," may be comforting intellectually, but it may do little to stabilize the emotions of the child. We dismiss the reality of holographic space! We forget how "real" the dream world is and that our perceptions create our reality. The world of the child is "magical" or "fluidly holographic" due to the blurring of their weakly formed boundaries. Children easily merge the holographic realities that adults see as separate. They feel more keenly their interconnectedness with all of the reality around them. Developmentally, we were once fully merged with the "realities" around us; individuation from these realities was a critical stage in our development. This natural individuation process is deeply impacted by trauma. As we shall see, at the moment of a trauma's induction, this individuation process is reversed. Let me explain.

Trauma is induced when our boundaries become permeable for a fraction of a second and our reality is fused with that of another. For an instant, our individuality is lost. For this very reason, individuation from a powerful and overwhelming scene of trauma, whether dream, flashback, or other anxiety producing experience, is an essential stage for the healing of trauma. Comparable to the trauma resolution process for an adult, the resolution for the child requires the presence of someone who shows interest in helping the wounded child and is willing to support the individuation. It is necessary, therefore, for someone to facilitate the child's resolution of the feelings of fear. This effort, ideally served by the parent, can assist in identifying the emotional need manifest in the dream. Through assistance in reframing the dream, the child learns of her resources, including her ability to foster safety; she acquires the tools needed to maintain safety for future needs. For a child, the reframing may simply require bringing Mom, Dad, or an imaginary protector or friend into the original scene to provide resolution. The corrected picture can then be taken, framed, and the colors moved through the area(s) of the body where the fear was present. Most professionals have never been trained in ways to help children resolve such nightmares or fears.

It is my goal to provide tools to facilitate healing within the various realms of holographic space. The tenets I share with you have been validated by my own experiences, both professional and personal. Several years ago, after a series of frightening dreams, I awoke with a message repeating itself in my mind: "Heal your dreams!" Intrigued as I was by this rather uncommon experience, I considered the implication of the message. Previously, I had dreamed that I was employing the trauma resolution process on myself within the dream, but I had never considered using it on myself after waking from a dream. Upon waking from my next frightening dream, I proceeded to identify the feeling that surfaced when I thought of the dream. I then defined its metaphorical form and proceeded to return to its point of origin – the dream itself (in this case). Upon returning to the holographic scene of the dream, I transformed the image from a scene of fear and hurt into one of serenity and consolation. Completing the scene, I framed it and placed it in the places in my body where I had felt the residual negative feelings from the dream. The nightmares ceased, and immediately I felt much calmer, no longer a "victim" of my dream states.

Having applied the technique with adult clients as well as adolescents, I believe that we can help younger children to transform their dreams of fear and pain into scenes of nurturing and safety – and who would be a more appropriate facilitator than their own parents or teachers? Trauma induction, more often than not, is related to the inability to utilize one's own resources to stop the overwhelming event from occurring. For the young child, the principal protective resource is Mom or Dad. Similarly, what is needed for the resolution of a childhood nightmare is a nurturing presence that can help transform a scene of pain and fear to one of safety. By entering holographic space with the child and helping her to heal frightening experiences, an incredible empowerment can occur. By helping children through such moments, a profound sense of safety and security can be created that will provide invaluable tools for dealing with future life traumas.

Although we are all, in some way, trauma survivors, many of us have come to live with the false perception that we are destined to be the victims of our traumas, flashbacks, and nightmarish dream states. This is not true. We are discovering that, just as we can readily change the past as it is encoded emotionally within our nervous system, so too can we change our dreams. As multidimensional beings continuously moving within the various levels of holographic space, we have the power to create and recreate our realities. This requires an "awakening" – a decisive movement from our "victimhood" on both conscious and subconscious levels. We are not intended to be prisoners of the traumas encoded in our nervous systems which manifest as disease, addiction, depression, nightmare, and flashback. Conscious awakening requires that we move beyond the false security of victimhood and stasis and move into realms that we thought were inaccessible – like the world of dreams, among other holographic spaces.

Recently I have discovered periods upon waking or just before falling asleep that seem to bridge both the conscious and subconscious minds – moments where every detail of the dream from which I just awoke is completely understood, moments where answers to the most complicated questions are available. Earlier in my life I experienced dreams so unfamiliar and peculiar that they frightened me. I now enjoy a great confidence and excitement over exploration of these previously elusive realms of consciousness. Dreams are, like traumas, occasions for exploring the power and magnificence of our multidimensional nature. They are opportunities for healing and for exercising our true creator potential. With the healing of traumas, the bridging of the "conscious" and "subconscious" minds may allow us to dispense with this duality of mind. In fact, it may be that the distinction between the conscious and subconscious minds is, itself, merely the by-product of our stored traumas. For now, with so many of our traumas held intact "below" ("sub," from the Latin) our surface consciousness, the distinction accurately reflects the challenge we face – the invitation to full, conscious awakening to health.

Chapter Fourteen

The Healing of Disease

One of the most remarkable results of my work with trauma survivors concerns the concept of "disease." Newtonian thinking left us with the impression that the majority of our physical complaints had their origins in the mechanistic workings of the physical body. Most of my clients readily attributed their headaches to their "sinus" problems, their neck pain to having "slept on it wrong last night," their back pain to some injury that simply "flared up" from time to time and just could not be fully relieved, their "chronic pain" to the car accident that left permanent nerve damage, etc. But the majority of trauma survivors discovered that they could resolve their physical pain. Most survivors found that their pain was a specific memory surfacing for conscious resolution. Though I am not currently working in a "traditional" hospital setting, but, rather, in a facility that focuses on the treatment of addictions, depression, trauma, and dual diagnosis, through observation and measurement I can report to you that over eighty percent of the "pains" that my clients have assumed to be physiological in origin are, in fact, memory fragments surfacing for healing. In fact, eighty percent is a conservative estimate. We have neglected the power and importance of "emotion" for so long that we have succumbed to the limitations of "five-sensory" thinking and the belief that all our diseases originate in some distortion in the physical body. My work with trauma survivors teaches me that this is not accurate. The reason for this is the simple fact that the majority of our physiological pain has its origins, not in a biologically induced distortion, but in forms of emotional trauma that imprint profoundly in the cells and fields of our bodies.

Scientists tell us that our bodies are one hundred percent memory – that diseases such as viruses afflict us by their capacity to seize control of the DNA of our cells and cause a change which then becomes replicated over and over until it is once again corrected by our own immune system. Our healing has always depended upon this mysterious capacity to alter or "correct" our cellular memory. With little understanding of this cellular memory, medical science has focused on biochemical intervention, leaving other approaches untouched. We possess far more influence over cellular memory, however, than we were led to believe. From our research, we now understand this "chain of command" from the mind to the brain, from the brain to the body, and from the body all the way down to the cellular-genetic-molecular level. In his work, The Psychobiology of Mind Body Healing, Ernest Rossi has highlighted this relationship. We have examined this chain of command in our discussions of trauma induction and the role of the Limbic-Hypothalamic-Pituitary-Adrenal Axis and its role in creating our "frozen scenes" or "state-dependent" memories at moments of trauma. Emotions clearly imprint in cellular memory at moments of trauma. I personally know this because I feel their site locations as my clients disclose their pain. In other words, the majority of our "diseases" are the by-product of our remarkable capacity to alter our states of consciousness which imprint at the cellular level. Our bodies mirror these profound changes in our consciousness as a way of helping us to maintain or restore balance. What emerges is the fact that the "physical" manifestation of what we call "disease" is typically the last stage in the trauma disclosure process.

Personal insights into the misunderstood nature of disease derived from observing my clients locating and accessing trauma memories through the cues received from pain or discomfort in the physical body. When they focused on the point of origin of the feeling, the cells which held the pain, they were able to access the memory and, in most cases, completely resolve the pain. All pains are a form of memory, as the medical profession has shown us. But we did not know that the majority of such pains have their origin in "traumatic" memories. (Remember that we are using the "broadened" understanding of the word trauma: any experience that causes state-bound encoding of an experience.) Upon resolution of my clients' memories – when their "trances" were corrected, the pains were gone! Residual pain frequently indicated a remaining memory. There were occasions when survivors experienced permanent physiological damage to the nervous system as a result of trauma. Nevertheless, when the emotional component of the trauma that caused the chronic injury was resolved, the pain, typically, diminished. Emotional trauma exacerbates chronic pain states. We now have the tools to distinguish between chronic physical pain and the pain somatically induced by trauma.

We are learning from shocking cases like Diedra (pp. 60-66). Diedra's body was permanently damaged by medical attempts at intervention, only for the pain to return fully intact because it was the "body memory" resulting from sexual abuse. Even when the nerves were surgically severed in her body, the pain remained intact and baffled the nation's leading kidney specialists and neurologists as to how pain could continue to manifest in an area of the physical body where the nerves were no longer functioning.

Serious damage has occurred as a result of the lack of knowledge about trauma induction – medical damage. We are greater than our physical bodies, and our capacity to hold trauma memories intact, despite medical interventions, confirms this. Every trauma that I have helped to resolve was, first, accessible through its physiological manifestation and the discomfort it created. To resolve the pain caused by trauma, removing or merely medicating the discomfort does not suffice. The latter merely delays the healing process. By actually focusing on our pain, we learn to utilize our natural ability to access cellular memory and to resolve the complex states of consciousness which are simply cueing us to their presence. I have worked with individuals possessing histories of congestive heart failure, cancerous tumors, chronic pain, unexplained tremors, pancreatitis, arthritis, urinary tract infections, colitis, peristaltic stoppage, tinnitus, recurrent migraines, panic attacks, PMS, etc. In each of these cases, specific memories were found which manifested in physiological symptoms. When their "symptoms" were honored as potential cues for greater healing, rather than something to be eliminated, remarkable outcomes were achieved. In most cases, the pains and symptoms that had defied medical treatment resolved in periods of time that the doctor's deemed "miraculous" – i.e., miraculous to those who failed to understand the dynamics of trauma induction and the inherent power that we each possess to heal our memories and their subsequent manifestations in our bodies.

A short time ago I was shopping in a favorite store when a former client greeted me with a hug, telling me about her recent life changes. She also showed me her hands. One hand was completely free of the swelling caused by arthritis while the swelling was reduced to one knuckle in the other and was continuing to diminish. Her healing came as a result of finding the courage to address her memories of childhood violence – all related to physical abuse from her father. Her own anger, which she was unable to express appropriately and safely at the time of the trauma, was encoded in the nerve centers of her hands. As she worked with the memories of her father's abuse, her hands became tightly fisted, and her knuckles, white. Soon after enacting the resolution during these sessions, there was visible improvement. She reported that the osteopathic physician who treated her called it a "miracle" and inquired about what she had done to produce such results. I have been awed by the manner in which memory resolution can so profoundly and instantaneously impact the physical body.

While in treatment, a client who was a minister began to experience chest pains and was rushed to the hospital, fearing a recurrence of his congestive heart failure of some years earlier. Absolutely nothing appeared in any of the tests. Upon returning to treatment, I helped him to focus on his symptoms and found a "black, heavy feeling around the outside of the heart" which had been present since his teens. When he focused on the feeling, he quickly returned to a scene in the kitchen when he was fourteen years old, with his father, drunk and in a "blackout," beating his mother and siblings. He had been taking boxing in school and punched his father so hard it knocked him to the floor.

His father never hit his mother or his siblings after that incident. The trauma, however, resulted from the tremendous remorse he felt about not "honoring his father and mother" as he had been taught, though he had little choice but to stop the abusive behavior. To have to strike the father he truly loved imprinted as a profound trauma in this boy's heart plexus. This "double bind" disclosed that his choice to become a minister was prompted by his urgent need to alleviate the persistent feeling of guilt that he had felt most of his life.

Recently, while visiting a friend in the hospital in Baton Rouge, she shared with me her suspicion that her abdominal blockage was related to unresolved grief issues. I offered to assist her investigation, whereupon we discovered a number of significant losses, the pain of which was encoded at "gut level" during her childhood. Quickly she was able to reframe the memories, notifying the cells of her body of the "corrected message" by establishing and substituting a new scene. She experienced full recovery and attributed the expediency of her recovery to the resolution of her grief issues.

Disease is defined as "a condition of an organism that impairs normal physiological functioning."[1] The traumas presenting in the lives of the individuals mentioned here succeeded in impairing this normal functioning. These memories fostered dis-ease. And while we know that the limbic-hypothalamic system functions wondrously to prevent us from being overwhelmed at moments of trauma, it also results in the repression of "T-cell" production which is responsible for protecting our bodies from illness. When, therefore, we freeze and encode trauma to stop our pain, we also slow T-cell production, thereby setting up the possibility that, unless the trauma is resolved, the areas of our nervous system most impacted by the trauma may manifest this distortion as illness. Our immune system is jeopardized. Whether an illness is trauma-induced or not, all illnesses are occasions for healing. It has been most exciting to participate with AIDS patients in treatment, addressing many of their long-unresolved traumas. After completing treatment, they telephone or write, reporting that, following their trauma resolution work, their T-cell counts "skyrocketed." Some were found to be "in remission," and there was difficulty finding the virus in their systems. Considering the amount of trauma evidenced in the average individual and the direct correlation between unresolved trauma and its manifestation as disease, I conclude that very few of us, if any, are operating with our immune systems at optimum capacity. It would appear that we may now have a powerful tool to facilitate the healing of diseases that were previously considered inexplicable or untreatable. The great gift is that trauma resolution will always enhance the functioning of the immune system.

The study of trauma resolution teaches us that the majority of our diseases are the creations of our quantum minds – arresting and encoding our painful perceptions to facilitate their resolution. Distortions imprinted in the cells and electromagnetic fields of our bodies during moments of trauma eventually surface, needing to be released. In a society devoted to the avoidance of all pain, how is our emotional body expected to get our attention to let us know that it is time to heal our distorted perceptions about life, reality, etc.? If, as quantum physics discloses, our perceptions create our reality, it is logical that these perceptions will manifest as real distortions – as "diseases." Diseases then become the cues to the healing of the emotional body and to accessing our inherent spiritual power – to alter our past and present states of consciousness. They serve as an invitation to wholeness.

As multidimensional beings we do, indeed, create our realities, consciously and subconsciously, and from this multidimensionality we can also create our diseases. The creation of disease, is, most often, a side-effect of the induction of trauma, which is largely subconscious and automatic. The majority of diseases are the creations of our wounded ego-states that are distorting our cellular memory and our electromagnetic fields. One psychiatrist with whom I worked informed me that her study of the profiles of women with breast cancer revealed commonalities. Frequently she found women who were in marriages where they felt "trapped" and financially dependent, unable to leave, whereupon they became angry at their partners and themselves. From my ability to feel and locate the emotional pain of trauma, I assure you that anger and resentment are routinely held in the chest area.

A recent case in point was Linda, a woman referred to me who had recurrent ovarian tumors. In working with her, I recognized that she matched the profile of "trapped, dependent, and angry," and

I detected anger and resentment in her chest area when she spoke of the severe physical and emotional abuse during her marriage. What amazed me, however, was the intensity of the pain that I felt above her right abdominal region. I commented on this to her and asked if she had any idea why the anger originating in her chest area might have centered or focused itself in her right ovary. Linda paused and said, "No, not really," but then suddenly looked up and said, "Well, wait a minute." A look of surprise dawned on her face after which she said, "You know, I think I know why this is happening … just as I finally got up my courage to leave this abusive marriage, … calling the lawyer and getting my finances ready, I got pregnant … and I got so angry at myself for doing that." Her anger was then redirected at herself – and, more specifically, at her reproductive organs, particularly her "right ovary," whence the recurrent tumors arose. She knew that the tumors were related to her "states of consciousness" because she had already been able to "make two of them go away," although "something kept them coming back," she stated. She felt much relieved after identifying this core trauma.

Linda also provided validation for another issue that I had pondered. She mentioned that, even with her cancer, she had been unable to stop smoking – even using the nicotine "patches." When asked where in her body she felt the need to smoke, without hesitation she indicated her chest-lung area. When she focused on the sensation she suddenly returned to the memory, at age seventeen, of the last time that her father physically abused her. She left home, never returned, and moved in with her best friend. It was only then that her anger, hurt and pain found consolation through smoking. She continued to explain that her smoking began that day as an act of rebellion, as satisfaction for finally being free of the abuse, and as a way of calming down and medicating her pain – a cold comfort celebration. Linda realized that this trauma had induced a number of emotional triggers which bound her to the smoking behavior, despite her conscious efforts to the contrary. She accessed the original scene, dialogued with her seventeen year old self, offered new ways of dealing with her need for safety and nurturing, and framed the scene. After moving this solution through her body, she was able to stop smoking with little difficulty. I have found that the majority of individuals who cannot stop smoking have similar memories where they are "psychologically bound" by their subconscious or wounded self to smoke as a way of alleviating some intense pain or as a reward for enduring or escaping the traumatic environment. These emotions are their greatest "triggers" to smoke or otherwise medicate. I have seen this as a standard phenomenon in the treatment of many addictions and illnesses. Trauma experiences have the power to "lock" certain behaviors into our psyche. Many addicts experience traumatic "using" episodes which encode profound feelings of shame. Subsequent use then triggers the earlier shame trauma and causes an intensification of the previous shame feelings, thereby leading to a greatly enhanced need to medicate again. This is the origin of the "shame spiral" described by countless trauma survivors. Similarly, feelings of guilt can "lock in" disease patterns because of the subconscious belief that I am "deserving" of this pain "because it's my fault." These assumptions are quite natural to a child whose nature is self-referencing.

The single, most exciting development in my trauma work in the last two years is the increase in my sensitivity to different types of electromagnetic distortions. This sensitivity has provided clues about the memory patterns that may underlie illnesses. Just over a year ago I had the opportunity to work with a cancer patient, Carrine, who was experiencing the recurrence of carcinoma after each surgery. Beginning our session with a scan of her body, focusing on the pain so evident at the tumor site near her solar plexus, I felt the pain suddenly shift to the top of her right leg; the pain from the "tumor site" was suddenly gone. We shifted focus to the pain in her leg, at which point she accessed a memory of being seven years old and having contracted an infection in her foot from innocently playing in an area that turned out to be a waste dump. Carrine's leg began to hurt and her father picked her up and carried her to the nearby hospital. Suddenly she became tearful. This, she stated, was the only time that she ever remembered her father holding her. The insight she gleaned from this memory was her subconscious perception that "you have to be sick to get the love you need." Carrine recognized that this belief was impeding her ability to resolve her illness. During a subsequent session, the pain from the main tumor site again shifted, and I felt the pain move to her left side below her ribs. She confirmed this shift. This time she accessed a memory of being five or six years old and being taken by her mother on a public bus to get treatment for a serious infection. Her mother had already worked a long day at another hospital and "looked so tired" that my client felt extremely guilty about being ill and inconveniencing her mother. Carrine processed how this belief prevented her from wanting to seek help and recover from her illness – she didn't want to inconvenience anyone. She remembered how it had felt when she had "burdened" her mother. We both realized that we were tracking the history of her resistance to getting help or getting well. She reframed the memory and dialogued with the wounded child-self that harbored these false beliefs, resulting in a complete alleviation of the pain.

From this client and many others, I discovered that many illnesses seem to have a memory history that can be mapped. In addition, the subconscious mind knows the entire sequencing, the order of resolution needed, and even how many memories can be addressed in a specific time frame. I found myself being cued by my client's pain and working with her through a series of memories that established her resistance and blockages to healing. The image that came to mind as we worked through these memories was that of the various magma channels of a volcano that contribute to the eventual eruption. By the time we become seriously ill, we are already in a state of eruption with a malfunctioning immune system. Sometimes it is too late to stop the eruption itself, as in the case of Carrine, above, who had lived with traumas impairing her efforts to heal. We often fail to heed the early warning signs that precede such an eruption and are left to manage the full blown crisis. It was surprising for both myself and Carrine to feel the pain from the main tumor site subside and "change location." Each time it switched, we accessed a relevant memory, as described above. At the end of each of these sessions, though she became tired from the work, she was very grateful and was completely pain free. Unfortunately, as with many illnesses, there is a need to staunch the magma flows in order that the eruption may be lessened or prevented; in her case, the cancer was too far advanced, though the alleviation of her pain and the healing that she accomplished was profound and exceedingly helpful.

With respect to outcomes, I have become somewhat "spoiled." I am accustomed to seeing the majority of my clients experience the complete alleviation of the physiological symptoms of the surfacing memory; this is simply the by-product of the resolution of the precipitating trance. If other symptoms or the same symptoms present themselves, this means that there is usually another or related memory that must yet be resolved for the hologram or metaphor to disappear. Upon resolution of this additional memory, the symptoms are usually gone. I can often gauge the effectiveness of the resolution process by the client's final scan of his body upon completion of the process. If any symptoms remain, they are usually different from the original metaphor and suggest another memory. In the majority of cases, there is no remaining physiological pain.

One of the most important concepts for our understanding of illness concerns the holographic nature of memory. As you may recall, the fragment of a holographic memory has the capacity to reproduce the whole. Because this is true, the unresolved emotional trauma from an experience could lead to the recurrence of the whole pain syndrome. In the case of Diedra (pp. 59-65), her pain was clearly emotional and holographic in its origins, encoded as pain in her left kidney region during the original abuse experiences. Even severing the nerves in her body did not stop the pain encoded from the memory. With the advent of holographic memory theory, psychology and medicine are no longer just related, they are inseparable at this level of sophisticated perception.

Recently I worked with Patti, a woman who was addicted to pain medications. She attributed her addiction to the chronic pain in her legs. She indicated to the facility's medical director who examined her upon admission, that she had been in a severe car accident. The physician stated that Patti was experiencing cramping, muscular pain, and circulatory problems related to her injury. Patti informed him that medical tests had confirmed nerve damage from her childhood accident. Over the years, all of her physicians had concurred. I met Patti for the first time while lecturing on the dynamics of trauma induction. During the session she was very restless, due to the pain, and was considering leaving treatment. She became hopeful when she learned that traumas could sustain or exacerbate pain in the body long after the trauma is over – and, on occasion, long after the physical body has healed. Her hope was to reduce the levels of her "chronic pain," thereby reducing her urge to medicate with narcotics. The following day Patti participated in my trauma resolution therapy group. Commencing the trauma resolution process, she immediately focused on the pain in her legs. She described it as a "heavy crushed feeling and a burning" in her legs. She stated that she was seven years old when she first felt the pain. When I asked about where she was when she first felt these sensations, I was surprised that she saw herself lying next to the highway, following a car accident. The location of the visual scene suggested that the moment of the trauma's encoding (T-1) actually occurred after the accident. So what, then, was the trauma? When I asked what happened next after she found herself beside the interstate, she stated that the cars just kept passing by and "no one would stop to help." "And what happens next," I asked, "when no one will stop and help?" She became tearful and replied: "I thought that I was going to die." The trauma itself – the moment of its encoding, was not about the accident, but about the fear that she would die when no one would stop and help her. She felt totally abandoned and frightened. During the original event, she encoded her terror of abandonment, accompanied in the scene by the crushing pain in her legs. In resolution, she reframed the memory to release feelings of terror, abandonment, and pain. Patti visualized bringing her injured seven year old self to the hospital in a more timely manner and resolved her fear and pain. She also needed to move a "green light" through her seven year old's legs to heal her pain. Upon obtaining the "corrected" scene, she saw a frame of "green and gold." Patti then moved the colors mentally through her legs. I felt a significant release of energy from the base of her spine. I then asked how her legs were feeling, expecting some residual pain from the "reported" nerve damage. She looked at me with a surprised expression on her face and declared: "It's gone – the pain … it's all gone." We were both equally surprised that the pain that had led to years of addiction to pain medications proved to be the result of a remaining emotional memory fragment. The pain that she had experienced was simply the somatic flashback of her traumatic memory surfacing for resolution. Please note that this case is not an exception; most car accidents, for instance, encode an emotional trauma component. The ignored emotional pain will continue to seek our attention by cueing us to the exact nature of the memory via the physical body. Resolution of the emotional component of memory will result in diminution of the pain; the degree will be determined by the incidence of any permanent injury to the nervous system. Whenever possible, we should, in an appropriate and timely manner, return to our traumatic memory in order to resolve the emotional component of our trauma – to determine how much is physiological damage and how much is simply the somatic memory of trauma. Much of what is "assumed" as "chronic pain" is due, in fact, to residual trauma memory surfacing from the subconscious. With the techniques we are developing, there is little to lose and much to gain by eliminating the possibility of emotional trauma as the source of the pain, prior to intrusive medical intervention. We may eventually see something of a reversal in the diagnostic processes, with trauma components being eliminated first.

Diseases, however, are not only the manifestations of trauma. There is also, for instance, a healing unto and through death that is mediated by diseases. These "terminal" illnesses are the agencies through which many of us continue our spiritual journey beyond this plane. As Michael Talbot discussed in his work, The Holographic Universe, death is simply a shift in our holographic consciousness, not the end of it.[2] As we learn to facilitate the healing of others, we are reminded in various ways that the outcomes are not ours to choose. Let us never forget that there is, ultimately, a healing unto and through death for each of us. I believe that death is, ultimately, a choice from the spiritual (soul) level as evidenced by the "pre-departure" behaviors of so many of our loved ones. I saw my mother discharged from the hospital "in remission" only to go home, rock in her favorite rocking chair for a few minutes, climb back into bed, and lose consciousness quite suddenly. She had insisted that she wanted to die peacefully at home and clearly knew that she was dying. Certain disease experiences will not be healed by "clearing" our traumas, for there are higher purposes at work. However, many illnesses that we deem "terminal" are lessons and opportunities for healing, for resolving trauma. Just as it took the deaths of millions of alcoholics over millennia for us to become conscious of the presence and nature of this disease, we are now becoming aware of our blindness about the pervasiveness and power of trauma within the nervous system. This awakening to the hidden trauma-based nature of many of our diseases will assist us in accessing and realizing our creator potential.

In his book entitled, <u>Quantum Healing</u>, Deepak Chopra speaks profoundly of the mind-body unity.[3] As exciting as his book was, I was disappointed at his statement that the mechanism of how a thought might defeat a cancer cell "might be unknowable."[4] What was more shocking to me was the fact that he had just described an excellent example of Holographic Memory Resolution, though the process was incomplete. In his book, Chopra cited the case of a sixty-one year old man who was diagnosed with throat cancer.[5] His disease was progressed to late stages – he could hardly swallow, and his weight was only ninety-eight pounds.[6] At that time in 1971, the patient met Dr. O. Carl Simonton, a radiologist at the University of Texas.[7] As Chopra pointed out, the patient's prognosis was not only poor, with the doctors giving him a five percent chance of surviving five years after treatment, but he appeared to be so weak that he seemed unlikely to respond well to radiation.[8] As a desperate attempt to support the radiation therapy, Dr. Simonton decided to try the use of supportive visualization, teaching the patient to visualize his cancer as vividly as possible.[9] The patient was, fortunately, encouraged to use his own mental imagery, rather than that supplied by the doctors. Visualizing his immune system as white blood cells successfully attacking the cancer cells, he swept them out of his body, leaving only healthy cells behind.[10] The patient stated that he envisioned his immune cells as a blizzard of white particles, covering the tumor like snow burying a black rock.[11] Dr. Simonton instructed the patient to go home and repeat this visualization throughout the day.[12] Within a short time, his tumor was shrinking, and within two months, the tumor was gone.[13] The patient then used this technique on his arthritis and remained both cancer and arthritis-free for a period of six years. Dr. Simonton was surprised at the turn of events and later sought to develop his approach into a visualization therapy, though his effort met with only limited success.[14] Since that time, we have learned much more about using our holographic perception. I will share these advances from my own experience.

Founded on the successful resolution of physical, mental, and emotional blockages, I hold that two essential components must be present. They include:

1. Authentic access of the client's personal, internal picture of the metaphorical form of the blockage. The mind readily provides the correct holographic perception for distortions in our system – like the "black rock" (color is especially powerful and helpful due to its relationship to frequency).

2. Use of a solution employing the resources provided by the client's subconscious mind. The client, while initially prompted by Simonton "from the outside," was allowed his own process. He then reached within his own subconscious mind for the "new scene" or transformational vehicle. Two important features emerge about this resolution: a) the use of color, which produces a change in frequency; in the case above, the patient visualized a change from the color black, located at the lower end of the electromagnetic spectrum, to the color white (the snow) at the top of the spectrum. b) The "emotional" correction or shift created by the patient's own choice of a beautiful scene of white snow; this transformed a scene of pain and fear (T-1) to a scene of beauty (T+1).

The "personalization" of the solution and the use of color to secure the transformation are essential. Two items missing from Simonton's approach were: 1) the "framing" of the new picture and its permanent placement at the location of the original tumor, and 2) the determination if the cancer itself was memory-based. Was any effort made to track the pain of the cancer tumor to its time and place of inception? Was trauma involved? This is probable from my experience. Without effective trauma resolution, a memory-based illness will recur to announce its irresolution. It appears that six years later, the cancer returned. I have found that, whenever an unhealthy scene is removed from the nervous system, the healthy counterpart must replace it or an attempt to fill it with something else will occur. Otherwise, we may experience recurrence, develop another illness, or switch addictions.

The ultimate key to the resolution of traumas resides in promoting the trauma survivor's own supercomputer to provide the intricate counter-metaphor that uniquely fits the original parameters of the wound (psychic wound) in the nervous system. Such a complex determination is certainly beyond any therapist or physician-guided visualization of what the "specialist" thinks should happen to bring about the client's healing. The solution must be the client's own. Frequently my clients hear me declare: "To heal yourself, you must access your metaphor, enter your scene, employ your personal solution, and use your frame to secure it in the original location and at the original moment of its induction (T-1). I have not the expertise to do this for you; I can only facilitate this process." My clients are encouraged to continue moving the picture/frame through the whole body to accelerate the release and to assure complete displacement of the "old memory" from the cells and fields of the body.

The study of the resolution of physical, emotional, verbal, sexual, and spiritual abuse has suggested that, at a moment of trauma, the nervous system became distorted to the degree that it "paused" or froze to prevent further overwhelm to the system. When it halted, it froze the impending threat within the holographic memory capacity of that system and encoded it as metaphor. This memory, manifest as an electromagnetic distortion, is corrected via the creation and placement of the "new scene." Traumas, as electromagnetic deficiencies or distortions, are perceived as dense, dark, heavy forms of energy when viewed holographically. The healing of trauma requires the restoration of the electromagnetic fields of the body – a return to the pre-trauma state of the nervous system. The use of color in the reframing of memories serves as a natural medium for reprogramming the cells and fields of the body. As physics teaches us, color , sound, and vibration are all frequency. Healing can occur through diverse agencies. However, if left unaddressed for long periods of time, these deficiencies will manifest their electromagnetically distorted natures, eventually taking their corresponding shape in the physical body. The forms of disease these traumas take have been the object of study by various authors. Louise Hay, for instance, having struggled with cancer, offers personal reflection into which emotional deficiencies predispose certain diseases.

In the healing process, it is the subconscious that already possesses the resources to direct us to the precipitant of the distortions as well as their solutions. By becoming conscious of our true nature as creators and healers, we learn to bring these infinite resources to bear on all levels, awakening to our true nature and potential to transform our intrapersonal and interpersonal realities, to manifest our spiritual nature. Diseases are occasions for us to reflect on our spiritual nature and to examine those beliefs and experiences that may need to change for us to realize our true potential. From the spiritual perspective, they are intended as occasions of empowerment. Once the lessons are learned, the disease experience is no longer needed.

It is fundamentally understood that the younger and less traumatized we are, the easier it is to incorporate these lessons. With children and adolescents, particularly, I learned that it is not always necessary to access the trauma memory itself to achieve resolution. Being younger and "less defended," they are able to simply replace the metaphorical form of a blockage with the color-frequency that resolves it. Readily they know the solution. Adults are able to do this in some circumstances. Many memories and distortions presenting in the physical body do not require conscious recall or awareness of the precipitant. It is sufficient to simply replace the container of pain or disease with the color-frequency that resolves it. I have worked with adolescents who, for instance, accessed no conscious memory of any specific event in association with the "pains" in their bodies, but who simply discarded the painful metaphors in a manner appropriate for them and replaced the memories with the color of their choice. This is often a simple but effective exercise for stress related symptoms – stress headaches, for instance. If the feelings cannot be "replaced" easily, I usually treat the symptoms as a cue for a memory and proceed accordingly. It is not uncommon for my clients to simply resolve one metaphor by replacement and to resolve another by actually entering the original scene. If we have already "worked on" and released the emotional pain of a trauma memory, often all that is left is the container or metaphor imprinted in the cellular memory of the body. This can be replaced with correct frequency (color). I do not make these determinations; the subconscious mind of my client chooses. Each of us desires to simply replace our trauma memories with the correct frequency, the easy solution, but for many of our memories, greater empowerment seems to be achieved or required by entering the original scene and reclaiming our power. Children and adolescents seem to be able to recover their power, more often than not, without having to access the original scene; they simply send in the correct frequency(ies) which they, usually, manifest very quickly. These techniques continue to evolve, and, I suspect, will modify even further to provide great new modalities for healing children.

A short time ago, all of my knowledge and expertise were subjected to scrutiny with a personal issue that arose. I began to experience a mysterious pain in my left abdominal region. Having no conscious memory about the nature of such a pain, I attempted simple "replacement" with color, which helped to decrease the pain, but did not resolve it. The pain returned. The electromagnetic fields in my hands also provided some relief, but, again, did not alleviate it. I considered the possibility that it was a physiological trauma of some sort and sought medical consultation. After routine tests, a "parasite" indigenous to Israel where I spent my archaeological days was identified and eliminated, but the pain remained. Additional tests including abdominal ultra-sounds, a colonoscopy, sixteen biopsies, and even a CAT scan, all of which produced no significant findings. The day after the CAT scan, however, I was sitting in my office and the pain became more intense. I decided to apply "full" technique on myself to enhance its effectiveness, including placement of my dominant hand over the dorsal point of my spine to enhance visualization (See Chapter Eight on Electromagnetic Fields). Suddenly I felt eleven sharp needle-like stabbing sensations in that site in my abdomen. The last jab caused me to jump from the chair. It felt like a needle went through my whole body. I asked myself how old I was, and heard: "two." When I asked where I was, I sensed: "in the hospital with bronchitis." When I asked what happened next, I saw a silver cylinder with another silver cylinder in it, with the picture of a needle moving in and out of the central cylinder. Was this the cause of the stabbing pains? I later learned that such syringes were in use in the late 1950's in hospitals. I reframed the scene to notify my two year old self that he was going to be OK and removed him from the scene. I moved four correcting colors through the site in my abdomen and felt the immediate alleviation of the pain. Later, I learned from my sisters that I had been in the hospital at age two and nearly died of bronchitis. This explained my terror of needles that endured until a fortunate encounter with a gentle dentist who treated me when I was high school age. I then realized that the injection I received during the CAT scan had triggered the actual memory. When I resolved the scene, that pain never returned.

We are all awakening to the presence of the voices within us, offering, by means of our memories and traumatic experiences, unique opportunities for healing and empowerment. With the advent of new data on trauma induction and encoding, we have come to recognize the pervasive presence of trauma and its impact on the individual and collective consciousness. If Gary Zukav is correct in his assessment, we have evolved predominantly from subconscious intentionality. With this predominance of the subconscious mind (at ninety-three percent) comes the admission that we have been following the dictates of our internalized traumas. Every human being has experienced and encoded traumas during life's unfolding. To the extent that these traumas have remained intact in our body's cells and electromagnetic fields, our autonomic nervous system, endocrine system, and immune system have been affected. As I emphasized earlier, we have known the impact of stress on these systems since the work of Hans Selye in the 1930's. This data, enlightened by our understanding of trauma-induction, suggests that few of us allow our immune system to function optimally. We may not comprehend, therefore, the full potential of the human immune system until we resolve the traumas we hold. Our recent work with AIDS patients gives us hope, however, for, upon resolution of their traumas, even without the support of medications, their T-Cell counts rose remarkably. The resolution of our traumas, therefore, holds great hope and may, for the first time, indicate to us the true capacity of the human immune system for healing. The outcome is contingent upon honest answers to the question that we must ask ourselves individually and collectively: How much trauma have we encoded in our nervous system?

Over the past seven years, I have been privileged to experience my own empowerment and to facilitate the empowerment of thousands of other trauma survivors who, like myself, have overcome life-threatening experiences and memories that haunted their existence and fostered illusions about themselves and others. Sometimes these traumas manifested as physical illness, but they also imprinted as spiritual trauma that blinded us to our true nature as creators. At times they left us with the perception that we were unlovable or that love was inaccessible. This was the greatest trauma. These old imprints can now be healed, and, as a result, so can the diseases that such belief distortions generate. The illnesses that manifest in our bodies correlate directly to our underlying belief systems. Our trauma moments create these false beliefs. Such distortions in our consciousness leave "gaps" or deficiencies in the cells and electromagnetic fields of our bodies and predispose us to recreate these distortions in our daily lives. The body is the manifestation of our minds, of our states of consciousness. As we learn to move fluidly within holographic space, we gain mastery over our states of consciousness – we discover our nature as creators and healers. To the extent that every fragment of holographic reality contains the whole, we possess a creator and healer within us. The requisite love, insight, and power are present within us; they are our birthright. There is immeasurable hope in the shifts of consciousness that are now occurring through our exploration of human healing potential.

Chapter Fifteen

Each morning we are born again.
What we do today is what matters most.

Buddha

Creating the Future
and Resolving the Past

A client taught me a most exciting use for the creative visualization techniques employed in this work. He arrived for a session stating that he had experienced no recurrence of any of the symptoms related to the memories that he had already resolved, but he had been experiencing fear and anxiety about returning home after inpatient treatment and held specific fears about relapse. He explained that the evening before, his anxiety increased. He tried to locate the feelings in his body, finding the source of the anxiety in his chest area. Based on the success of his previous memory resolution experiences, he decided to create the picture of the future that he needed in order to avoid relapse. He visualized himself driving past his favorite bar on the main street of town without reacting – remaining sober and emotionally present to his family. He reported that he then created the following scene: He took a picture of "a sober and peaceful life in recovery," framed the picture in the colors of his choice, and moved the colors of the frame through his body where the anxiety was felt. He stated that he immediately experienced relief – the anxiety was gone, and he now was "OK" about returning home. This use of imaging assisted him in predisposing his mind and body for a new way of life upon his return home from treatment. With this "future adaptation" of the reframing process, I assist my clients in articulating and creating for themselves the environment that they need to support their recovery. I invite them to utilize the colors of these "anticipated realities" to help anchor their vision of recovery into their current life and to help shape the circumstances around them into the lifestyle they seek. "When you feel distracted from your recovery program," I remind them, "you need only think of the color of the frame of your 'recovery picture' and move the color through your body to feel centered and focused." My clients have found this anchoring technique quite helpful. If we employ this reframing technique to resolve the past, can we not also use it to create the future that we desire?

Since this experience, I have had the opportunity to use the technique to help Olympic contenders remove trauma-induced obstacles to their success and to create their desired outcomes. I must admit that I was surprised when I saw the amount of emotional and physical trauma that was induced during the competition in the 1996 Olympic Games. From my work with athletes, I became aware that we can encode trauma in our bodies by pushing ourselves so hard physically that we cause injury – ignoring our emotional needs and warning signs about over extension and disrespect of our bodies. The emotional sensitivity of our nervous system will not allow us to abuse our bodies without encoding this emotional self-violation in metaphorical form in the nerve centers involved. We may be able to condition ourselves mentally to perform to our satisfaction, but if we abuse ourselves emotionally, we will leave a lasting, negative impact on our physical bodies. Remember that emotional traumas get our attention by presenting themselves to our consciousness through physical pain. I see this often with football injuries that continue to present as pain years later, although the physical injury site actually is healed. The individual does not realize that the old "aches and pains" from his athletic days are the encoded memory fragments of his mental and emotional self-abuse. Our nervous systems are too sensitive to be treated carelessly or recklessly because we simply must achieve some mental goal. It may be easier to achieve unbelievable athletic feats when we disassociate ourselves from our bodies, but we often induce trauma as we do this. Now we are learning to honor the remarkable sensitivity of our emotional bodies. If we do not, the body will notify us later of the abuse we induced, as we discussed in the previous chapter on the healing of diseases.

Long ago I heard reports that the Russians utilized visualization techniques to foster athletic improvement. Over the past few years, students interested in sports psychology have begun to study and express interest in adapting Holographic Memory Resolution to the athletic field. From watching the Olympics and Olympic trials, it is quite clear that many Olympic hopefuls suffer from limitations imposed by traumas induced from both home and the athletic arena itself. I have no doubt that the techniques that we are developing can be used to resolve anxieties and limitations to improve personal performance and foster success. The physiology of the body changes rapidly when memories are resolved. Persons with chronic neck, back, and shoulder pain suddenly find themselves pain free because they took the time to access and resolve the memory that created their suffering.

Of the various uses for these powerful holographic visualization techniques, the most rewarding and powerful application involves the facility of the human mind to employ this technique to resolve issues pertaining to grief and death. Earlier in this work I spoke of those theorists who refer to death as a simple shift to another level of holographic consciousness. Just as flashbacks, nightmares and traumas are "altered states" or holographic shifts that are readily accessible to us, so, too, are grief issues.

Our subconscious mind is continuously open to the higher spiritual realms and dimensions of reality, particularly in the Theta states of sleep, self-hypnosis, and deep meditation. The impact of Newtonian thinking on spirituality created a terrible duality that left many of us with the feeling that the spiritual realm was separate and inaccessible. Our "solidity" bound us to the laws and rules of the material plane. On the contrary, as holographic beings of light, we possess the capacity to move fluidly, when unencumbered by traumas and damaging beliefs, within the realm of the holographic mind. It is this ability which makes the resolution of grief issues readily attainable.

One case that taught me a great deal about our multidimensionality was the case of "Jamie." Jamie was a seventeen year old who had experienced severe trauma, losing nearly all of his family members in separate, unrelated accidents. Among the first, and most traumatic of these, was the death of his mother when he was nine years old. Before I knew anything of his history, and before I could begin the verbal process with him, I undertook an initial scan of his body and felt a potent knife-like pain emanating from his heart region; my hand nearly went numb. When I asked Jamie to describe his feelings as we began, he stated, "I feel sad."

"When you feel this sadness, where do you feel this physically?" I asked.

"In my heart," he responded.

"And what's it like – this sadness inside your heart area?" I inquired.

"Does it have a shape or a size?" I questioned.

"It's a sharp stabbing pain," he stated.

"And is there anything else about it?" I invited.

"It's cold," he stated bluntly.

"And how old might you be when you first feel a cold stabbing pain on the inside of your heart like that?" I asked quietly.

"I'm nine."

"And can you see where you are when you're nine years old and you're feeling sad like that?"

"I'm in the yard," he responded.

"And what happens when you're in the yard, and you're nine?" I asked.

"People are coming and going, and I know that something is wrong – I'm afraid that it's about my mom 'cause she's been in the hospital with cancer for so long ... then my aunt comes and tells me that she's died."

"And what happens then when she tells you that?" I encouraged gently.

"I just feel numb, and I keep playing in the yard," he stated.

"And what needs to happen with this memory, Jamie? ... (pause) What would you like to see happen for that younger part of yourself who felt so shocked and numb? Do we need to talk to Mom since you didn't get to say 'goodbye'?"

"Yeah, I'd like to do that," he said quietly. "They didn't take me much to the hospital the weeks before she died," he added.

"Let's do that then … if you could see your mother in your mind's eye today, can you see how she looks?" I inquired softly and tentatively.

"I can see stairs ... I see her now (his eyes becoming tearful) ... I saw her in a picture in my head after she died ... she was at the top of these stairs ... she's at the top now and wants me to come up," he answered.

"So take all the time that you need to do that," I stated and paused. "How does she look?" I inquired.

"Beautiful … peaceful and happy, but concerned," he described.

"Is there anything that you'd like to tell her?" I asked.

"Yeah, a lot!" he said.

"Then take all the time you need to tell her all the things that you've wanted to tell her ... you can do that silently if you're more comfortable ... (silent pause) ... and see if there's anything that she wants to tell you too," I added. Jamie sat in silence, while I tracked the rapid movement of his eyes.

He nodded, indicating that it was all right now.

"Is there anything else you'd like to do ... do you need to give her a hug?" I invited.

"We're already hugging," he stated.

"Then let's take a picture of the two of you together the way you'd like to remember ... (pause) and keep in mind that this is a living picture that you can return to whenever you need to; let me know when you have that picture the way you want it," I continued.

"OK; I have it," he responded.

"Is there anything else you need to do with this picture?" I inquired.

"No," he stated, "but she told me that I have to go back down the stairs – that it's not time yet, but that she'll be watching over me." He smiled.

I felt chills run down my back. "When you're ready, let's put a beautiful frame around the picture the way you'd like to remember it," I suggested.

"OK! I have it. It's a brilliant white light – like the light around her," he stated.

"Let's move that brilliant white light through your body, especially through your heart where the sharp, sad pain used to be – to let your body know that you and Mom are OK now ... and that anytime you need to you can return to that picture in your mind and feel her love and presence watching over you."

After some minutes he stated, "OK – I've done it."

"How does your body feel now?" I asked.

"Peaceful," he confirmed.

"When you think of your mom now, how do you feel?" I asked.

"I can see the picture in my mind – I feel good," he declared.

Jamie and I then processed his experience. He talked about how he had a "vision" of his mom after her death and saw her at the top of these "weird stairs." As a nine year old he did not understand their meaning, but now that he had the new picture, he felt that he understood and felt "good " about the vision. Jamie was easily able to access and utilize his holographic nature – his spiritual resources for healing and resolution. I have rarely encountered anyone unable to visualize a loved one when the subconscious mind deems it appropriate. This type of resolution experience is more "interactive" and moves beyond the limitations of our traditional space and time perceptions. As you can imagine, the spontaneous details frequently hold surprises for the therapist. Many ask if this type of experience is "real" and can be trusted. I am convinced that this experience comes at the prompting, the healing exigencies, of the client's own subconscious mind and carries the strongest healing potential that I have yet witnessed. I have not seen any of its "fruits" to be negative or to hinder anyone's spiritual beliefs. If anything, I have seen the "mutual" healing that seems to be evidenced for both parties present in the scene. If our loved ones can watch over us after their "transition," as I firmly believe, then there is a type of spiritual healing that occurs for both parties when their deaths or the traumas they caused us no longer contribute to our addictions, depression, dysfunction, or disease.

One of the most surprising events during the initial development of this technique occurred when one of my more actively "intuitive" clients was accessing and dialoguing with a part of herself that had experienced a childhood trauma. While she was dialoguing with the younger, "wounded" part of herself, this intuitive child-self suddenly commented on the presence of a rose-colored light that was reportedly standing next to me. "It's your mother," she later confirmed. My mother had died in 1983, yet I was aware that she continued to "assist" me in my life and was often present. I had not expected my client's own holographic space to overlap into my own. After the experience, I realized that my client simply possessed a highly developed capacity to see and move within holographic space. This reality, as you may glean, is not merely a subjective one.

Carl Jung frequently spoke of our unconscious access to spiritual reality. Ignatius Loyola emphasized the utilization of all of our senses to enter into meditative states. This form of meditation or multidimensional thinking has proved to be among my own most powerful experiences. After the retreat experience that I had at La Storta, Italy, (where Ignatius had his vision to reform the Catholic church and establish the Jesuit Order) I learned that, preparing myself with yoga and entering with all of my senses into the eternal truths and accounts presented in the scriptures, the accounts themselves transcended their original context – space and time, and became "alive" in present time. I came to understand that the metaphorical language of spiritual literature provides a gateway to access the unlimited resources of Spirit which are not bound by any space or time limitations. We can bring light to the past, present, or future. The message of the "Divine Incarnation" or "Indwelling" posited in the spiritual literature of many cultures announces that it is by the bridge now existing between the conscious and the subconscious minds that the divine is made accessible to us. The holographic capacity to shift our consciousness to promote healing is readily available. Within our subconscious minds we have continuous access to the unlimited resources of spirit, as Carl Jung pointed out to us. The spiritual limitations that we have experienced until the present are not so much the product of our "moral" failures as they are the product of the limitations imposed by the exile from our own subconscious resources caused by trauma. These traumas, as you may recall, are usually frozen and stored automatically by the subconscious. Our capacity to deal with and move within holographic space promises healing from flashback, nightmare, and even the unresolved pain of "death." All types of losses become occasions to exercise our holographic consciousness to resolve blockages to wholeness and integration. The "deaths" of loved ones become an opportunity for spiritual growth by calling upon our ability to move and communicate within holographic space. Individuals living in certain Native American cultures consciously choose the moment of their transition and deliberately "shut down" the systems of their bodies, making a peaceful "transition" in the location of their choosing. Death becomes the consummate experience for manifesting our ability to alter consciousness and to move within holographic space. At long last we are coming to a conscious participation in this creative process of play within holographic space. As to the true extent and nature of this ability, I suspect we have only begun to "awaken."

Chapter Sixteen

Happiness is what we feel when our biochemicals of emotion,
the neuropeptides and their receptors, are open and flowing
freely. It is a scientific fact that we can feel what others feel
– emotional resonance. The oneness of all life is based on
this simple reality. Our molecules of emotion are all vibrat-
ing together.

Candace Pert (1997)

Conclusions

Never in my life have I been more excited or hopeful about who we are and our ability to heal and transform our physical, mental, emotional, and spiritual realities. This work is simply a starting point – an opportunity to begin transcending illusions that were imprinted upon us but which can now be relinquished to reveal our true identities. I know that it will be my lifelong adventure to teach and empower others about this remarkable resource that has been revealed through my experience with trauma. And I know that I shall be helpful in offering some "teaching tools" along the way. Yet, in summary, what is the main lesson to be gleaned from all of this discussion about trauma?

The journey beyond trauma begins, for each of us, with an inner awareness or realization that our "survival" has been built on specific experiences that have shaped for us a certain view of reality. Such a life perspective, constructed not from our choosing as magnificent creators of reality, but dictated from trauma – from moments of radical powerlessness and fear of extinction – created reaction not empowerment. Instead of discovering and becoming excited about our power to manifest beauty and divinity, we, as individuals and as a society, become ensnared in a victim mentality. Such a mentality is addictive and self-limiting. It imposes certain illusions about self, relationships, Higher Power, human nature, the world, emotion, diseases – about the very nature of love.

My personal efforts to move through these limitations revealed commonalities shared by many – a great illusion that we have borne from time immemorial and which we, only now, are becoming capable of relinquishing. As the immensity of this illusion emerged, it was my hope that I could help to liberate others from similar constraints. And the process began with my own inner search.

Amidst the profound sense of insecurity that I internalized from others as a child, a vision of the world was created that necessitated the employment of certain psychological defenses – of a means to counter the overwhelming feelings of aloneness and isolation. From my experience and my work with countless trauma survivors, I know now that this created a desperate attachment – a kind of addiction to a certain view of reality. This finite view of reality developed in response to specific crises that befell during my development. Within my subconscious mind, as is true for each trauma survivor, the overwhelming life experiences which I was not able to integrate remained alive and potent – preserved in the cells and fields of my body. I was to learn that my consciousness itself was constrained by these frozen moments which, at an early age, produced a diminished sense of self – an illusory sense of smallness and fear. Given the dominant influence of these powerful memories stored in my subconscious, I lived much of my life, as my father had, with the feeling that some life-threatening aloneness was only seconds away, threatening to burst my carefully constructed bubble of security. As a result of these "false" perceptions, my life became more a matter of "burying the treasure" so as not to lose it. Although there were wonderful, inspirational, and joyful moments in my development, there frequently remained a mysterious threatening cloud nearby to mar any experience. My stewardship of power was off to a rather slow start. My energies were primarily spent to prevent further abandonment, aloneness, and emptiness. I also discovered that I was not alone in my distrust of reality or in my efforts to cope with it.

In our efforts to survive our internalized traumas, our conscious minds find distraction and build carefully constructed illusions of fulfillment as success, power, wealth, conquest, freedom from pain, orgasm, worship, body-beautiful, popularity, academic achievement, satiation, religiosity, and futurism, to name only a few of our options. We can also hide behind the images of victimhood, blame, powerlessness, disease, and "accident" as a way of maintaining our fragile and limited view of reality, choosing to remain unconscious and conveniently secure within our well-constructed and well-defined parameters. These defenses, we tell ourselves, will prevent any untimely "near-emotional-death experiences" from surfacing without due planning or warning. Living within our carefully created view of reality offers the illusion of completeness, but, as you can sense, it is remarkably burdensome and tiring. It drains our power and dilutes our truth. It is only when our illusions of completeness are recognized, challenged, or threatened that we begin to move beyond "survival mode" into our true potential. Those very experiences of pain that we have spent most of our lives avoiding turn out to be the fertile field, the opportunity to move from our illusions into our true place as "creators."

Suddenly we begin to realize that, from the outset, we possessed the perfect backdrop to move us toward our own empowerment – our parents (and the others who participated in our care). My father, for instance, as such a burdened trauma survivor, with his shyness and inability to express love openly, gave me the best experience of love he could in the midst of his own tortured psyche. He became the perfect teacher and motivator for moving me through the lessons of trauma. Through his eyes I was able to see the impact of trauma on the soul. With the help of my mother's intuition, I could also feel the dense energetic influence of trauma. I began to realize how intricate and perfect is the plan for our individual and collective evolution.

Our subconscious minds (our spiritual, Higher Selves, souls, etc.) consistently seek to awaken us to the illusions which are constraining us. This great purpose reaches out to us and, more often than not, because of our "avoidant" natures, does so through our pain. Countless times I have facilitated trauma resolution work with individuals who suddenly realize that the tightness in their legs that has kept them from sleeping soundly for the last forty-two years has simply been a powerful unresolved incident of emotional abandonment presenting itself for healing. In our haste to maintain our "comfortable," illusory view of reality, we have commonly ceased listening to ourselves and become entrapped in our own "secure" world-view. It took living with other trauma survivors for me to become willing to break through the false security offered by these powerful illusions. Freud called them defense mechanisms. It does not help that there are whole systems whose raison d'etre is to maintain such illusions of power. It is, in fact, the resultant cycle of self-addiction to our carefully constructed views of reality and our illusions that we must escape. This challenge is a spiritual one.

The most profound impact of trauma on our lives can be termed "spiritual." From the deepest layers of our psyche we have undertaken a search for wholeness and fulfillment. Our initial search was built upon the promises and examples of our parents, our ancestors, our mythologies, our religions, and our societies. There was an unspoken expectation that they would provide a universe of order and comfort. With the advent of trauma in our personal and collective histories, the promised order began to dissipate, and a picture of a much more fragile universe came into play. This, for many of us, was a kind of "theological trauma" – that is, it challenged the purported foundation of all security – our image or conception of the creative Source or "God." At first this challenge did not emerge as an intellectual one. It was actually mediated by our first "gods," our parents or primary caregivers, who, despite their best efforts, precipitated and transferred to us, in varying degrees, their intergenerational and collective illusions or traumas. Much of this pre-programming occurred long before the age of reason or language and was stored in our subconscious. The protective powers of our minds then allowed us to compartmentalize our painful states of consciousness in order to protect us from discomfort and disorientation; this served a profound spiritual, emotional service and laid the foundation for the healing process. We subconsciously utilized our internal resources which allowed us to freeze our (space and time) perceptions so well that they were sufficiently contained until such time as we would be strong, ready, safe, "awake" enough to consciously transform them. We are now reaching the level where our mass consciousness is increasing awareness of buried traumas and is beginning to bridge the subconscious barriers put in place at the instant the traumas were induced. It is no accident that my own introduction to the trauma field and my personal impetus for recovery occurred as a direct result of my exposure to addictions. This was the societal Pandora's Box which, with the recognition of alcoholism as a disease in the 1950's, opened the door to the understanding of the more subtle levels of trauma in such areas as "codependency," eating disorders, sexual addiction, etc. It revealed to us a societal trauma and a disease that "robbed us of will-power" – an experience that separated us from our intentionality. And it is also no accident that this knowledge paralleled the development of "Family Systems Theory" in the 1950's. We have all seen the progression: a disclosure of the nature of dysfunctional systems that foster emotional repression and result in unhealthy and compulsive coping mechanisms, addictions, relationship problems, and dis-empowerment, even disease. Currently all of our attention is drawn to issues of trauma and "repressed memories." It also "conveniently" coincides with the emergence of psychoneuroimmunology, the new mind-body science, and the convergence between science and spirituality. Much attention is now being drawn by these various disciplines to the power of the mind to store trauma, to alter its states of consciousness, to change the cellular, molecular, and even the genetic functioning of the cells of the body. There is some resistance to this nexus, to this new exploration, particularly by traditional systems of power founded on Newtonian physics. There is also a resistance manifest in our collective consciousness. As stated earlier in this work and affirmed by Gary Zukav in <u>The Seat of the Soul</u>, in the whole of human history, our dominant path, up to this point in time, has been "unconscious" evolution from our buried, "unconscious intentionality" (See p. 243). Unconscious intentionality is created by the desperate voices of our wounded selves struggling to stay alive in the midst of overwhelming pain. Their essential intent is to stop us from moving forward in time and into the face of imminent danger or death (at T: the moment of trauma); they do not want to move forward in time. With compassion, we can now understand and gently offer new solutions.

What becomes painfully apparent from my work with so many trauma survivors is that we, as human beings, have evolved through the dominance of our (ninety-three percent) subconscious, trauma-laden minds, wondering all the while why we could not transform our personal, interpersonal and global lives into the "Eden" that it was purported to be. Hopeful beyond measure is the fact that the key to breaking through our constricting and spiritually inhibiting illusions of separation is now manifesting. Many of us already feel this collective surge to access and resolve the "unfinished business" from our past, as it is stored in our subconscious. But to those of us that have and are still "acting out" the compartmentalized traumas or horrors of our childhood, this imminent shift triggers fear and defensiveness. The idea of being able to scientifically confirm, prove, access, recall, feel, and resolve memory with such precision triggers both great hope and great fear. This is understandable, for our predominant coping mechanism for the psycho-spiritual pain we hold within has been dissociation. Rather than integrate and heal those traumatized, addicted or "acting out" parts of our culture, we have, more often than not, responded by compartmentalizing and ostracizing them from our memory and consciousness – as though "out of sight, out of mind" would solve the dilemma. We have reacted in this way with our culture's endorsement. The Russian author Dostoevsky suggested that the measure of "civilization" of a culture is to be found by observing how it treats its prisoners. In our culture, we disassociate them from ourselves. If we wish to transform ourselves as a society, we might do well to begin with the justice system, including the prison and juvenile detention systems and their treatment of the human spirit. We have often settled for "justice" instead of seeking "healing." One of my former coworkers from my ministry days, Sister Helen Prejean (depicted in the film "Dead Man Walking") has already begun this task. Dissociative attempts to exterminate our societal traumas will never bring us healing.

As inherently spiritual beings, we are, in fact, connected on a profound level to all that shares consciousness. As a result, we each experience the upsurge of our forgotten and repressed states of mind. Through continuous media stimulation, the "triggers" are all around us to remind us of our individually and collectively repressed memories. These triggers produce for many, a strong, subconscious defense response. And, oftentimes, the defense is to shadows that are only glimpsed.

The spiritual key to moving beyond our fear and internal resistance, however, resides in the fact that, behind such experiences of trauma, each of us possesses, in our subconscious, a far more powerful memory or bridge which promises healing and wholeness beyond our imagining. If there is one message that could summarize what I have gleaned from my experience as a trauma survivor, it is the remarkable capacity that we possess to transform and to infinitely exceed the confines and constraints that have been spiritually, emotionally, mentally, and physically placed upon us by "trauma." In reality, our subconscious minds, in cooperation with the spiritual resources of our unconscious, facilitated the "creation" and storage of our traumas within us to allow our ego to expand sufficiently to allow the healing and integration of these "traumas" as learning experiences, advancing us on our soul's journey. To the unconscious mind (Higher Self) that transcends the limitations of time and space, our traumas are all lessons of spirit. They are occasions to challenge our holographic consciousness to expand and to become excited at its emergent power as "creator." It is the moment of quickening for consciousness.

The most wonderful part of working through my own traumas has been the emergence of this power as creator. It is no accident that I can now access and feel the electromagnetic forms of my emotions and those of others. This gift took form once I realized that I am more than the "object" which my traumas taught me to be. It is no accident that these natural healing abilities so often begin to manifest when our sexual-divine-creator (procreator) energy is released from the containers of the subconscious to which it was confined during the freezing of our abuse experiences. It is no accident that the ministers of many religious systems have lost touch with their own inherent healing abilities from the repression of the "kundalini" energy – the healing energy which is also our creative, sexual energy. Within the Catholic priesthood, there were many of us who sought to turn celibacy into a container-lifestyle, whereby we would never have to address our unresolved sexuality or abuse issues; "maybe," we thought, "we could just be non-sexual!" In the natural order there is no non-sexuality without non-creativity. And, when I speak of sexuality, if you are only thinking in terms of "genitality," you are reducing a profound energy to a narrow band of sensory perception and pleasure associations. I refer to the purest "tantra" of the East – the conversion of our life-force energy for love and service. The dimensions and impact of our sexuality go far beyond the notion of genitality. It is no accident that so many of those who are sexually addicted also present with religious addiction. Spiritual energies are intimately connected with the sexual energies of our bodyminds. There is no escaping this truth.

Once we have come to locate and recognize the containers which prevent us from moving into what we know from our inner spiritual awareness to be possible, we can begin integrating and learning those spiritual lessons which our traumas offer. Had it not been for my abuse experiences, these words would not be before you. There is a tremendous empowerment when we give ourselves enough trust to step beyond the confining view of reality that we reassure ourselves is safety. The safety offered by avoiding or ignoring the subconscious is fragile, indeed. The unconscious (Higher Self, soul, etc.) will always work to help us safely and gently bridge this avoidance by recreating the blockages or patterns over and over until we choose to recognize and respond to them. The unconscious will increase the pressure if the hints go unaddressed. The emotional body will cause us to feel discomfort in a specific location in our body in order to draw our attention to the trauma or blockage. The mental body will begin to send messages telling us in no uncertain terms that something is wrong with us. In the end, if we have failed to attend to these increasingly urgent communications, the physical body will manifest the presence of the blockage as "disease." Our diseases are no accidents; our headaches are no accidents.

The realization, however, that we can, within seconds, move into "quantum thinking" and access those dimensions of ourselves in which the blockages and precipitating memories are stored, is extremely healing and unbelievably empowering. I have rarely encountered anyone who could not learn to use this ability to accelerate the healing process. As holographic beings, there are virtually unlimited options to advance our healing. This is not to say that there is no resistance or even choice involved in approaching our traumas. Resistance has long served to protect us in its own, albeit misled, way from "death" and overwhelm. We owe a profound debt to those parts of our consciousness that, despite limited access to resources and protection, managed to sustain us long enough to obtain help and resolution. The real challenge has been to avoid over-attachment or addiction to these temporary measures. Among the sources of resistance to our healing are the following:

◆ Resistance, first and foremost, comes from the subconscious, wounded ego-states themselves. Our wounded ego-states believe that, if the event is accessed and proceeds forward, there will be no one there to help them, and they will die, as originally feared. This is the impact of our having encoded the trauma at "T-1" – the instant just prior to the worst part of the trauma; to the wounded ego-state, one second forward in time and we are facing death. Now, years later, this is obviously an illusion, although it certainly may not feel so when the trauma memory is triggered. The "truth" is that we have already survived and are now adults who are qualified and capable of understanding what happened to those wounded parts of ourselves as well as loving them into wholeness. Sometimes, however, the fear that is triggered when our memories approach can overpower our rational (seven percent) minds and lead us to "postpone" accessing our memories until we feel that we will no longer be overwhelmed. This is particularly true when we have been recreating or "acting out" our traumas in current time and there is danger of retraumatization. Living with an alcoholic spouse after having been severely abused by alcoholic parents often makes the need for change feel threatening, overwhelming, and even impossible to face. Safety is a primary requirement for trauma resolution to proceed. Our mental, emotional, spiritual and physical bodies will, nevertheless, speak more and more loudly when we remain powerless in our lives. Such impotence is not our nature or destiny.

◆ A second form of resistance to healing is related to the old belief that we have to "re-live" our memories and the horrible feelings in order to resolve them. As we have seen in this work, our trauma memories are the protective act of our higher consciousness and need not be feared. We need only return to "T-1," as we have seen throughout this work, to achieve resolution.

♦ A more surprising form of resistance to the resolution of our traumas is the realization that we do, indeed, have the power to heal our past. Our past only hurts us because of the emotional pain and power it continues to hold over us. This awareness often triggers great fear for a more subtle reason. One of the most important lessons of any effective memory resolution is the fact that I have the ability to "take my power back" from those persons or situations that occasioned its loss. This implies that I have the ability to take responsibility for my reality. The fear that emerges is often due to the misperception that taking responsibility means taking blame or blaming loved ones. There need be no blame in this issue of trauma – neither self nor others. Blaming keeps us stuck in the trauma; it states that there is still unresolved trauma stored in my system that is yet to be healed. Blame indicates that there remain unresolved feelings of anger, resentment, pain, etc., stored in my body about the traumatic experience. Effective resolution of the memory releases me from this connection or need to blame. Blaming also allows me to keep my "victim role" intact and to maintain my addiction to my comfortable, accustomed view of the world that has "so unjustly wronged me" – poor me! Blaming takes the focus away from the oft frightening prospect of personal empowerment and allows us distraction from the fear about our ability to move forward. As trauma survivors we question our ability to wield power in a nurturing or responsible manner. We grow attached to our ways of coping with this fear. Remember that we are "creatures of habit" and that we become easily addicted to our finite view of reality.

♦ A final source of resistance is the feeling: "I'm already too tired to face these overwhelming feelings and memories." I frequently see this in trauma survivors who have attempted, over many years, numerous trauma resolution therapies. They have become disheartened by approaches that failed, in the end, to provide resolution for their memories. Some achieved a significant degree of resolution in affect, but the "cellular memory" was untouched, leaving the pain syndrome intact. Others were misled to repeatedly relive the traumatic experiences under the impression that the painful affect would release when its power was exhausted; failing to address the T-1 encoding properly, the survivor became exhausted while the memory remained intact! Some, therefore, have "therapy trauma," as I call it, getting the false message from the ineffective therapy that complete resolution will not happen. Even the "crisis debriefing" approaches used to deal with large-scale trauma have often left survivors with messages about the assured recurrence of flashbacks but with little guidance as to how to resolve them. I noted this in working with the senior staff of TWA regarding the Flight 800 disaster. It is exhausting when we must fend off the continuous attempts of our bodies, minds, and spirits to bring these burdens to the surface because we know of no way to resolve them. Some of our "exhaustion," therefore, is due to our ignorance about the options now available to us. If we can but trust ourselves sufficiently to enter the scene and "take our power back" from those who disempowered us, we will have more energy than we have ever known. I often have to coax my more "exhausted" clients to devote a few minutes to see if we can reframe a memory that they have already borne overlong.

The key to this healing process is the realization of what we have to gain by risking entry into these seeming bottomless, unfathomable waters of our subconscious minds. We risk losing our diseases, our low self-esteem, our destructive marriages, our wonderfully faithful, reliant and ever-present addictions, our depression, our abuse of ourselves and our children, our spiritual emptiness, our need to be in control, and everything else that threatens our pseudo-security. We are now learning to heal ourselves and others in ways that do not require a re-experiencing or retraumatization. We are, at the same time, discovering that we are multidimensional beings who have the capacity to alter our states of consciousness in order to facilitate healing. This experience teaches us much more than simply how to resolve trauma. The dissolution of our "containers of consciousness," our traumas, is offering us a taste of spiritual and emotional intimacy that was only glimpsed in past generations. There is a profound intimacy ensured for those willing to move beyond the familiar role of victim.

Science and spirituality are forming a nexus, joining hands to communicate the same truth: we have the power within us to heal and transform our reality. We have the knowledge and ability now to heal the individual and collective subconscious that has held us trapped from our true nature as creators. The Newtonian-based models are failing rapidly and giving way to technologies that do not foster illusions of separateness, but, rather, encourage intimacy with all that is. Although this process begins with the "selves within" – with acknowledgment of the integration possible between our own ego-fragments, it then expands to others – to our "other-selves." Among our most precious lessons, we are now recognizing that "you" and "I" are not so separate. We are learning of our ability to transcend the limitations of space and time. We discover that we are continuously in a dynamic exchange of energy that extends beyond the spatio-temporal illusions. Even as we read this, we unite on a profound level of awareness, of Truth. The barriers that allowed us to ignore those parts of ourselves, each other, our environment and planet – they all vanish in favor of a promise of intimacy and expansion that leaves us breathless. With our traumas intact, we have never been able to answer the question as to who we really are – who we may have been intended to be from the perspective of the "Divine Mind" which encompasses all. What is our "creative" potential? Neither have we known what an optimally functioning immune, endocrine, or autonomic nervous system is capable of creating for us in terms of health. We are capable of healing the diseases and distortions which we created out of trauma.

In closing, I remind you of your power as a creator, a power that we share. If, as I now believe, our universe (and much more) is holographic, then we are expressions of the Creator and we contain the whole, in some manner. It is our spiritual adventure to explore this. From my holographic experiences, I have no doubt that we, our senses, our bodies, our bodyminds, our consciousness, our universe are all holographic. The implication is that each of us is an individuated expression of the One Mind which creates all. The vision of figures like Teilhard de Chardin, who saw the divine macrocosm in the microcosm, and Mother Theresa, who saw Christ in all people, regardless of religion, is not so far-fetched from this perspective. We are the holographic containers (fragments) of a singular reality and intentionality which is offering us, through our very nature, an opportunity to experience reintegration with the whole – in other words, to return home. We are mystical; we are light. We are interconnected in ways we never imagined. I have learned much about this through feeling the consciousness – feeling the actual emotional pain stored in the bodymind of others – feeling the energy borne in the lessons of another place and time.

We can use our abilities to facilitate our mutual healing and evolution. We are not returning home alone. In fact, given the emergence of this holographic model – the model of the multidimensional self, we have never been less alone. Divinity is suggested in each and every "fragment" of our consciousness. Every holographic trauma memory, by its nature, contains the divine – the potential to resolve or return home. Though these holographic scenes of trauma were overlaid with emotional pain that left us feeling out of touch with the "bigger picture," they always contained the key for returning home. I refer to one of my favorite movies, based on the book by L. Frank Baum: "The Wizard of Oz. " In this remarkable film which introduced many of us to the "power of color," we heard a singular message: "If I had told you that you had the power in the beginning, you wouldn't have believed me ... you had to learn this for yourself." Such is the wiser path of empowerment, though it certainly has not always felt pleasant. Such is the nature of our earthly adventure.

I thank you, my "trauma friends," for granting me the privilege of sharing your experiences, for by your presence in my life, you have revealed this process and this power to me. Remember always, beneath the pain, what you "contain." I thank you – for you, in the midst of your pain, come as teachers – to teach yourself of your own nature and power, and to help awaken this awareness in others – like myself. In our sharing and "merging," you have also felt the truth of what I say. It changes our ways of learning and knowing! May you embrace your multidimensionality – your ability to go beyond the limitations imposed by traumas, imposed by the intentions of other people and systems from other places and times. Learn to live and ride within your ability to perceive non-physicality. Accept the challenge to enter your pain and emerge on the other side. Tap into your spiritual strength to move beyond the illusions created by the intense feelings you still carry from unresolved traumas. From the standpoint of the unconscious or Higher Self, these are simply occasions provided to expose your nature as creator. From the perspective of the subconscious, they are aspects of yourself that remain trapped in other times and places until the healer appears – you. From the level of the conscious mind, these wounded selves may first appear as a physical pain – in your eyes, neck, stomach, legs, etc.. Perhaps they will manifest as an irritating pattern or mental message that recurs in your life. You may have a disease which is presenting you with the greatest invitation that you have ever received. These experiences are all gateways to empowerment. I have seen and felt them open through the willingness of the trauma survivors who have allowed me to join them in their quest for freedom. I have felt the low frequency energy move out of the bodymind and have felt the calm and peace which replaced it.

I have worked with individuals referred for trauma work from Hazelden, Springbrook, Sierra Tucson, the Mayo Clinic, M.D. Anderson, the Betty Ford Clinic, and a variety of other treatment centers throughout the country. They came with symptoms such as migraines, insomnia, lupus, and cancer, being told by their referring physicians, psychiatrists, psychologists, and therapists that recovery from their illnesses was directly impacted by their unresolved traumas. We are awakening! The emergent field of "psychoneuroimmunology" is an indication that we are coming to recognize the potency of the bodymind and its traumas, and their subsequent manifestation as dis-ease.

Within this work I have presented cases that have baffled the best "medical specialists" in the country. Knowledge about the dynamics we have discussed within this work could have facilitated the clients' healing process. In some trauma cases, this lack of awareness resulted in permanent physical damage, in contradiction of the sworn service of the Hippocratic oath: "Primum, non nocere" – "First, do no harm." The lessons of trauma have implications for all of us. Let us attend to the voices of the emotions stored within – let us attend to our feelings! There is an urgency to the message contained in this work. It has a profound spiritual import, and it will also have immense repercussions on our medical profession as the resistance diminishes. This is imminent for the medical profession, because, beyond all the ethereal reasons, the insurance companies love methods that work – and this works. It is functional reality.

This book focuses on trauma as the invitation to recognize the healer within us. Its more powerful purpose is to assist us in recalling our multidimensional nature as spiritual beings – as beings of light, who are now finding ourselves more at home with the advent of quantum physics and the heightened attentiveness to spirituality. We are being reborn at the nexus of spirituality and physics. There is a wonderful, unique energy present here.

If that which I have shared has resonated within you, has tapped your awareness of the creative potential you hold to transform your reality, the sharing has served its purpose. Perhaps it has roused the radiant child, the healer, the wise one, the tantra, the intuitive, the nurturer, or the mystic within. How old are you when you first feel this? In the end, there are no "new" lessons. You are your own teacher. All is remembrance! Re-member who you really are beneath the illusions. I remember you. Thank you for helping me to remember who I am (in the Biblical sense). I hope that I have served you similarly. Enjoy the exploration! Rejoice in the journey!

> *Come to the edge, he said.*
> *They said: We are afraid.*
> *Come to the edge, he said.*
> *They came.*
> *He pushed them ...*
> *And they flew.*
>
> *Guillaume Apollinaire (1888-1918)*

Notes

CHAPTER ONE: FOCUS

1. William Faulkner, cited by Timothy Hatcher, in a workshop entitled: "Body-Mind Unity,"presented at C.P.C. Meadow Wood Hospital in Baton Rouge, Louisiana, October, 1991.
2. "Healing Touch" is a modified version of the electromagnetic field technique called "Therapeutic Touch" developed by Dora Kunz at New York University. Healing Touch includes modifications from such influences as the healing work of Dr. Brugh Joy, Rosalyn Bruyere, and Native American cultures.

CHAPTER TWO: THE JOURNEY OF EMPOWERMENT

1. This notion of the profound interrelationship between rational thought and emotion was discussed in an article by Michael Lemonick, entitled "Glimpses of the Mind," in Time, July 17, 1995, pp. 44-52.

CHAPTER THREE: HOLOGRAPHIC SPACE

1. W. Brugh Joy, Joy's Way (New York: G.P. Putnam's Sons, 1979) p. 45.
2. Michael Talbot, The Holographic Universe (New York: Harper Collins Publishers, 1991), p. 1.
3. Talbot, p. 1.
4. Talbot, p. 2.
5. Umberto Eco, Semiotics and the Philosophy of Language (Bloomington: Indiana University Press, 1984), p. 89.

6. This definition of metaphor is derived from Eco's discussion of metaphor in terms of synecdoche and metonymy. See Umberto Eco, p. 90.
7. Ernest L. Rossi, The Psychobiology of Mind-Body Healing (New York: W.W. Norton & Company, Inc., 1986), p. 37.
8. Rossi, pp. 37-41. Rossi's work provides the most advanced synthesis to date of how stress and trauma manifest in the body via the limbic-hypothalamic system.
9. Rossi, p. xiv-xvi.
10. Rossi, p. xvi.
11. Rossi, p. xvi.

CHAPTER FOUR: TRAUMA METAPHORS

1. Ernest L. Rossi, The Psychobiology of Mind-Body Healing (New York: W.W. Norton & Company, Inc., 1986), p. 38.
2. Rossi, p. xvi.
3. Rossi, p. xvi.
4. Donna S. Dimski et al., "Renal Autotransplantation in the Loin Pain Hematuria Syndrome: A Cautionary Note," American Journal of Kidney Diseases, 20, No. 2 (August 1992), p. 180.
5. Dimski, p. 181.
6. Dimski, p. 181.
7. Dimski, p. 181.
8. Dimski, p. 181.
9. Dimski, p. 181.
10. Dimski, p. 181.
11. Dimski, p. 181.
12. Dimski, p. 181.
13. Dimski, p. 181.
14. Dimski, p. 181.
15. Dimski, p. 181.
16. Chris Griscom, Ecstasy is a New Frequency (Santa Fe: Bear and Company, 1987), p. 105.
17. See Louise Hay, Heal Your Body (Carson: Hay House, Inc., 1988), pp. 1ff.

CHAPTER FIVE: THE DYNAMICS OF TRAUMA INDUCTION

1. Chris Griscom discusses the issue of the sensitivity evidenced in the profiles of alcoholics in her work: Ecstasy is a New Frequency, (Santa Fe: Bear and Company, 1987), p. 76.
2. David Grove, Healing the Wounded Child Within (Edwardsville: David Grove Seminars, 1989), p. 10.

CHAPTER SIX: "TRIGGERS"

1. Julian Hawthorne et al., eds., The Literature of All Nations (Chicago: E.R. DuMont, 1901), I, p. 7.
2. Cited in Barbara Brennan, Hands of Light (New York: Bantam Books, 1988), p. 25.

CHAPTER EIGHT: THE ELECTROMAGNETIC KEY

1. The "perineural" cells are those which contain bundles of nerve fibers surrounded by an exterior layer of connective tissue. See Rosalyn Bruyere, Wheels of Light (Sierra Madre: Bon Productions, 1989, p. 54, note 47.
2. Ernest L. Rossi, The Psychobiology of Mind-Body Healing (New York: W.W. Norton & Company, Inc., 1986), p. 21.
3. Rossi, p. 20.
4. Rossi, p. 20.
5. Rossi, pp. 21-22.
6. Rossi, p. 20.
7. Rossi, pp. 21-22.
8. Rossi, p. 21.
9. Rossi, p. 24.

CHAPTER NINE: THE PHYSICS OF THE SOUL

1. See Thomas S. Kuhn, "The Structure of Scientific Revolutions," International Encyclopedia of Unified Science, II, No. 2 (1962), p. 1.
2. Kuhn, p. 6.
3. Kuhn, p. 6.
4. Kuhn, p. 144.
5. Kuhn, p. 147.
6. Kuhn, pp. 151-152.
7. Stephen F. Mason, A History of the Sciences (New York: Collier Books, 1962), p.198.
8. Mason, p. 206.
9. Barbara Brennan, Hands of Light (New York: Bantam Books, 1988), p. 20.
10. Janet Macrae, Therapeutic Touch (New York: Alfred A. Knopf, 1992), p. 3.
11. Macrae, p. 3.
12. Dora Kunz et al., "Fields and their Clinical Implications," in Dora Kunz, Spiritual Aspects of the Healing Arts (Wheaton, Ill.: Theosophical Publishing House, 1985). Cited in Macrae, p. 3, note 3.
13. Brennan, p. 27.
14. Brennan, p. 27.
15. Brennan, p. 28.

CHAPTER TEN: THE HIERARCHY OF HEALING

1. For a more detailed presentation of the distinctions between the various bodies, see Barbara Brennan, Hands of Light (New York: Bantam Books, 1988), pp. 41-54, and Chris Griscom, Ecstasy is a New Frequency (Santa Fe: Bear and Company, 1987), pp. 8-46.

2. A "hierarchy" is defined as "a group of persons or things arranged in order of rank, grade, class, etc. See, "Hierarchy," Webster's New World Dictionary (New York: Simon and Schuster, 1984), p. 661.

3. Roberto Assagioli, Psychosynthesis: A Manual of Principles and Techniques (New York: The Viking Press, 1971). Cited in Morton T. Kelsey, The Other Side of Silence (New York: Paulist Press), 1976), pp. 269-270.

4. Kelsey, p. 270.

5. See Louise Hay's numerous works including: Heal Your Body (cf. bibliography), You Can Heal Your Life, The Power is Within You; see also Deepak Chopra, Quantum Healing (New York: Bantam Books, 1989).

6. "Mind," The American Heritage Dictionary (Boston: Houghton Mifflin Company, 1987), p. 435.

7. "Mens," The New Collegiate Latin and English Dictionary (New York: Bantam Books, 1966), p. 181.

8. Griscom, p. 9.

9. Study of the dynamics of trauma induction suggests that more generic forms of "meditation" do not necessarily address the specificity of the defenses induced at the moment of freezing — the moment of trauma. Meditation, however, often assists by bringing the blockage into focus, into conscious awareness and by building other recovery resources. "Meditation" that facilitates the necessary bridging of the conscious and subconscious minds can enable the actual resolution of the original trauma.

10. Griscom, p. 12.

11. Griscom, p. 12.

CHAPTER ELEVEN: THE SPIRITUAL IMPLICATIONS OF TRAUMA

1. See Gershen Kaufman, "On Shame, Identity and Dynamics of Change." Paper presented in Symposium, D.L. Grummon, Chairman. Papers in Memory of Bill Kell: Issues on Therapy and the Training of Therapists. Symposium presented at the Meeting of the American Psychological Association in New Orleans, La.: August, 1974.

2. Kaufman, p. 1.

3. Kaufman, p. 1.

4. John Bradshaw, Healing the Shame that Binds You (Deerfield Beach, Florida: Health Communications, Inc., 1988); see Figure 3.1: "Layers of Defense Against The Agony of Internalized Shame."

CHAPTER TWELVE: RECOVERING SPIRITUAL AWARENESS

1. Barbara Brennan, Hands of Light (New York: Bantam Books, 1988), p. 20.
2. Brennan, p. 20.
3. Brennan, p. 20.
4. See Gary Zukav, The Dancing Wu Li Masters (New York: Bantam Books, 1980).
5. Zukav, pp. 305-306.
6. Zukav, p. 308.
7. Talbot, p. 291.
8. Talbot, pp. 290-291.
9. Talbot, p. 291.
10. Talbot, p. 291.
11. Talbot, p. 291.
12. Talbot, p. 1.
13. Talbot, p. 2.
14. Talbot, p. 2
15. Talbot, p. 2.
16. Talbot, pp. 2-3
17. Talbot, p. 3.
18. Bernie Siegel, Love, Medicine, and Miracles (New York: Harper & Row, 1986). Cited in Talbot, p. 6.
19. "Homeostasis," The American Heritage Dictionary (Boston: Houghton Mifflin Company, 1987), p. 332.
20. Talbot, p. 21.
21. Talbot, p. 21.
22. Talbot, p. 21.
23. Julian Hawthorne et al., eds., The Literature of All Nations (Chicago: E.R. DuMont, 1901), I, p. 7.
24. See Anne Wilson Schaef, When Society Becomes an Addict (San Francisco: Harper and Row Publishers, 1987).
25. Kaufman, On Shame, Identity, and Dynamics of Change, p. 2.
26. Kaufman, p. 1.
27. Harville Hendrix, Getting the Love You Want (New York: Harper Perennial, 1988), p. 1.
28. Gary Zukav, The Seat of the Soul (New York: Simon and Schuster, Inc., 1989), p. 137.
29. See Viktor E. Frankl, Man's Search for Meaning (New York: Simon and Schuster, Inc., 1963).
30. Frankl, p. 163.
31. Yogiraj Vethathiri Maharishi, Physical Exercises for Health and Longevity (Madras: Vethathiri Publications, 1982).

32. See Janet Macrae, <u>Therapeutic Touch</u> (New York: Alfred A. Knopf, 1992). "Healing Touch" is a similar therapeutic modality sponsored and taught by the American Holistic Nurses Association and drawing from the experience and contributions of Rosalyn Bruyere, Brugh Joy, Barbara Brennan, Janet Mentgen, and others. Dorothea Hover, R.N., Ed.D., recently informed me that she is currently in the process of publishing the first text on "Healing Touch."

33. Lyall Watson, <u>Lifetide: The Biology of Consciousness</u>. Cited in Brennan, p. 27.

34. Swami Rama, <u>Living with the Himalayan Masters</u> (Honesdale, Pennsylvania: Himalayan International Insitute of Yoga Science and Philosophy, 1989), p. 263.

35. Alcoholics Anonymous, <u>Alcoholics Anonymous</u> (New York: Alcoholics Anonymous World Services, Inc.), p. 59.

36. Robert Odom, Your <u>Companion to Twelve Step Recovery</u> (Carson, Ca.: Hay House, Inc., 1994), pp. 152-153.

CHAPTER THIRTEEN: THE HEALING OF DREAMS

1. See Patricia Garfield, <u>The Healing Power of Dreams</u> (New York: Simon and Schuster, 1991).

2. Garfield, pp. 60-74.

CHAPTER FOURTEEN: THE HEALING OF DISEASE

1. "Disease," The <u>American Heritage Dictionary</u> (Boston: Houghton Mifflin Company, 1987), p. 204.

2. See Deepak Chopra, <u>Quantum Healing</u> (New York: Bantam Books, 1989).

3. Chopra, p. 28.

4. Chopra, p. 27.

5. Chopra, p. 27.

6. Chopra, p. 27.

7. Chopra, p. 28.

8. Chopra, p. 28.

9. Chopra, p. 28.

10. Chopra, p. 28.

11. Chopra, p. 28.

12. Chopra, p. 28.

13. Chopra, p. 28.

Bibliography

Alcoholics Anonymous. <u>Alcoholics Anonymous</u>. New York: Alcoholics Anonymous World Services, Inc., 1952.

Assagioli, Roberto. <u>Psychosynthesis: A Manual of Principles and Techniques</u>. New York: The Viking Press, 1971.

Bradshaw, John. <u>Healing the Shame that Binds You</u>. Deerfield Beach, Fla.: Health Communications, Inc., 1988.

Brennan, Barbara. <u>Hands of Light</u>. New York: Bantam Books, 1988.

Bruyere, Rosalyn. <u>Wheels of Light</u>. Sierra Madre: Bon Productions, 1989.

Chopra, Deepak. <u>Quantum Healing</u>. New York: Bantam Books, 1989.

Dimski, Donna, et al. "Renal Autotransplantation in the Loin Pain-Hematuria Syndrome: A Cautionary Note." <u>American Journal of Kidney Diseases</u>, 20, No. 2 (August 1992), 180-186.

"Disease." <u>The American Heritage Dictionary</u>. Boston: Houghton Mifflin Company, 1987.

Eco, Umberto. <u>Semiotics and the Philosophy of Language</u>. Bloomington: Indiana University Press, 1984.

Faulkner, William. Quoted by Timothy Hatcher and Leslie Todd Petrie. "Body-Mind Unity." A Workshop Presented at C.P.C. Meadow Wood Hospital. Baton Rouge, La.: October, 1991.

Franki, Viktor E. <u>Man's Search for Meaning</u>. New York: Simon and Schuster, Inc., 1963.

Garfield, Patricia. The Healing Power of Dreams. New York: Simon and Schuster, Inc., 1991.

Griscom, Chris. Ecstasy is a New Frequency. Santa Fe: Bear and Company, 1987.

Grove, David. Healing the Wounded Child Within. Edwardsville: David Grove Seminars, 1989.

Hatcher, Timothy, and Leslie Todd Petrie. "Body-Mind Unity." A Workshop presented at C.P.C. Meadow Wood Hospital. Baton Rouge: October, 1991.

Hawthorne, Julian, et al., eds. The Literature of All Nations. 10 vols. Chicago: E.R. DuMont, 1901.

Hay, Louise. Heal Your Body. Carson, Ca.: Hay House, 1988.

_____. You Can Heal Your Life. Carson Ca.: Hay House, 1987.

_____. The Power is Within You. Carson Ca.: Hay House, 1988.

Hayward, Susan. A Guide for the Advanced Soul. Hong Kong: Mandarin Offset, 1986.

Hayward, Susan & Malcolm Cohen. A Bag of Jewels. Hong Kong: Mandarin Offset, 1991.

Hendrix, Harville. Getting the Love You Want. New York: Harper Perennial, 1988.

"Hierarchy." Webster's New World Dictionary. New York: Simon and Schuster, 1984, 661.

"Homeostasis." The American Heritage Dictionary. Boston: Houghton Mifflin Company, 1987, 332.

Joy, W. Brugh. Joy's Way. New York: G.P. Putnam's Sons, 1979.

Kaufman, Gershen. "On Shame, Identity and Dynamics of Change." Paper Presented in Symposium, D.L. Grummon, Chairman. Papers in Memory of Bill Kell: Issues on Therapy and the Training of Therapists. Symposium Presented at the Meeting of the American Psychological Association. New Orleans: August, 1974.

Kelsey, Morton. The Other Side of Silence. New York: Paulist Press, 1976.

Kuhn, Thomas S. "The Structure of Scientific Revolutions." International Encyclopedia of Unified Sciences, 1962, II, No. 2.

Kunz, Dora, and E. Peter. "Fields and their Clinical Implications." In Kunz, Spiritual Aspects of the Healing Arts. Wheaton, Ill.: Theosophical Publishing House, 1985.

Lemonick, Michael. "Glimpses of the Mind." In Time, July 17, 1995, 44-52.

Macrae, Janet. Therapeutic Touch. New York: Alfred A. Knopf, 1992.

Maharishi, Yogiraj Vethathiri. Physical Exercises for Health and Longevity. Madras: Vethathiri Publications, 1982.

Mason, Stephen. A History of the Science. New York: Collier Books, 1962.

"Mens." The New Collegiate Latin and English Dictionary. New York: Bantam Books, 1966 , 181.

"Mind." The American Heritage Dictionary. Boston: Houghton Mifflin Company, 1987, 435.

Odom, Robert. Your Companion to Twelve Step Recovery. Carson, Ca.: Hay House, 1994.

Rama, Swami. Living with the Himalayan Masters. Honesdale, Pennsylvania: Himalayan International Institute of Yoga Science and Philosophy, 1989.

Rossi, Ernest. The Psychobiology of Mind-Body Healing. New York: W.W. Norton & Company, Inc., 1986.

Schaef, Anne Wilson. When Society Becomes an Addict. San Francisco: Harper and Row Publishers, 1987.

Siegel, Bernie. Love, Medicine and Miracles: Lessons Learned About Healing from a Surgeon's Experience with Exceptional Patients. Harper and Row Publishers, 1986.

Talbot, Michael. The Holographic Universe. New York: Harper Collins 1991.

Watson, Lyall. Lifetide: The Biology of Consciousness. New York: Simon and Schuster, 1987.

Zukav, Gary. The Dancing Wu Li Masters. New York: Bantam Books, 1988.

_____. The Seat of the Soul. New York: Simon and Schuster, Inc., 1989.

Invocation

The atmosphere around us is being purified by the Divine Presence;
The atmosphere around us is purified by the Divine.
The Divine Energy descends upon us and enters our bodies and souls.
The Divine Light enters my body; I am purified, blessed, and healed.
I am protected by this force and from the Source in all my activities, day and night in all places.
I am one with all that is.
I am one with the Divine Mind.

Yogiraj Vethathiri Maharishi

Lightbearer's "Our Father"

Prime Creator, Intelligent Infinity, the One Source of All,
Which dwells in perfect balance,
Sacred is the vibration of the Logos.
May the plan of our Higher Selves be realized as we
*   surrender to the Divine within.*
May we manifest our place in the plan.
May we experience all we need to overcome.
Teach us to release and empty that we may be filled.
Guide us through the shadows of our fears,
*   that we may be freed of the illusions of separation.*
For ours is the wisdom, the power, and the glory,
Beyond time and space,
So be it!

Anonymous
Modified, Baum 1996

Mrs. Booth's dog
Stay at Dee's at 12 ish.